Biosimilars
Design and Analysis
of Follow-on Biologics

Chapman & Hall/CRC Biostatistics Series

Editor-in-Chief

Shein-Chung Chow, Ph.D.
Professor
Department of Biostatistics and Bioinformatics
Duke University School of Medicine
Durham, North Carolina

Series Editors

Byron Jones
Biometrical Fellow
Statistical Methodology
Integrated Information Sciences
Novartis Pharma AG
Basel, Switzerland

Jen-pei Liu
Professor
Division of Biometry
Department of Agronomy
National Taiwan University
Taipei, Taiwan

Karl E. Peace
Georgia Cancer Coalition
Distinguished Cancer Scholar
Senior Research Scientist and
Professor of Biostatistics
Jiann-Ping Hsu College of Public Health
Georgia Southern University
Statesboro, Georgia

Bruce W. Turnbull
Professor
School of Operations Research
and Industrial Engineering
Cornell University
Ithaca, New York

Chapman & Hall/CRC Biostatistics Series

Adaptive Design Methods in Clinical Trials, Second Edition
Shein-Chung Chow and Mark Chang

Adaptive Design Theory and Implementation Using SAS and R
Mark Chang

Advanced Bayesian Methods for Medical Test Accuracy
Lyle D. Broemeling

Advances in Clinical Trial Biostatistics
Nancy L. Geller

Applied Meta-Analysis with R
Ding-Geng (Din) Chen and Karl E. Peace

Basic Statistics and Pharmaceutical Statistical Applications, Second Edition
James E. De Muth

Bayesian Adaptive Methods for Clinical Trials
Scott M. Berry, Bradley P. Carlin,
J. Jack Lee, and Peter Muller

Bayesian Analysis Made Simple: An Excel GUI for WinBUGS
Phil Woodward

Bayesian Methods for Measures of Agreement
Lyle D. Broemeling

Bayesian Methods in Health Economics
Gianluca Baio

Bayesian Missing Data Problems: EM, Data Augmentation and Noniterative Computation
Ming T. Tan, Guo-Liang Tian,
and Kai Wang Ng

Bayesian Modeling in Bioinformatics
Dipak K. Dey, Samiran Ghosh,
and Bani K. Mallick

Biosimilars: Design and Analysis of Follow-on Biologics
Shein-Chung Chow

Biostatistics: A Computing Approach
Stewart J. Anderson

Causal Analysis in Biomedicine and Epidemiology: Based on Minimal Sufficient Causation
Mikel Aickin

Clinical Trial Data Analysis using R
Ding-Geng (Din) Chen and Karl E. Peace

Clinical Trial Methodology
Karl E. Peace and Ding-Geng (Din) Chen

Computational Methods in Biomedical Research
Ravindra Khattree and Dayanand N. Naik

Computational Pharmacokinetics
Anders Källén

Confidence Intervals for Proportions and Related Measures of Effect Size
Robert G. Newcombe

Controversial Statistical Issues in Clinical Trials
Shein-Chung Chow

Data and Safety Monitoring Committees in Clinical Trials
Jay Herson

Design and Analysis of Animal Studies in Pharmaceutical Development
Shein-Chung Chow and Jen-pei Liu

Design and Analysis of Bioavailability and Bioequivalence Studies, Third Edition
Shein-Chung Chow and Jen-pei Liu

Design and Analysis of Bridging Studies
Jen-pei Liu, Shein-Chung Chow,
and Chin-Fu Hsiao

Design and Analysis of Clinical Trials with Time-to-Event Endpoints
Karl E. Peace

Design and Analysis of Non-Inferiority Trials
Mark D. Rothmann, Brian L. Wiens,
and Ivan S. F. Chan

Difference Equations with Public Health Applications
Lemuel A. Moyé and Asha Seth Kapadia

Chapman & Hall/CRC Biostatistics Series

Biosimilars
Design and Analysis
of Follow-on Biologics

Shein-Chung Chow

Duke University School of Medicine
Durham, North Carolina, USA

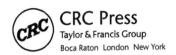

CRC Press
Taylor & Francis Group
Boca Raton London New York

CRC Press is an imprint of the
Taylor & Francis Group, an **informa** business
A CHAPMAN & HALL BOOK

CRC Press
Taylor & Francis Group
6000 Broken Sound Parkway NW, Suite 300
Boca Raton, FL 33487-2742

First issued in paperback 2019

ISBN-13: 978-1-4665-7969-9 (hbk)
ISBN-13: 978-0-367-37972-8 (pbk)

Library of Congress Cataloging-in-Publication Data

Chow, Shein-Chung, 1955-
    Biosimilars : design and analysis of follow-on biologics / Shein-Chung Chow.
        pages cm. -- (Chapman & Hall/CRC biostatistics series ; 60)
    Includes bibliographical references and index.
    ISBN 978-1-4665-7969-9 (hardback) 1. Pharmaceutical biotechnology. 2. Pharmaceutical biotechnology industry. 3. Drugs--Generic substitution. 4. Pharmaceutical policy. 5. Biological products. I. Title.

    RS380.C45 2014
    615.1'9--dc23   2013012926

Visit the Taylor & Francis Web site at
http://www.taylorandfrancis.com

and the CRC Press Web site at
http://www.crcpress.com

Contents

Preface

Biologic drug products are therapeutic moieties that are manufactured using a living system or organism. These are important life-saving drug products for patients with unmet medical needs. They also comprise a growing segment in the pharmaceutical industry. In 2007, for instance, worldwide sales of biological products reached $94 billion, accounting for about 15% of the pharmaceutical industry's gross revenue. Meanwhile, many biological products face losing their patents in the next decade. Attempts have been made therefore to establish an abbreviated regulatory pathway for approval of biosimilar drug products, that is, follow-on (or subsequent entered) biologics of the innovator's biological products in order to reduce cost. However, due to the complexity of the structures of biosimilar products and the nature of the manufacturing process, biological products differ from traditional small-molecule (chemical) drug products. Although the concepts and principles for bioequivalence and interchangeability could be the same for both chemical generics and biosimilar products, scientific challenges remain for establishing an abbreviated regulatory pathway for approval of biosimilar products due to their unique characteristics.

This book is intended to be the first book entirely devoted to the design and analysis of biosimilarity and drug interchangeability and includes tests for comparability in important quality attributes at critical stages of manufacturing processes of biological products. It covers most of the statistical issues that one may encounter in biosimilar studies under various study designs at different stages of research and development of biological products. The goal of this book is to provide a useful desk reference and describe the state of the art to (1) scientists and researchers engaged in pharmaceutical/clinical research and development of biological products, (2) those in government regulatory agencies who have to make decisions in the review and approval process of biological regulatory submissions, and (3) biostatisticians who provide statistical support to the assessment of biosimilarity and drug interchangeability of biosimilar products. I hope that this book can serve as a bridge among the pharmaceutical/biotechnology industry, government regulatory agencies, and academia.

The scope of this book is restricted to scientific factors and practical issues related to the design and analysis of biosimilar studies that are commonly seen in biosimilar research and development. Also, since regulatory requirements for assessment of biosimilar products between the European Medicines Agency (EMA) and the United States Food and Drug Administration (FDA) are similar but slightly different, this book primarily focuses on regulatory requirements from FDA. The book contains 17 chapters. Chapter 1 provides a background of pharmaceutical/clinical development of biosimilar products and describes commonly seen scientific factors and practical issues in biosimilar clinical research and development. Chapter 2 reviews past experience for generic approval of small-molecule drug products. Chapter 3 summarizes regulatory requirements for assessment of biosimilar products (or follow-on biologics) and includes a review of recently published FDA draft guidances on biosimilar products. Criteria for assessment of biosimilarity, which are available in the regulatory guidances/guidelines and/or literature, are described in Chapter 4. Chapter 5 introduces statistical methods for assessing average biosimilarity based on the concept of relative distance between a test product and a reference product as compared to the distance between the reference product and itself. Chapter 6 proposes a general approach based on biosimilarity index (reproducibility probability) for the assessment of biosimilar products. Chapter 7 explores the relationship between the concept of testing non-inferiority and testing for equivalence. Chapter 8 deals with statistical tests for assessment of biosimilarity in variability of biosimilar products. Formulas or procedures for sample size calculations for comparing variabilities under a crossover design or a parallel design with or without replicates are given in Chapter 9. Chapter 10 studies the impact of variability on biosimilarity limits for assessing biosimilar products. Chapter 11 investigates the feasibility/applicability of the assessment of interchangeability (in terms of the concepts of switching and alternating among biosimilar products) and describes useful study designs that address switching and/or alternation in biosimilar studies. The issue of immunogenicity in biosimilar studies is examined in Chapter 12. Chemistry, manufacturing, and control (CMC) requirements for biological products in regulatory submission are discussed in Chapter 13. Chapter 14 provides statistical methods for testing comparability of important quality attributes at various critical stages of a manufacturing process of biosimilar products. Stability design and analysis of biosimilar products are dealt with in Chapter 15. Chapter 16 discusses statistical tests for assessment of biosimilarity using biomarker data. Current issues for assessing biosimilarity and interchangeability of biosimilar products are discussed in the Chapter 17.

From Taylor & Francis Group, I would like to thank David Grubbs for providing me the opportunity to work on this book. I wish to express my gratitude to my wife Annpey Pong, PhD, for her understanding, constant encouragement, and support during the preparation of this book. I thank Laszlo Endrenyi, PhD, of the University of Toronto for his constructive comments and editing, which have led to a significant improvement of the book. I would also like to thank colleagues from the Statistical Scientific Advisory Board (SSAB) on Biosimilars (sponsored by Amgen, Inc.), Amgen, Inc., the Department of Biostatistics and Bioinformatics, Duke Clinical Research Institute (DCRI), Duke Clinical Research Unit (DCRU), and the Center for AIDS Research (CFAR) of Duke University School of Medicine as well as many friends from academia, the pharmaceutical industry, and regulatory agencies for their support and discussions during the preparation of this book.

Finally, the views expressed are those of the author and not necessarily those of Duke University School of Medicine. I am solely responsible for the contents and errors of this book. Any comments and suggestions will be very much appreciated.

Shein-Chung Chow, PhD

School of Medicine
Duke University
Durham, North Carolina

1

Introduction

1.1 Background

In the United States (U.S.), for small-molecule drug products, when an innovative (brand-name) drug product is going off patent, pharmaceutical and/or generic companies may file an abbreviated new drug application (ANDA) for the approval of the generic copies of the brand-name drug. In 1984, the United States Food and Drug Administration (FDA) was authorized to approve generic drug products under the *Drug Price Competition and Patent Term Restoration Act*, which is also known as the *Hatch-Waxman Act*. For the approval of generic (small-molecule) drug products, the FDA requires that evidence of *average* of bioavailability, which is measured in terms of the rate and extent of drug absorption, be provided through the conduct of bioequivalence studies. As indicated by Chow and Liu (2008), the assessment of bioequivalence as a surrogate for evaluation of drug safety and efficacy is based on the so-called *Fundamental Bioequivalence Assumption* that if two drug products are shown to be bioequivalent in average bioavailability, it is assumed that they will reach the same therapeutic effect or that they are therapeutically equivalent. Many practitioners interpret that approved generics and the brand-name drug can, in most cases, be used interchangeably since they are therapeutically equivalent. Under the Fundamental Bioequivalence Assumption, regulatory requirements (e.g., FDA guidances), study design (e.g., a standard two-sequence, two-period crossover design), acceptance criteria (e.g., the 80/125 rule based on log-transformed data), and statistical methods (e.g., Shuirmann's two one-sided tests procedure or the confidence interval approach) for the assessment of bioequivalence have been well established over the past several decades (see, e.g., Schuirmann, 1987; FDA, 2001, 2003; Chow and Liu, 2008).

Unlike small-molecule drug products, a generic version of a biological products is only a similar biological drug product (SBDP) in comparison with the originator biological product. It should be noted that the SBDPs are *not* like the small-molecule generic drug products, which are usually referred to as containing *identical* active ingredient(s) as the innovative drug product. The concept for the development of SBDPs, which are made of living cells or organisms, is very different from that of the (small-molecule) generic drug products. The SBDPs are usually referred to as *biosimilars* by the European Medicines Agency (EMA) of the European Union (EU), *follow-on biologics* (FOB or FoB) by the U.S. FDA, and subsequent entered biologics (SEB) by the Health Canada. Throughout this book, unless otherwise stated, the term biosimilars or follow-on biologics will be used. Note that experience with biosimilar development worldwide can be found in McCamish and Woollett (2011).

Webber (2007) defines follow-on (protein) biologics as products that are intended to be *sufficiently similar* to an approved product to permit the applicant to rely on certain existing scientific knowledge about the safety and efficacy of an approved reference product. It should be noted that the generic (small-molecule) drug products are fundamentally different from biosimilar (large-molecule) drug products. For example, biosimilar products are made of living cells and have heterogeneous structures (usually mixtures of related molecules) which are difficult to characterize. In addition, biosimilar products are often variable and sensitive to environmental conditions such as light and temperature. A small change or variation at any critical stage of a manufacturing process of a biological product could result in a drastic change in clinical outcomes. Thus, the current standard methods for bioequivalence assessment of generic drug products may not be appropriate for the assessment of biosimilar products due to these fundamental differences.

On March 23, 2010, the *Biologics Price Competition and Innovation* (BPCI) *Act* (as part of the Affordable Care Act) was written into law, which has given the FDA the authority to approve similar biological drug products. As indicated in the BPCI Act, a biosimilar product is defined as a product that is *highly similar* to the reference product notwithstanding minor differences in clinically inactive components and there are no clinically meaningful differences in terms of safety, purity, and potency. However, little or no discussion regarding how similar is considered highly similar is given in the BPCI Act. As stated in Subsection 351(k)(4), a biological product is considered to be *interchangeable* with the reference product if (1) the biological product is biosimilar to the reference product; and (2) it can be *expected* to produce the same clinical result in *any given patient*. In addition, for a biological product that is administered more than once to an individual, the risk in terms of safety or diminished efficacy of alternating or switching between use of the biological product and the reference product is not greater than the risk of using the reference product without such alternation or switch. Thus, by definition, there is a clear distinction between biosimilarity and interchangeability. In other words, biosimilarity does not imply interchangeability, which is much more stringent. The BPCI Act also states that if a test product is judged to be interchangeable with the reference product, then it may be substituted, even alternated, without a possible intervention, or even notification, of the health care provider. However, as noted earlier, interchangeability is expected to produce the *same* clinical result in *any given patient*, which can be interpreted as that the same clinical result can be expected in *every single patient*. In reality, conceivably, lawsuits may be filed if adverse effects are recorded in a patient after switching from one product to another.

Following the passage of the BPCI Act, in order to obtain input on specific issues and challenges associated with the implementation of the BPCI Act, the U.S. FDA conducted a 2 day public hearing on the *Approval Pathway for Biosimilar and Interchangeability Biological Products* held on November 2–3, 2010, at the FDA in Silver Spring, Maryland. Several scientific factors were raised and discussed at the public hearing. These scientific factors included criteria for assessing biosimilarity, study design and analysis methods for the assessment of biosimilarity, and tests for comparability in quality attributes of the manufacturing process and/or immunogenicity (see, e.g., Chow et al., 2010). These issues primarily focused on the assessment of biosimilarity. The issue of interchangeability in terms of the concepts of alternating and switching was also mentioned and discussed. The discussions of these scientific factors have led to the development of regulatory guidances. On February 9, 2012, the U.S. FDA circulated three draft guidances on the demonstration of biosimilarity for comments. These draft guidances are

1. Scientific Considerations in Demonstrating Biosimilarity to a Reference Product (FDA, 2012a)
2. Quality Considerations in Demonstrating Biosimilarity to a Reference Protein Product (FDA, 2012b)
3. Biosimilars: Questions and Answers Regarding Implementation of the BPCI Act of 2009 (FDA, 2012c)

Subsequently, the FDA hosted another public hearing on the discussion of these draft guidances at the FDA on May 11, 2012.

As patents of a number of biological products are due to expire in the next few years, the subsequent production of follow-on products has aroused interest within the pharmaceutical industry as biosimilar manufacturers strive to obtain part of an already large and rapidly growing market. The potential opportunity for price reductions versus the originator biological products remains to be determined, as the advantage of a slightly cheaper price may be outweighed by the hypothetical increased risk of side effects from biosimilar molecules that are not exact copies of their originators. In this chapter, we shall focus not only on the fundamental differences between small-molecule drug products and biological products but also on practical issues surrounding the assessment of biosimilar products, including scientific factors on biosimilarity, drug interchangeability, quality, and comparability in manufacturing process, and clinical efficacy and side effects.

The rest of this chapter is organized as follows. In the next section, fundamental differences between small-molecule drug products and biological drug products are briefly described. Section 1.3 provides a brief summary of the current regulatory requirements for the approval of biosimilars in the

European Union and the United States. The concepts and corresponding issues regarding biosimilarity, drug interchangeability, and the quality and comparability in the manufacturing process are discussed in Sections 1.4, 1.5, and 1.6. Note that basic concepts and issues are briefly introduced here. These basic concepts and issues will be discussed in greater detail in later chapters. The aim and scope of the book are given in the last section of this chapter.

1.2 Fundamental Differences

Biosimilars are fundamentally different from small-molecule generic drugs. Some of the fundamental differences between biosimilars and generic drugs are summarized in Table 1.1. As can be seen from the table, for example, small-molecule drug products are made by chemical synthesis, while large-molecule biologics are made of living cells or organisms. Small-molecule drug products have well-defined structures which are easy to characterize, while biosimilars have heterogeneous structures with mixtures of related molecules which are difficult to characterize. Small-molecule drug products are usually relatively stable, while biosimilars are known to be variable and very sensitive to environmental conditions such as light and temperature. A small change or variation during the manufacturing process may translate to a drastic change in clinical outcomes (e.g., safety and effectiveness). Small-molecule drug products which are often taken orally are generally prescribed by general practitioners, while biosimilars which are usually injected are often prescribed by specialists. In addition, unlike small-molecule drug products, biosimilars may induce unwanted immune responses which may cause a loss of efficacy or change in their safety profile. Moreover, with differences

TABLE 1.1

Fundamental Differences between Chemical Drugs and Biologics

Chemical Drugs	Biologics
Made by chemical synthesis	Made of living cells or organisms
Defined structure	Heterogeneous structure Mixtures of related molecules
Easy to characterize	Difficult to characterize
Relatively stable	Variable Sensitive to environmental conditions such as light and temperature
No issue of immunogenicity	Issue of immunogenicity
Usually taken orally	Usually injected
Often prescribed by a general practitioner	Usually prescribed by specialists

in the size and complexity of the active substance, important differences also include the nature of the manufacturing process.

As indicated by Kuhlmann and Covic (2006), biological products are usually recombinant-protein molecules manufactured in living cells. Thus, manufacturing processes for biological products are highly complex and require hundreds of specific isolation and purification steps. As a result, in practice, it is impossible to produce an *identical* copy of a biological products, as changes to the structure of the molecule can occur with changes in the production process. Since a protein can be modified during the process (e.g., a side chain may be added, the structure may have changed due to protein misfolding, and so on), different manufacturing processes may lead to structural differences in the final product, which result in differences in efficacy and safety, and may have a negative impact on the immune responses of patients. It should be noted that these issues may also occur during the post-approval changes of the innovator's biological products.

Biosimilar products are not generic products since they are *not* identical to their originator products. Thus, biosimilars should not be brought to market using the same procedure applied to generics. This is partly a reflection of the complexities of manufacturing and safety and efficacy controls of biosimilars when compared to their small-molecule generic counterparts (see, e.g., Chirino and Mire-Sluis, 2004; Schellekens, 2004; Crommelin et al., 2005; Roger and Mikhail, 2007). Instead, for investigating biological products, including biosimilars, the state-of-the-art of analytical procedures should be applied.

1.3 Regulatory Requirements

For the approval of biosimilars in the EU community, the EMA has issued a new guideline describing general principles for the approval of similar biological medicinal products, or biosimilars. The guideline is accompanied by several concept papers that outline areas in which the agency intends to provide more targeted guidance (EMA, 2003a,b, 2006a–g). Specifically, the concept papers discuss approval requirements for several classes of human recombinant products containing erythropoietin, human growth hormone, granulocyte-colony stimulating factor, and insulin. The guideline consists of a checklist of documents published to date relevant to the data requirements for biological pharmaceuticals. It is not clear what specific scientific requirements will be applied to biosimilar applications. In addition, it is not clear how the agency will treat the innovator data contained in the dossiers of the reference product. The guideline provides a useful summary of the biosimilar legislation and previous EU publications, but it provides few answers to the issues.

On the other hand, for the approval of follow-on biologics in the United States, its path depends on whether the biological products is approved under the United States Food, Drug, and Cosmetic Act (US FD&C) or if it is licensed under the United States Public Health Service Act (US PHS). As indicated, some proteins are licensed under the PHS Act, while some are approved under the FD&C Act. For products approved under a New Drug Application (NDA, under the US FD&C Act), generic versions of products can be approved under an ANDA, for example, under Section 505(b)(2) of the FD&C Act. For products that are licensed under a Biologics License Application (BLA, under the US PHS Act), there exists no abbreviated BLA. As pointed out by Woodcock et al. (2007), for the assessment of similarity of follow-on biologics, the FDA would consider the following factors:

1. The robustness of the manufacturing process
2. The degree to which structural similarity could be assessed
3. The extent to which the mechanism of action was understood
4. The existence of valid, mechanistically related pharmacodynamic (PD) assays
5. Comparative pharmacokinetics (PK)
6. Comparative immunogenicity
7. The amount of available clinical data
8. The extent of experience with the original product

A typical example would be the recent regulatory approval of Omnitrope (somatropin), which was approved in 2006 under Section 505(b)(2) of the FD&C Act. Omnitrope was approved based on the following evaluations:

1. Physicochemical testing that established highly similar structure to Genotropin
2. New non-clinical pharmacology and toxicology data specific to Omnitrope
3. PK, PD, and comparative bioavailability data
4. Clinical efficacy and safety data from comparative controlled trials and from long-term trials with Omnitrope
5. Vast clinical experience and a wealth of published literature concerning the clinical effects (safety and effectiveness) of human growth hormone

The approval of Omnitrope was based on an ad hoc, case-by-case review of an individual biosimilar application. In practice, there is a strong industrial interest and desire for the regulatory agencies to develop review standards and an approval process for biosimilars instead of an ad hoc, case-by-case review of individual biosimilar applications. For this purpose, the FDA has established three committees to ensure consistency in the FDA's regulatory approach and guidance to applicants regarding development programs for proposed biosimilar biological products which are intended for submission under the new section 351(k) of the PHS Act. The three committees involve the two centers of FDA which actively review submissions on new biosimilars: the Center for Drug Evaluation and Research (CDER) and the Center for Biologics Evaluation and Research (CBER). The committees to review applications for biosimilars are the CDER/CBER Biosimilar Implementation Committee (BIC), the CDER Biosimilar Review Committee (BRC), and the CBER Biosimilar Review Committee. The CDER/CBER BIC will focus on the cross-center policy issues related to the implementation of the BPCI Act. The CDER BRC and CBER BRC committees are responsible for considering applicant requests for advice about proposed development programs for biosimilar products, reviewing Biologic License Applications (BLAs) that are submitted under section 351(k) of the PHS Act, and managing related issues. Thus, the CDER BRC (CBER BRC) review process steps include the following:

1. An applicant submits a request for advice.
2. Internal review team meeting.
3. Internal CDER BRC (or CBER BRC) meeting.
4. Internal post-BRC meeting.
5. CDER (CBER) meeting with the applicant.

As mentioned earlier, the FDA has circulated, on February 9, 2012, three draft guidances on the assessment of biosimilar products. The first draft guidance regarding scientific considerations is intended to assist sponsors in demonstrating that a proposed therapeutic protein product is biosimilar to a reference product for the purpose of a submission for a marketing application under section 351(k) of the PHS Act. The second draft guidance on quality considerations describes the Agency's current thinking on the factors to consider when demonstrating that a proposed protein product is highly similar to a reference product. Specifically, the guidance is intended to provide recommendations to applicants on scientific and technical information on the chemistry, manufacturing, and controls (CMC) section of a marketing application for a proposed biosimilar product. The third draft guidance provides answers to common questions from sponsors interested in developing proposed biosimilar products, biologics license application (BLA) holders, and other interested parties regarding FDA's interpretation of the BPCI Act.

It should be noted that the three draft guidances do not describe the FDA's current position on drug interchangeability. In order to obtain public input and comments on the draft guidances and drug interchangeability, the FDA also hosted a public hearing at FDA on May 11, 2012. The thinking on drug interchangeability in terms of the concepts of switching and alternating was explored while some useful study designs and statistical methods were proposed and discussed at the public hearing. More details regarding individual regulatory requirements for assessing biosimilarity of biosimilar products from the EU, the United States, and Japan and a discussion regarding the comparison and harmonization of these regulatory requirements are given in Chapter 3.

1.4 Biosimilarity

1.4.1 Definition and Basic Principles

As indicated earlier, the BPCI Act defines a biosimilar product as a product that is *highly similar* to the reference product, notwithstanding minor differences in clinically inactive components. There are no clinically meaningful differences between a biosimilar and an originator biological product in terms of safety, purity, and potency. Based on this definition, we would interpret that a biological medicine is biosimilar to a reference biological medicine if it is highly similar to the reference in *safety, purity,* and *potency*. Here purity may be related to some important *quality* attributes at critical stages of the manufacturing process, and potency has something to do with the *stability* and *efficacy* of the biosimilar product. However, little or no discussion regarding how similar is considered highly similar (or how close is considered sufficiently close) was mentioned in the BPCI Act.

The BPCI Act seems to suggest that a biosimilar product should be highly similar (sufficiently close) to the reference drug product in all spectrums of good drug characteristics such as identity, strength (potency), quality, purity, safety, and stability as described in the U.S. Pharmacopeia and National Formulary (see, e.g., USP/NF, 2000). In practice, however, it is almost impossible to demonstrate that a biosimilar product is highly similar to the reference product in *all* aspects of good drug characteristics in a *single* study. Thus, to ensure that a biosimilar product is highly similar to the reference product in terms of these good drug characteristics, different biosimilar studies may be required. For example, if safety and efficacy are the concern, then a clinical trial must be conducted to demonstrate that there are no clinically meaningful differences in terms of safety and efficacy between a biosimilar product and the innovator biological product. On the other hand, to ensure that important quality attributes are highly similar, critical stages of the manufacturing process, assay development/validation, process control/validation, and product specification of the reference product should be necessarily established through the conduct of relevant studies. In addition, studies need to be conducted for testing the comparability in the manufacturing process (raw materials, in-use materials, and end-product) between the biosimilars and the reference product. This is extremely important because biological products are known to be sensitive to small changes or variations in environmental factors such as light and temperature, during the manufacturing process. In some cases, if a surrogate endpoint such as PK, PD, or a genomic marker is predictive of the primary efficacy/safety clinical endpoint, then a PK/PD or genomic study may be used to assess biosimilarity.

The current regulatory requirements are guided on a case-by-case basis by the following basic principles:

1. The extent of the physicochemical and biological characterization of the product
2. The nature or possible changes in the quality and structure of the biological product due the changes in the manufacturing process (and their unexpected outcomes)
3. Clinical/regulatory experiences with the particular class of the product in question
4. Several factors that need to be considered for biocomparability

Most recently, in its recent draft guidance on *Scientific Considerations in Demonstrating Biosimilarity to a Reference Product*, the FDA has suggested that considerations and reviews of biosimilarity should be based on the totality-of-the-evidence. This indicates that the FDA is interested in demonstrating *global* similarity in all aspects related to safety, purity, and potency of the biosimilar products.

1.4.2 Criteria for Bioequivalence/Biosimilarity

The BPCI Act defines a biosimilar product as a biological product that is highly similar to the reference drug product. However, no criteria for assessing biosimilarity were mentioned in the Act. Statistically, one could refer to as *similarity* between two drug products as similarity in average, variability, or distribution of the response of a specific study endpoint of interest. In practice, the assessment of similarity in the average of the response of a specific study endpoint is often considered. A typical example is the assessment of average bioequivalence in terms of drug absorption (which is measured by the study endpoint of area under the blood or plasma concentration time curve or maximum concentration) for the regulatory approval of generic drug products. In this book, unless otherwise stated, we shall focus on the biosimilarity in the *average* response of the study endpoint of interest in a given biosimilar study. More details regarding the bioequivalence experience for small-molecule drug products are discussed in the next chapter.

In practice, the terms of biosimilarity (similarity), bioequivalence (equivalence), comparability, biocomparability, and consistency are alternately used in biopharmaceutical/biotechnology research and development. For comparisons between drug products, some criteria for the assessment of bioequivalence (e.g., the comparison of drug absorption profiles), similarity (e.g., the comparison of dissolution profiles), and comparability or consistency (e.g., comparisons between manufacturing processes) are available in either regulatory guidelines/guidances or the literature. These criteria, however, can be classified into the following categories:

1. Absolute change versus relative change
2. Aggregated versus disaggregated criteria
3. Moment-based versus probability-based criteria
4. Scaled versus unscaled criteria
5. Weighted versus unweighted criteria

In what follows, these categories of criteria are briefly reviewed. While the criteria have been applied to bioequivalence studies, they are equally relevant to investigations of biosimilarity.

1.4.2.1 Absolute Change versus Relative Change

In clinical research and development, for a given study endpoint, post-treatment absolute change from baseline or post-treatment relative change (% change) from a baseline is usually considered for comparisons between treatment groups. A typical example would be the study of weight reduction in an obese patient population. In practice, it is not clear whether a clinically meaningful difference in terms of absolute change from the baseline can be translated to a clinically meaningful difference in terms of relative change from the baseline. Sample size calculations based on power analysis in terms of absolute change from the baseline or relative change from the baseline could lead to a very different result.

For generic approval, current U.S. regulation adopts a one size-fits-all criterion based on *relative change* for bioequivalence assessment. In other words, we conclude (average) bioequivalence between a test product and a reference product if the 90% confidence interval for the ratio of geometric means of the primary endpoint (e.g., a PK response such as the area under the blood or plasma concentration time curve) between the two drug products is (in%) completely within 80% and 125%. Note that regulatory agencies suggest that a log-transformation be performed before data analysis for the assessment of bioequivalence.

1.4.2.2 Aggregated versus Disaggregated Criteria

As indicated by Chow and Liu (2008), bioequivalence can be assessed by evaluating differences, *separately*, in averages, intra-subject variabilities, and variance due to subject-by-formulation interaction between drug products. Individual criteria for the assessment of differences in averages, intra-subject variabilities, and variance due to subject-by-formulation inter-action are referred to as *disaggregated criteria*. If the criterion is a single summary measure composed of these individual criteria, it is called an *aggregated criterion*.

For the assessment of bioequivalence in average bioavailability (ABE), most regulatory agencies recommend the use of a disaggregated criterion based on average bioavailability. That is, bioequivalence is concluded if the average bioavailability of the test formulation is within (80%, 125%) that of the reference formulation, with a certain assurance. Note that the EMA (2001) and WHO (2005) use the same equivalence criterion of 80%–125% for the log-transformed PK responses such as the area under the blood or plasma concentration time curve (AUC).

Aggregated criteria for population bioequivalence (PBE) and individual bioequivalence (IBE) were presented in an FDA guidance (FDA, 2001). PBE and IBE will be discussed in greater detail in Chapter 4. It is noted here only that both procedures rely on aggregated criteria. PBE evaluates *jointly* the differences between the means and between the total variances of the two drug products. (Total variances are the sums of the between- and within-subject variances.) Similarly, IBE assesses *jointly* the differences between the means and between the intra-subject variances as well as the variance com-ponent of the subject-by-product interaction (FDA, 2001). These examples of aggregated criteria will be considered later.

For aggregated criteria, the FDA proposes the use of an individual bio-equivalence (IBE) criterion (IBC) for addressing drug switchability and population bioequivalence (PBE) criterion (PBC) for addressing drug pre-scribability (FDA, 2001). For the assessment of IBE, the IBC, denoted by θ_I, can be expressed as

$$\theta_I = \frac{\delta^2 + \sigma_D^2 + \sigma_{WT}^2 - \sigma_{WR}^2}{\max\{\sigma_{W0}^2, \sigma_{WR}^2\}},\tag{1.1}$$

where

$\delta = \mu_T - \mu_R, \sigma_{WT}^2, \sigma_{WR}^2, \sigma_D^2$ are the true differences between means, the intra-subject (within-subject) variabilities of the test product and the reference product, and the variance component due to subject-by-formulation interaction between drug products, respectively

σ_{W0}^2 is a scale parameter specified by the user

Similarly, the PBC for the assessment of PBE, denoted by θ_P, suggested in the FDA guidance (FDA, 2001) is given by

$$\theta_P = \frac{\delta^2 + \sigma_{TT}^2 - \sigma_{TR}^2}{\max\{\sigma_{T0}^2, \sigma_{TR}^2\}},\tag{1.2}$$

where

σ_{TT}^2, σ_{TR}^2 are the total variances for the test product and the reference product, respectively

σ_{T0}^2 is a scale parameter specified by the user

A typical approach is to construct a one-sided 95% confidence interval for $\theta_I(\theta_P)$ for the assessment of individual (population) bioequivalence. If the one-sided 95% upper confidence limit is less than the bioequivalence limit of $\theta_I(\theta_P)$, we then conclude that the test product is bioequivalent to that of the reference product in terms of individual (population) bioequivalence. More details regarding individual and PBE can be found in Chow and Liu (2008).

1.4.2.3 Moment-Based versus Probability-Based Criteria

Schall and Luus (1993) proposed the moment-based and probability-based measures for the expected discrepancy in PK responses between drug products. The moment-based measure compares the expectation of the (squared) difference between responses of the test and reference products (*T* versus *R*) with that of the (squared) difference between two administrations of the reference formulation (*R* versus *R'*). The probability-based approach makes the same comparison but utilizes the probabilities for occurrence of such differences. Details of the approaches will be provided in Chapter 4. The moment-based measure suggested by Schall and Luus (1993) is based on the following expected mean-squared differences:

$$d(Y_j;Y_{j'}) = \begin{cases} E(Y_T - Y_R)^2 & \text{if } j = T \text{ and } j' = R \\ E(Y_R - Y_R')^2 & \text{if } j = R \text{ and } j' = R. \end{cases} \quad (1.3)$$

For some pre-specified positive number *r*, one of the probability-based measures for the expected discrepancy is given as (Schall and Luus, 1993)

$$d(Y_j;Y_{j'}) = \begin{cases} P\{|Y_T - Y_R| < r\} & \text{if } j = T \text{ and } j' = R \\ P\{|Y_R - Y_R'| < r\} & \text{if } j = R \text{ and } j' = R. \end{cases} \quad (1.4)$$

$d(Y_T; Y_R)$ measures the expected discrepancy for some PK metric between the test and reference formulations, and $d(Y_R; Y_R')$ provides the expected discrepancy between the repeated administrations of the reference formulation. The role of $d(Y_R; Y_R')$ in the formulation of the bioequivalence criteria is to serve as a control. The rationale is that the reference formulation should be bioequivalent to itself. Therefore, for the moment-based measures, if the test formulation is indeed bioequivalent to the reference formulation, then $d(Y_T; Y_R)$

should be very close to $d(Y_R;Y_R')$. It follows that if the criteria are functions of the difference (or ratio) between $d(Y_T;Y_R)$ and $d(Y_R;Y_R')$, bioequivalence is concluded if they are smaller than some pre-specified limit. On the other hand, for probability-based measures, if the test formulation is indeed bioequivalent to the reference formulation, as measured by $d(Y_R;Y_R')$, then comparison $d(Y_T;Y_R)$ should not be much larger. As a result, bioequivalence is concluded if the criterion based on the probability-based measure is larger than some pre-specified limit.

Chow et al. (2010) compared the moment-based criterion with the probability-based criterion for the assessment of bioequivalence or biosimilarity under a parallel group design. The results indicate that the probability-based criterion is not only much more stringent but also sensitive to small changes in variability. This justifies the use of the probability-based criterion for the assessment of biosimilarity if a certain level of precision and reliability of biosimilarity is desired.

1.4.2.4 Scaled versus Unscaled Criteria

Scaled criteria are usually referred to as criteria that are adjusted for the intra-subject variability of the reference product or for the therapeutic index. For example, the IBC criterion, to be discussed in Chapter 4, is adjusted, depending on the circumstances, either for a constant variance or for the within-subject variability. The PBC criterion is adjusted correspondingly and thereby becomes also a scaled criterion. Scaled criteria adjusting for the variability of the reference product do not penalize good generic or biosimilar products having smaller variability.

As indicated by the FDA, a drug product is considered a highly variable drug if its intra-subject coefficient of variation (CV) is higher than or equal to 30%. It should be noted that, by applying the regulatory criterion for average BE, it may be difficult to demonstrate bioequivalence or biosimilarity between highly variable test and reference drug products. Alternatively, Haidar et al. (2008) described a procedure using scaled average bioequivalence (SABE) for the assessment of bioequivalence for highly variable drug products. The procedure has been, in effect, adopted by the FDA for bioequivalence assessment of highly variable drug products. As a result, SABE has attracted much attention for possible application for the assessment of biosimilarity of follow-on biologics since biological products are usually highly variable.

1.4.2.5 Weighted versus Unweighted Criteria

Weighted criteria are aggregated criteria with different weights of each component (e.g., of the difference between means and of the variance components). For example, the three components of IBE (the difference between the means, the difference between the within-subject variances, and the variance component for the subject-by-product interaction) may be considered to have differing weights. However, this could further complicate an already complicated criterion. In practice, it is a challenging question to select an appropriate weight for each component, which will then have an impact on the assessment of bioequivalence or biosimilarity. Besides, it is difficult to interpret the selected weights for each component since there are masking effects among differences in means and variance components (Chow, 1999). Note that assessments of biosimilarity assessments are based on the totality-of-the-evidence. The FDA seems to suggest a weighted criterion or weighted scoring system (across different functional areas or domains) for global similarity.

In summary, for the assessment of bioequivalence of small-molecule drug products, the FDA recommends aggregated, moment-based, scaled, and unweighted criteria based on relative change. This has led to SABE for average bioequivalence of highly variable drug products and also, earlier, to the criteria for IBE and PBE. For the assessment of biosimilarity, on the other hand, Chow et al. (2010) suggested a disaggregated, probability-based, scaled, and weighted criterion based on relative distance (the distance between "T versus R" and "R versus R") being considered. This has led to the development of the (totality) biosimilarity index for the assessment of biosimilarity and drug interchangeability, which are further discussed in Chapter 6 (biosimilarity) and Chapter 11 (interchangeability).

1.4.3 Biosimilarity versus Non-inferiority

As indicated in the 2012 FDA draft guidance on *Scientific Considerations in Demonstrating Biosimilarity to a Reference Product,* in some cases, a one-sided test (non-inferiority design) may be appropriate for comparing safety and effectiveness and also advantageous as it could generally allow for a smaller sample size than an equivalence (two-sided) design (see, e.g., Chow et al., 2008). The FDA draft guidance provided the following example. If doses of the reference product higher than those recommended in its labeling do not create safety concerns, then a one-sided test may be sufficient for comparing the efficacy of certain protein products. The FDA draft guidance indicated that it is generally important to demonstrate that a proposed product has no more risk in terms of safety and immunogenicity than the reference product. For this purpose, a one-sided test may also be adequate in a clinical study which evaluates immunogenicity or other safety endpoints, as long as it is clear that lower immunogenic or other adverse events would not have implications for the effectiveness of a protein product. For a non-inferiority design, the FDA draft guidance indicated that a non-inferiority margin should be pre-specified with scientific justification.

The approaches of non-inferiority, superiority, equivalence, and similarity will be presented in detail in Chapter 7.

Statistically, testing for non-inferiority includes testing for equivalence and testing for superiority. In practice, we may test for equivalence or test for superiority once the non-inferiority has been established. Thus, non-inferiority does not imply equivalence. It should be noted that testing for non-inferiority/superiority is often employed based on a one-sided test procedure at the 5% level of significance, which is equivalent to a two-sided test procedure at the 10% level of significance. In practice, it is suggested that a one-sided test procedure at the 2.5% level of significance should be applied for testing non-inferiority; it is equivalent to a two-sided test procedure at the 5% level of significance. Similarly, testing for superiority includes testing for equivalence and testing for non-inferiority. In other words, we may test for equivalence or test for non-inferiority if we fail to reject the null hypothesis of non-superiority. It should also be noted that superiority does not imply equivalence. In practice, it is also suggested that a one-sided test procedure at the 2.5% level of significance, which is equivalent to a two-sided test procedure at the 5% level of significance, should be used for testing superiority.

Since non-inferiority is regarded as one-sided equivalence, we may consider establishing *non-inferiority* first and then test for *non-superiority* for the assessment of biosimilarity by utilizing the concept of *asymmetric* equivalence limits (α). This proposal deals with distinct values of α_1 and α_2 rather than $\alpha_1 = \alpha_2$. This enables us to adopt flexible biosimilarity criteria. However, the selection of the non-inferiority margin and the choices of α_1 and α_2 are controversial issues. Consideration of spending functions could be helpful. In any case, consensus among the regulatory agency, pharmaceutical/biotechnology industry, and academia should be reached based on appropriate and valid scientific/statistical justification. More details regarding testing for non-inferiority versus testing for equivalence or similarity are given in Chapter 7.

1.4.4 Practical Issues

In practice, the following questions are often asked when assessing biosimilarity between biosimilars and an innovative drug product.

How similar is considered highly similar?—Current criteria for assessment of bioequivalence may, in some cases, be useful for determining whether a biosimilar product is similar to a reference product. However, they do not provide additional information regarding the *degree* of similarity. As indicated in the BPCI Act, a biosimilar product is defined as a product that is *highly similar* to the reference product. However, little or no discussion regarding the degree of similarity for achieving *highly similar* was provided. It may well be that, in addition to the demonstration of similarity, on the average, of a study endpoint, demonstration of similarity in variability of a study endpoint should also be considered for achieving *highly similar* as defined in the BPCI Act.

What criteria should be used for assessing biosimilarity?—As indicated earlier, several criteria for the assessment of similarity are available in the published regulatory guidelines/guidances and the literature. The question regarding what criteria should be considered for assessing biosimilarity has become interesting. However, no systematic comparisons have been undertaken among these criteria in terms of their relative advantages and limitations. In practice, it is of interest to investigate

1. Whether these criteria will lead to the same conclusion?
2. Which criterion is superior (or more efficient) in comparison with others for a fixed sample size?
3. Can these criteria translate to one another?
4. Which criterion is telling the truth?

Further research is needed in order to address these questions.

Is a one-size-fits-all criterion feasible?—The use of one size-fits-all criterion for bioequivalence assessment has been criticized in the past several decades. The major-criticism is that it ignores the variability associated with the response. In practice, it would be difficult, if not impossible, to demonstrate, with the usual criterion for average bioequivalence, that a test product is bioequivalent to a reference product if the reference product is highly variable. The one size-fits-all criterion is also criticized for penalizing good products having lower variability. Thus, it has been suggested that the one-fits-all criterion be flexible by adjusting for the intra-subject variability of the reference product and/or the therapeutic window whenever possible. This has led to the approach of the SABE criterion which can be applied to the assessment of bioequivalence for highly variable drug products. Since most biological products are considered highly variable, the application of SABE for assessment of biosimilar products is being studied (see, e.g., Zhang et al., 2013).

Should similarity in variability or distribution of response be considered?—As discussed earlier, the one size-fits-all criterion, based on the average response of the study endpoint, suffers from the following disadvantages:

1. It ignores the variability associated with the response
2. It may penalize good products with lower variability

The use of SABE for highly variable drugs is an attempt to fix the problem. In practice, it is of interest to establish similarity in variability or distribution for the response of the study endpoint for achieving the ultimate goal of high similarity (see, e.g., Chow and Liu, 2010). For this purpose, many authors have explored the potential application of IBE or PBE to assess biosimilarity (see, e.g., Hsieh et al., 2010). Hsieh et al. (2010) suggested that the similarity in variability of the response of the study endpoint be evaluated because the assessment of similarity in variability is more stringent than that for assessing the biosimilarity in average and, consequently, a higher degree of similarity can be achieved.

What endpoints should be used for the assessment of biosimilarity?—As indicated in the BPCI Act, a biosimilar product should not only be highly similar to that of a reference product but also there should be no clinically meaningful differences in terms of the drug characteristics of safety, purity, and potency. Thus, an easy answer to this question would depend upon which good drug characteristics one would like to show high similarity. For example, if we are to show that there are no clinically meaningful differences in terms of safety and potency (efficacy), then clinical endpoints for safety and efficacy should be used for the assessment of biosimilarity.

Should a clinical trial always be conducted?—If one would like to show that the safety and efficacy of a biosimilar product are highly similar to those of the reference product, then a clinical trial may be required. In some cases, clinical trials for the assessment of biosimilarity may be waived if there is substantial evidence that surrogate endpoints or biomarkers are predictive of the clinical outcomes. On the other hand, clinical trials are required for the assessment of drug interchangeability in order to show that the safety and efficacy between a biosimilar product and a reference product are similar in any given patient of the patient population under study.

What if a biosimilar product turns out to be superior to the reference product?—It should be noted that superiority (including both statistical superiority and clinical superiority) is not biosimilarity. Thus, if a biosimilar product has been shown to be superior to the reference product, then it is suggested that it should be considered as a new biological product. Thus, it is a controversial issue that a biosimilar product should go through the lengthy regulatory review/approval process for similar indications if it is shown to be superior to the innovative product.

Is there a unified approach for the assessment of biosimilarity?—Chow et al. (2010) proposed a unified approach, which is referred to as the biosimilarity index, for the assessment of biosimilarity. The method of biosimilarity index is robust with respect to criteria for biosimilarity and the study design used. The proposed biosimilarity index can be extended to a totality biosimilarity index, which can be used to provide the totality-of-the-evidence across functional areas or domains for the assessment of biosimilarity as suggested in the FDA draft guidance on scientific considerations. More details regarding the development and application of the biosimilarity index for assessing biosimilarity can be found in Chapter 6.

1.5 Interchangeability of Biological Drug Products

As indicated in the Public Health Act Subsection 351(k)(4), that is, in Subsection (k)(4) of the BPCI Act, the term *interchangeable* or *interchangeability* in reference to a biological product means that the biological product may be substituted for the reference product without the intervention of the health care provider who prescribed the reference product. Along this line, in what follows, the definition and basic concepts of interchangeability (in terms of switching and alternating) are given.

1.5.1 Definition and Basic Concepts

As stated in the Public Health Act Subsection 351(k)(4), a biological product is considered to be interchangeable with the reference product if (1) the biological product is biosimilar to the reference product, and (2) it can be expected to produce the same clinical result in *any given patient*. In addition, for a biological product that is administered more than once to an individual, the risk in terms of safety or diminished efficacy of alternating or switching between use of the biological product and the reference product is not greater than the risk of using the reference product without such alternation or switch.

Thus, by the definition of the BPCI Act, there is a clear distinction between biosimilarity and interchangeability. In other words, biosimilarity does not imply interchangeability which is much more stringent. According to the BPCI Act, if a test product is judged to be interchangeable with the reference product, then it may be substituted, even alternated, without a possible intervention, or even notification, of the health care provider. However, interchangeability is expected to produce the *same* clinical result in *any given patient*, which can be interpreted as expecting the same clinical result in *every single patient*. In reality, conceivably, lawsuits may be filed if adverse effects are recorded in a patient after switching from one product to another.

It should be noted that when the FDA declares the biosimilarity of two drug products, it may not be assumed that they are interchangeable. Therefore, labels ought to state whether for a follow-on biologic which is biosimilar to a reference product, interchangeability has or has not been established. However, payers and physicians may, in some cases, switch products even if interchangeability has not been established.

1.5.2 Switching and Alternating

Unlike the interchangeability of small-molecule drug products (in terms of prescribability and switchability) (Chow and Liu, 2008), the FDA has slight perception of drug interchangeability for biosimilars. From the FDA's perspective, interchangeability includes the concepts of switching and alternating between an innovative biological products (R) and its follow-on biologics (*T*). The concept of switching involves the switch from not only "*R* to *T*" or "*T* to *R*" (narrow sense of switchability) but also "*T* to *T*" and "*R* to *R*" (broader sense of switchability). As a result, in order to assess switching, biosimilarity for "*R* to *T*," "*T* to *R*," "*T* to *T*," and "*R* to *R*" needs to be assessed based on some biosimilarity criteria under a valid study design.

On the other hand, the concept of alternating is referred to as either the switch from *T* to *R* and then switch back to *T* (i.e., "*T* to *R* to *T*") or the switch from *R* to *T* and then switch back to *R* (i.e., "*R* to *T* to *R*"). Thus, the difference between "the switch from *T* to *R*" or "the switch from *R* to *T*" and "the switch from *R* to *T*" or "the switch from *T* to *R*" needs to be assessed for addressing the concept of alternating.

1.5.3 Study Design

For the assessment of bioequivalence for chemical drug products, a standard two-sequence, two-period (2 × 2) crossover design is often considered, except for drug products with relatively long half-lives. Since most biosimilar products have relatively long half-lives, it is suggested that a parallel-group design should be considered. However, the parallel-group design does not provide independent estimates of variance components such as inter-subject and intra-subject variabilities and the variability due to subject-by-product interaction. Thus, it is a major challenge for assessing biosimilarity and interchangeability (in terms of the concepts of switching and alternating) of biosimilar products under parallel-group designs.

For the assessment of switching, a switching design should allow the assessment of biosimilarity for the switch from "*R* to *T*," "*T* to *R*," "*T* to *T*," and "*R* to *R*" in order to determine whether there is a risk when a switch occurs. For this purpose, Balaam's 4 × 2 crossover design, that is, *TT*, *RR*, *TR*, *RT*, may be useful. Similarly, for addressing the concept of alternating, a two-sequence, three-period dual design, that is, *TRT*, *RTR*, may be useful since the designs allow the assessment of the switch from *T* to *R* and then back to *T*, that is, "*T* to *R* to *T*" and from *R* to *T* and then back to *R*, that is, "*R* to *T* to *R*." For addressing both concepts of switching and alternating for drug interchangeability of biosimilars, a modified Balaam's crossover design, that is, *TT*, *RR*, *TRT*, *RTR*, is recommended.

More details and further discussions regarding the design and analysis of drug interchangeability in terms of switching and alternating are given in Chapter 11.

1.5.4 Remarks

With small-molecule drug products, bioequivalence generally reflects therapeutic equivalence. Drug prescribability, switching, and alternating are generally considered reasonable. With biological products, however, variations are often higher (other than PK factors may be sensitive to small changes in conditions). Thus, often only parallel-group design rather than crossover kinetic studies can be performed. It should be noted that very often, with follow-on biologics, biosimilarity does *not* reflect therapeutic comparability. Therefore, switching and alternating should be pursued with extreme caution.

1.6 Scientific Factors

Following the passage of the BPCI Act, in order to obtain input on specific issues and challenges associated with the implementation of the BPCI Act, the U.S. FDA conducted a 2 day public hearing on the *Approval Pathway for Biosimilar and Interchangeability Biological Products* held on November 2–3, 2010, at the FDA in Silver Spring, Maryland, United States. In what follows, some of the scientific factors and practical issues are addressed.

1.6.1 Fundamental Biosimilarity Assumption

Similar to the Fundamental Bioequivalence Assumption for the assessment of bioequivalence, Chow et al. (2010) proposed the following Fundamental Biosimilarity Assumption for follow-on biologics:

> *When a biosimilar product is claimed to be biosimilar to an innovator's product based on some well-defined product characteristics, it is therapeutically equivalent, provided that the well-defined product characteristics are validated and are reliable predictors of safety and efficacy of the products.*

For the chemical generic products, the well-defined product characteristics are the exposure measures for early, peak, and total portions of the concentration–time curve. The Fundamental Bioequivalence Assumption assumes that equivalence in the exposure measures implies therapeutical equivalence. However, due to the complexity of the biosimilar drug products, one has to verify that some validated product characteristics are indeed reliable predictors of safety and efficacy. It follows that the design and analysis of studies for the evaluation of similarity between a biosimilar drug product and an innovator product are substantially different from those for the chemical generic products.

1.6.2 Consistency in Manufacturing Process/Quality Control

Tse et al. (2006) proposed a statistical quality control (QC) method to assess a proposed index to test the consistency between raw materials (which are from different resources) and/or between final products manufactured by different manufacturing processes. The consistency index is defined as the probability that the ratio of the characteristics (e.g., potency) of the drug products produced by two different manufacturing processes is within a pre-specified limit of consistency. The consistency index close to 1 indicates that the characteristics of the drug products from the two manufacturing processes are almost identical. The idea for testing consistency is to construct a 95% confidence interval for the proposed consistency index under a sampling plan. If the constructed 95% confidence lower limit is larger than a pre-specified QC lower limit, then we claim that the final products produced by the two manufacturing processes are consistent.

Let U and W be characteristics of the drug products from two different manufacturing processes, where $X = \log U$ and $Y = \log W$ follow normal distributions with means μ_X, μ_Y and variances V_X, V_Y, respectively. Similar to the idea of using $P(X < Y)$ to assess reliability in statistical QC (Church and Harris, 1970; Enis and Geisser, 1971), Tse et al. (2006) proposed the following probability as an index to assess the consistency between the two different manufacturing processes:

$$p = P\left(1-\delta < \frac{U}{W} < \frac{1}{1-\delta}\right),$$

where $0 < \delta < 1$ and is defined as a limit that allows for consistency. Tse et al. (2006) refer to p as the consistency index. Thus p tends to 1 as δ tends to 1. For a given δ, if p is close to 1, characteristics U and W are considered to be nearly identical. It should be noted that a small δ implies the requirement of high degree of consistency between the characteristics U and W. In practice, it may be difficult to meet this narrow specification for consistency. Tse et al. (2006) proposed the following QC criterion. If the probability that the lower limit $LL(\hat{p})$ of the constructed $(1 - \alpha) \times 100\%$ confidence interval of p is larger than or equal to a pre-specified QC lower limit, say, QC_L, exceeds a pre-specified number β (say $\beta = 80\%$), then we claim that U and W are consistent or similar. In other words, U and W are consistent or similar if $P(QC_L \leq LL(\hat{p})) \geq \beta$, where β is a pre-specified constant.

1.6.3 Biosimilarity in Biological Activity

Pharmacological or biological activity is an expression describing the beneficial or adverse effects of a drug on living matter. When the drug is a complex chemical mixture, this activity is exerted by the substance's active ingredient or pharmacophore but can be modified by the other constituents. The main kind of adverse biological activity is a substance's toxicity. Activity is generally dosage-dependent and it is not uncommon to have effects ranging from beneficial to adverse for one substance when going from low to high doses. Activity depends critically on the fulfillment of the ADME (absorption, distribution, metabolism, and elimination) criteria.

Biosimilarity refers to comparisons between a reference product and a biosimilar product (the new EU "pharmaceutical review" legislation published on April 30, 2004, amended the EU community code on medicinal products to provide for the approval of biosimilars based on fewer preclinical and clinical data than had been required for the original reference product.)

The complexity of the protein and knowledge of its structure–function relationships determine the types of information needed to establish similarity.

1.6.4 Similarity in Size and Structure

In practice, various in vitro tests such as the assessments of the primary amino acid sequence, charge, and hydrophobic properties are performed to compare the structural aspects of biosimilars with their originator molecules. However, it is a concern whether in vitro tests can be predictive of biological activity in vivo due to the fact that there are significant differences in biological activity despite similarities in size and structure. Besides, it is difficult to assess biological activity adequately as few animal models are able to provide data that can be extrapolated for an accurate and reliable prediction of biological activity in humans. Thus, controlled clinical trials remain the most reliable means of demonstrating therapeutic similarity between a biosimilar molecule and the originator product.

1.6.5 Issues of Immunogenicity

The immune system consists of a diverse and complex set of cells and organs that have complicated interactions with each other and with other physiological systems. These complexities make the detection and evaluation of drug-induced immunogenicity difficult. The use of biosimilar products could have unwanted immune responses. An unwanted immune reaction could result in a clinical consequence of severe life-threatening conditions. Thus, the assessment of potential immunogenicity on the immune system is an important component of the overall evaluation of the safety (toxicity) of biosimilar products. However, although immunogenicity findings could indict a biosimilar product for some types of clinical investigations or certain indications, these findings appear to be rare (FDA, 2002).

Since all biological products are biologically active molecules derived from living cells and have the potential to evoke an immune response, immunogenicity is probably the most critical safety concern for the assessment of biosimilarity of follow-on biologics. The immune responses to biological products can lead to loss in efficacy and change in safety profile such as

1. Anaphylaxis
2. Injection site reactions
3. Flu-like syndromes
4. Allergic responses

The risk of immunogenicity can be reduced through stringent testing of the products during their development. More details regarding issues on immunogenicity are provided in Chapter 12.

1.6.6 Comparability/Consistency of Manufacturing Processes

Unlike small-molecule drug products, biological products are made of living cells. Thus, manufacturing of biological products is a very complicated process, which involves the steps of

1. Cell expansion
2. Cell production (in bioreactors)
3. Recovery (through filtration or centrifugation)
4. Purification (through chromatography)
5. Formulation

A small discrepancy at each step (e.g., purification) could lead to a significant difference in the final product, which might cause drastic change in clinical outcomes. Thus, process control and validation play an important role for the success of the manufacturing of biological products. In addition, since at each step (e.g., purification) different methods may be used at different biological manufacturing processes (within the same company or at different biotech companies), tests for consistency are necessarily performed. Note that at the step of purification, the following chromatography media or resin are commonly considered:

1. Gel filtration
2. Ion exchange
3. Hydrophobic interaction
4. Reversed phase normal phase
5. Affinity

Thus, at each step of the manufacturing process, primary performance characteristics should be identified, controlled, and tested for consistency for process control and validation.

Issues involving the comparability and the assessment of consistency for manufacturing processes are presented in Chapter 14.

1.6.7 Other Practical Issues

There are many critical attributes of a potential patient's response to follow-on biologics. For a given critical attribute, valid statistical methods are necessarily to be developed under a valid study design and a given set of criteria for similarity, as described in the previous section. Several areas can be identified for developing appropriate statistical methodologies for the assessment of biosimilarity of follow-on biologics. These areas include, but are not limited to

Reference standards—For the development of biosimilar products, any information regarding the reference product is critical because the assessment of biosimilarity and interchangeability may heavily depend upon the performance of the reference product. We shall refer to the performances of the reference product in various functional areas as *reference standards*. In practice, the sponsors of biosimilar products usually have limited information regarding the reference product even if the reference product has expired (not much information is available in public). In this case, how to establish reference standards (or the baseline) for comparison has become very critical (Davis et al. 2009). In practice, it is suggested that a study comparing the reference product to itself be considered, in a three-arm investigation consisting of a test product, a reference product, and the other reference product, in order to establish the baseline or reference standards for a valid and reliable assessment of the biosimilar product. Note that in these cases, the same reference product may come from either different batches of the same manufacturing process or different manufacturing processes (sites or countries).

Criteria for biosimilarity—In addition to the issue regarding what criteria for biosimilarity should be used (in terms of average, variability, or distribution), the following questions are of particular interest to scientists/researchers in the subject area. First, should a one size-fits-all criterion be applied to different functional areas (or domains) for achieving the totality-of-the evidence between biosimilars and the innovative product? If the answer to this question is negative, then what degrees of similarity at different functional areas (or domains) should be considered? For some functional areas, the degree of similarity could have less impact on the clinical outcomes as compared to others. In this case, what weights should be used for achieving the totality-of-the-evidence when assessing biosimilarity?

Criteria for interchangeability—In practice, drug interchangeability (in terms of IBE for switchability for small-molecule drug products) is recognized to be related to the variability due to subject-by-drug product interaction. However, it is not clear whether the criterion for interchangeability should be based on the variability due to subject-by-product interaction or on the variability due to subject-by-product interaction adjusted for intra-subject variability of the reference drug. Moreover, for the assessment of interchangeability (in terms of the concepts of switching and alternating) of biosimilar products, it is not clear (1) whether the criterion based on the variability due to subject-by-drug interaction for small-molecule drug products can be applied directly to biosimilar products, and (2) how the criterion based on the variability due to subject-by-drug product relates to the relative risk with and without alternating and switching of biosimilar products.

Bridging studies for assessing biosimilarity—As most studies of biosimilars are conducted using a parallel design rather than a replicated crossover design, independent estimates of variance components such as for within subjects and the variability due to subject-by-drug interaction are not possible. In this case, bridging studies may be considered.

Other practical issues include (1) the use of a percentile method for the assessment of variability, (2) comparability in biologic activities, (3) sample size determination for immunogenicity studies with extremely low incidence rates, (4) QC/assurance in manufacturing processes (see, e.g., ICH, 1996, 1999, 2005), (5) stability testing for multiple lots and/or multiple laboratories (see, e.g., ICH, 1996), (6) the potential use of sequential testing procedures and multiple testing procedures, and (7) assessing biosimilarity using a surrogate endpoint or biomarkers such as genomic data (see, e.g., Chow et al., 2004).

More discussion of the aforementioned practical issues can be found in the last four chapters (CMC requirements, stability analysis, assessing biosimilarity using biomarker data, and current issues). Further research is needed in order to address the aforementioned scientific factors and practical issues recognized at the FDA Public Hearings (November 2–3, 2010 and May 11, 2012) and Public Meeting for User Fees (December 16, 2011).

1.7 Aim and Scope of the Book

This book is intended to be the first book entirely devoted to the design and analysis for the development of follow-on biologics. It focuses on the assessment of biosimilarity and of interchangeability of biosimilars as well as on tests for the comparability in the manufacturing processes of biological products. It covers the statistical issues that may be encountered in biosimilar studies under various study designs, at the various stages of research and development of biological products. It is my goal to provide a useful desk reference and the state-of-the-art examination of the subject area to scientists and researchers engaged in pharmaceutical/clinical research and the development of biological products, those in government regulatory agencies who have to make decisions in the review and approval process of biological regulatory submissions, and to biostatisticians who provide the statistical support to the assessment of biosimilarity and drug interchangeability of biosimilars and related issues regarding the QC/assurance and test for the comparability in the manufacturing processes for biological products. I hope that this book can serve as a bridge among scientists in the pharmaceutical/ biotechnology industry, government regulatory agencies, and academia.

The scope of this book covers statistical issues that are commonly encountered for the assessment of biosimilarity and drug interchangeability of follow-on biologics. In this chapter, the definitions, regulatory requirements, and scientific factors regarding biosimilarity and drug interchangeability have been discussed. In the next chapter, past experience for bioequivalence assessment for small-molecule drug products is briefly described. Chapter 3 summarizes regulatory requirements for the assessment of biosimilar products (or follow-on biologics). Also included in this chapter is a review of recently published FDA draft guidances on biosimilar products. Criteria for the assessment of biosimilarity which are available in the regulatory guidances/guidelines and/or the literature are described in Chapter 4. Chapter 5 introduces statistical methods for assessing average biosimilarity based on the concept of relative distance between a test product and a reference product as compared to the reference product versus itself. Chapter 6 proposes a general approach based on a biosimilarity index (reproducibility probability) for the assessment of biosimilar products. Chapter 7 explores the relationship between the concept of testing non-inferiority and testing for equivalence. Chapter 8 provides some statistical tests for the assessment of biosimilarity in variability of biosimilar products. Formulas and procedures for sample size calculations for comparing variabilities under a crossover design or a parallel design with or without replicates are given in Chapter 9. Chapter 10 studies the impact of variability on biosimilarity limits for assessing biosimilar products. Chapter 11 investigates the feasibility/applicability for the assessment of interchangeability (in terms of the concepts of alternating and switching among biosimilar products). The issue of immunogenicity in biosimilar studies is examined in Chapter 12. CMC requirements for biological products in BLA (Biologic Licence Application) submissions are discussed in Chapter 13. Chapter 14 provides statistical methods for testing comparability in manufacturing processes of biosimilar products. Stability design and analysis of biosimilar products are given in Chapter 15. Chapter 16 discusses statistical tests for the assessment of biosimilarity using biomarker data. Current issues for assessing biosimilars are discussed in the last chapter.

For each chapter, whenever possible, examples are included to illustrate the described statistical methods for the assessment of biosimilarity and drug interchangeability. In addition, if applicable, topics for future research are provided. All computations in this book are performed using version 9.20 of SAS. Other statistical packages such as *R* and *S*-plus can also be applied.

2

Bioequivalence Experience for Small-Molecule Drug Products

2.1 Background

As indicated in the previous chapter, when an innovative small-molecule drug product is going off patent, brand-name pharmaceutical and generic companies may file an abbreviated new drug application (ANDA) for approval of the generic copies of the innovative drug product. The innovative drug product is usually referred to as the brand-name drug product or *reference* product. A generic copy is a drug product identical to the reference drug which is the subject of an approved new drug application (NDA) with regard to active ingredient(s), route of administration, dosage form, strength, and conditions of use. Generic copies of the reference product are called *test* products. For the approval of generic drug products, the U.S. Food and Drug Administration (FDA) as well as other regulatory authorities require that evidence of bioequivalence in average bioavailability be provided through the conduct of pharmacokinetic (PK) bioequivalence studies. The assessment of bioequivalence in average bioavailability is usually referred to as the assessment of average bioequivalence (ABE). The assessment of bioequivalence as a surrogate endpoint for the evaluation of drug safety and efficacy is based on the *Fundamental Bioequivalence Assumption* that if two drug products are shown to be bioequivalent in average bioavailability, it is assumed that they are therapeutically equivalent. Note that, in clinical practice, many practitioners interpret that approved generic drug products can be used interchangeably since they are therapeutically equivalent to the brand-name drug.

For the approval of generic drug products, the FDA requires that bioequivalence studies be conducted for comparing drug absorption profiles between the test product and the reference product in terms of some PK parameters such as the area under the blood and/or plasma concentration–time curve (AUC) and maximum or peak concentration (C_{max}). AUC and C_{max} are the primary PK responses for measuring the extent and rate of drug absorption. In practice, we claim that a test drug product is bioequivalent to a reference drug product if the 90% confidence interval for the ratio of geometric means of the primary PK parameter (in %) is totally within the bioequivalence limits of (80%, 125%). The confidence interval for the ratio of geometric means of the primary PK parameters is obtained based on log-transformed data.

The purpose of this chapter is to provide a comprehensive summarization of experience in bioequivalence assessment of small-molecule drug products. In the next section, the process for the assessment of bioequivalence of generic approval for small-molecule drug products is given. Section 2.3 discusses the issue of drug interchangeability in terms of population bioequivalence (PBE) for addressing drug prescribability and individual bioequivalence (IBE) for drug switchability. Current thinking of FDA on the assessment of highly variable drug products is given in Section 2.4. Practical issues and frequently asked questions when assessing the bioequivalence of small-molecule drug products are discussed in Section 2.5 and Section 2.6, respectively. Brief concluding remarks are given in the last section of this chapter.

2.2 Process for Bioequivalence Assessment

The process of bioequivalence assessment starts with the so-called *Fundamental Bioequivalence Assumption* followed by the conduct of a bioequivalence study under a valid study design, appropriate statistical methods for the assessment of ABE, and then regulatory submission, review, and approval.

2.2.1 Fundamental Bioequivalence Assumption

As indicated by Chow and Liu (2008), bioequivalence studies are necessarily conducted under the Fundamental Bioequivalence Assumption, which constitutes legal basis (from the *Hatch-Waxman* Act) for regulatory review and approval of small-molecule generic drug products. The Fundamental Bioequivalence Assumption states that

> *If two drug products are shown to be bioequivalent, it is assumed that they will reach the same therapeutic effect or that they are therapeutically equivalent.*

In practice, bioequivalence in drug absorption has been interpreted as the confidence interval for the ratio of means (of drug absorption) being within the bioequivalence limits. An alternative would be to show that the tolerance intervals (or a distribution free model) overlap sufficiently. Under the previously mentioned Fundamental Bioequivalence Assumption, many practitioners interpret that generic drug products and the innovative drug product can be used interchangeably (i.e., that they can be freely switched within patients) because they are therapeutically equivalent. The FDA and other regulatory authorities, however, do not indicate that

(1) approved generic drug products and the innovative drug products can be used interchangeably, and (2) approved generic drug products can be used interchangeably. The FDA and other regulatory authorities only indicate that an approved generic drug product can be used as a substitute to the innovative drug product.

To protect the exclusivity of an innovative (or brand-name) drug product, the sponsors of the innovator drug products will usually make every attempt to prevent generic drug products from being approved by the regulatory agencies such as the FDA. One of the strategies is to challenge the Fundamental Bioequivalence Assumption by filing a *citizen petition* with scientific/clinical justification. In the United States, upon the receipt of a citizen petition, the FDA has legal obligation to respond within 180 days. It, however, should be noted that the FDA will not suspend or withhold the review/approval process of a generic submission of a given brand-name drug even if a citizen petition is under review within the FDA.

In spite of the Fundamental Bioequivalence Assumption, one of the controversial issues is that bioequivalence may not necessarily imply therapeutic equivalence and therapeutic equivalence does not guarantee bioequivalence either. The assessment of ABE for generic approval has been criticized to be based on legal/political considerations rather than scientific arguments. In the past several decades, many sponsors/researchers have made attempts to challenge this assumption without success. More discussions regarding the Fundamental Bioequivalence Assumption are given in Section 2.5.1.

2.2.2 Study Design

As indicated in the *Federal Register* (Vol. 42, No. 5, Sec. 320.26 (b) and Sec. 320.27 (b), 1977), a bioavailability study (single-dose or multi-dose) should be crossover in design, unless a parallel or other design is more appropriate for valid scientific reasons. Thus, in practice, a standard two-sequence, two-period (or 2×2) crossover design is often considered for a bioavailability or bioequivalence study. Denote by T and R the test product and the reference product, respectively. Thus, a 2×2 crossover design can be expressed as (TR, RT), where TR is the first sequence of treatments and RT denotes the second sequence of treatments. Under the (TR, RT) design, qualified subjects who are randomly assigned to sequence 1 (TR) will receive the test product (T) first and then cross over to receive the reference product (R) after a sufficient length of wash-out period. Similarly, subjects who are randomly assigned to sequence 2 (RT) will receive the reference product (R) first and then cross over to receive the test product (T) after a sufficient length of wash-out period.

One of the limitations of the standard 2×2 crossover design is that it does not provide independent estimates of intra-subject variabilities since each subject receives the same treatment only once. In the interest of assessing intra-subject variabilities, the following alternative crossover designs for comparing two drug products are often considered:

Design 1: Balaam's design—i.e., (TT, RR, RT, TR)

Design 2: Two-sequence, three-period dual design—e.g., (TRR, RTT)

Design 3: Four-period design with two sequences—e.g., (TRRT, RTTR)

Design 4: Four-period design with four sequences—e.g., (TTRR, RRTT, TRTR, RTTR)

Note that the aforementioned study designs are also known as higher-order crossover designs. A higher-order crossover design is defined as a crossover design with the number of sequences or the number of periods larger than the number of treatments to be compared.

For comparing more than two drug products, a Williams' design is often considered. For example, for comparing three drug products, a six-sequence, three-period (6×3) Williams' design is usually considered, while a 4×4 Williams' design is employed for comparing four drug products. Williams' design is a variance stabilizing design. More information regarding the construction and good design characteristics of Williams' designs can be found in Chow and Liu (2008).

Note that when designing a bioequivalence study, the question regarding "What length of wash-out is considered sufficient enough in order to wear off the possible residual effect that might be carried over from one period to the next?" is often asked. For immediate-release (IR) drug products, the FDA suggests at least 5.5 half-lives of the reference product be used, while 8.5 half-lives should be considered for controlled-release (CR) drug products. Regarding blood sampling, it is suggested that more sampling around C_{max} be considered. The sampling should cover at least three half-lives in order to characterize the blood or plasma concentration–time curve, which is often used to derive model-independent PK responses such as the area under the blood or plasma concentration–time curve (AUC) and the maximum concentration (C_{max}).

2.2.3 Power Analysis for Sample Size Calculation

As indicated in Chow and Liu (2008), formulas for sample size calculations under a given $p \times q$ crossover design can be obtained based on the evaluation of power curve of Schuirmann's two one-sided tests procedure. For this purpose, we define the following quantities:

$$\theta = \frac{\mu_T - \mu_R}{\mu_R},$$

$$CV = \frac{s}{\mu_R}$$

$$[-\delta\mu_R, \delta\mu_R] = \text{The bioequivalence limits,}$$

$t(\alpha, v) =$ The upper αth quantile of a t distribution with v degrees of freedom,

where
 μ_T and μ_R are the average bioavailabilities of the test and reference products, respectively

 s denotes the square-root of the mean square error from the analysis of variance table of the given crossover design

Note that θ is the ratio of the difference in average bioavailability between the two products and the average reference bioavailability, while CV stands for the coefficient of variation for the reference product. Because the power curves of Schuirmann's two one-sided tests procedure are symmetric about zero, in the section, we shall only present the formulas for the case where $\theta \geq 0$.

Let n_i be the number of subjects in each sequence i having the same value n, and F_v denote the cumulative distribution function of the t distribution with v degrees of freedom. Then, under an additive model, the power function $P_k(\theta)$ of the Schuirmann's two one-sided tests procedure at the α nominal level for design k as described in previous subsection can be obtained as

$$P_k(\theta) = F_{v_k}\left(\left[\frac{\delta - \theta}{CV\sqrt{b_k/n}}\right] - t(\alpha, v_k)\right)$$

$$- F_{v_k}\left(t(\alpha, v_k) - \left[\frac{(\delta + \theta)}{CV\sqrt{b_k/n}}\right]\right) \quad \text{for } k = 1, 2, 3, 4,$$

where

$$v_1 = 4n - 3, \quad v_2 = 4n - 4, \quad v_3 = 6n - 5, \quad v_4 = 12n - 5$$

$$b_1 = 2, \quad b_2 = \frac{3}{4}, \quad b_3 = \frac{11}{20}, \quad b_4 = \frac{1}{4}$$

Hence, the exact formula for determination of n required to achieve a $1 - \beta$ power at the α nominal level for the design k when $\theta = 0$ is given by

$$n \geq b_k\left[t(\alpha, v_k) + t\left(\frac{\beta}{2}, v_k\right)\right]^2\left(\frac{CV}{\delta}\right)^2 \quad \text{for } k = 1, 2, 3, 4,$$

and if $\theta > 0$, the approximate formula for n is

$$n \geq b_k\left[t(\alpha, v_k) + t(\beta, v_k)\right]^2\left(\frac{CV}{\delta - \theta}\right)^2 \quad \text{for } k = 1, 2, 3, 4.$$

For the multiplicative model, consider (0.8, 1.25) to be the bioequivalence limits of μ_T/μ_R and denoted by δ, where μ_T and μ_R are the median bioavailabilities of the test and reference products, respectively (Hauschke et al., 1992). Also, let ln denote the natural logarithm. Similarly, the sample size required for achieving a $1 - \beta$ power at the α level of significance for the design k after the logarithmic transformation is determined by the following formulas:

$$n \ge b_k \left[t(\alpha, v_k) + t\left(\frac{\beta}{2}, v_k\right) \right]^2 \left(\frac{CV_k}{\ln 1.25} \right)^2 \quad \text{if } \delta = 1$$

$$n \ge b_k [t(\alpha, v_k) + t(\beta, v_k)]^2 \left(\frac{CV_k}{\ln 1.25 - \ln \delta} \right)^2 \quad \text{if } 1 < \delta < 1.25$$

and

$$n \ge b_k [t(\alpha, v_k) + t(\beta, v_k)]^2 \left(\frac{CV_k}{\ln 0.8 - \ln \delta} \right)^2 \quad \text{if } 0.8 < \delta < 1$$

$$\text{for } k = 1, 2, 3, 4.$$

Note that in the formulas provided earlier, β is the probability of a type II error concluding bioinequivalence when in fact the two products are bioequivalent. $\delta, CV_k = \sqrt{\exp(\sigma_k^2) - 1}$, the coefficient of variation in the multiplicative model, and σ^2, the residual (within-subject) variance of the logarithmically transformed characteristics, can usually be obtained from previous studies. However, because the degrees of freedom are usually unknown, an easy way to find the sample size is to enumerate n (see, also, Chen et al., 1997).

2.2.4 Statistical Methods

As indicated earlier, ABE is claimed if the geometric means ratio (GMR) of average bioavailabilities between test and reference products is within the bioequivalence limits of (80%, 125%) with 90% assurance based on log-transformed data. Along this line, commonly employed statistical methods are the confidence interval approach and the method of interval hypotheses testing. For the confidence interval approach, a 90% confidence interval for the ratio of geometric means of a primary PK response such as AUC or C_{max} is obtained under an analysis of variance model. We claim bioequivalence if the obtained 90% confidence interval (in%) is totally within the bioequivalence limits of (80%, 125%).

For the method of interval hypotheses testing, the interval hypotheses are

$$H_0 : \text{Bioinequivalence versus } H_a : \text{Bioequivalence} \qquad (2.1)$$

Note that the aforementioned hypotheses are usually decomposed into two sets of one-sided hypotheses. The first set of hypotheses is to verify that the average bioavailability of the test product is not too low, whereas the second set of hypotheses is to verify that average bioavailability of the test product is not too high. Under the two one-sided hypotheses, Schuirmann's two one-sided tests procedure is commonly employed for testing ABE (Schuirmann, 1987).

In practice, other statistical methods are sometimes considered such as Westlake's symmetric confidence interval approach, the exact confidence interval based on Fieller's theorem, Chow and Shao's joint confidence region approach, Bayesian methods, and nonparametric methods such as the Wilcoxon–Mann–Whitney two one-sided tests procedure, a distribution-free confidence interval based on the Hodges–Lehmann estimator, and bootstrap confidence interval (Chow and Liu, 2008).

2.2.5 Remarks

Although the assessment of ABE for generic approval has been in practice for years, it has the following limitations:

1. It focuses only on the population average.
2. It ignores the distribution of the metric.
3. It does not provide independent estimates of intra-subject variability (ISV) and ignores the subject-by-formulation interaction.

Many authors criticized that the assessment of ABE does not address the question of drug interchangeability and it may penalize drug products with lower variability.

As indicated by the regulatory agencies, a generic drug can be used as a substitute for the brand-name drug if their bioequivalence has been demonstrated. Current regulations do not indicate that two generic copies of the same brand-name drug can be used interchangeably, even though they are bioequivalent to the same brand-name drug. Bioequivalence between generic copies of a brand-name drug is not required. Note that in practice, it is possible that there can be drift: one product is bioequivalent but with a slightly smaller response (parameter) than the innovator product and the other bioequivalent but with a slightly larger response (parameter) than the innovator product. Consequently, the difference could be large enough that the products are not bioequivalent. Thus, one of the controversial issues in the assessment of ABE is whether these approved generic drug products can be used interchangeably and safely.

2.3 Issue of Drug Interchangeability

Basically, interchangeability of small-molecule drug products can be considered either as drug prescribability or drug switchability. These concepts were much discussed in the 1990s and early 2000s. They are still valuable and important. However, the FDA and other regulatory agencies do not encourage at present their use and implementation.

Drug prescribability is defined as the physician's choice for prescribing an appropriate drug product for his/her new patients between a brand-name drug product and a number of generic drug products that have been shown to be bioequivalent to the brand-name drug product. The underlying assumption of drug prescribability is that the brand-name drug product and its generic copies can be used alternatively in terms of the efficacy and safety of the drug product. Drug prescribability, therefore, involves the administration of either drug product to a new patient. Drug switchability, on the other hand, is related to the switch from a drug product (e.g., a brand-name drug product) to an alternative drug product (e.g., a generic copy of the brand-name drug product) within the same subject, whose concentration of the drug product has been titrated to a steady, efficacious, and safe level. As a result, drug switchability is considered more critical than drug prescribability in the study of drug interchangeability for patients who have been on medication for a while. Drug switchability, therefore, is exchangeability within the same subject.

Note that in practice many use the terms interchangeability and switchability synonymously. (Another term used, in this context, is substitutability.) These terms are meant to replace, in a given patient, the administration of one drug product by another. Thus, these usages refer to subjects to whom the drug has already been administered and who are not naïve to it. The recent Canadian document is an example of the widespread usage of these terms. Also noteworthy is the definition of interchangeability in the *Biologics Price Competition and Innovation* (BPCI) Act of 2010, Section 7002: "(3) The term 'interchangeable' or 'interchangeability,' in reference to a biological product that is shown to meet the standards described in subsection (k)(4), means that the biological product may be substituted for the reference product without the intervention of the health care provider who prescribed the reference product."

2.3.1 Population Bioequivalence for Drug Prescribability

As indicated in Chow and Liu (2008), ABE can guarantee neither drug prescribability nor drug switchability. Therefore, the assessment and implementation of bioequivalence should take into consideration drug prescribability and drug switchability. To address drug interchangeability, it is recommended that PBE and IBE be considered for testing drug prescribability and drug switchability, respectively. More specifically, the FDA recommended that PBE be applied to new formulations, additional strengths, or new dosage forms in NDAs, while IBE should be considered for ANDA or AADA (abbreviated antibiotic drug application) for generic drugs (FDA, 2001).

To address drug prescribability, the FDA proposed the following aggregated, scaled, moment-based, one-sided criterion:

$$PBC = \frac{(\mu_T - \mu_R)^2 + (\sigma_{TT}^2 - \sigma_{TR}^2)}{\max(\sigma_{TR}^2, \sigma_{T0}^2)} \leq \theta_P,$$

(2.2)

where

μ_T and μ_R are the means of the test drug product and the reference drug product, respectively

σ_{TT}^2 and σ_{TR}^2 are the total variances of the test drug product and the reference drug product, respectively

σ_{T0}^2 is a constant that can be adjusted to control the probability of passing PBE

θ_P is the bioequivalence limit for PBE

The numerator on the left-hand side of the criterion is the sum of the squared difference between the population averages and of the difference in total variance between the test and reference drug products which measure the similarity for the marginal population distribution between the test and the reference drug products. The denominator on the left-hand side of the criterion is a scaling factor that depends upon the variability of the drug class of the reference drug product. The FDA guidance suggests that θ_P be chosen as

$$\theta_P = \frac{(\log 1.25)^2 + \varepsilon_P}{\sigma_{T0}^2},$$

(2.3)

where ε_P is guided by the consideration of the variability term $\sigma_{TT}^2 - \sigma_{TR}^2$ added to the ABE criterion. As suggested by the FDA guidance, it may be appropriate that ε_P be chosen as 0.02. For the determination of σ_{T0}^2, the guidance suggests the use of the so-called population difference ratio (PDR), which is defined as

$$PDR = \left[\frac{E(T - R)^2}{E(R - R')^2} \right]^{1/2}$$

$$= \left[\frac{(\mu_T - \mu_R)^2 + \sigma_{TT}^2 + \sigma_{TR}^2}{2\sigma_{TR}^2} \right]^{1/2}$$

$$= \left[\frac{PBC}{2} + 1 \right]^{1/2}.$$

(2.4)

Therefore, assuming that the maximum allowable PDR is 1.25, substitution of $(\log 1.25)^2/\sigma_{T0}^2$ for PBC without an adjustment of the variance term approximately yields $\sigma_{T0} = 0.2$.

2.3.2 Individual Bioequivalence for Drug Switchability

Similarly, to address drug switchability, the FDA recommended the following aggregated, scaled, moment-based, one-sided criterion:

$$\text{IBC} = \frac{(\mu_T - \mu_R)^2 + \sigma_D^2 + (\sigma_{WT}^2 - \sigma_{WR}^2)}{\max(\sigma_{WR}^2, \sigma_{W0}^2)} \leq \theta_I, \tag{2.5}$$

where

σ_{WT}^2 and σ_{WR}^2 are the within-subject variances of the test drug product and the reference drug product, respectively

σ_D^2 is the variance component due to subject-by-drug product interaction

σ_{W0}^2 is a constant that can be adjusted to control the probability of passing IBE

θ_I is the bioequivalence limit for IBE

The FDA guidance suggests that θ_I be chosen as

$$\theta_I = \frac{(\log 1.25)^2 + \varepsilon_I}{\sigma_{W0}^2}, \tag{2.6}$$

where ε_I is the variance allowance factor, which can be adjusted for sample size control. Note that the FDA guidance suggests $\varepsilon_I = 0.05$.

For the determination of σ_{W0}^2, the guidance suggests the use of an individual difference ratio (IDR), which is defined as

$$\text{IDR} = \left[\frac{E(T - R)^2}{E(R - R')^2} \right]^{1/2}$$

$$= \left[\frac{(\mu_T - \mu_R)^2 + \sigma_D^2 + (\sigma_{WT}^2 + \sigma_{WR}^2)}{2\sigma_{WR}^2} \right]^{1/2}$$

$$= \left[\frac{\text{IBC}}{2} + 1 \right]^{1/2}. \tag{2.7}$$

Therefore, assuming that the maximum allowable IDR is 1.25, substitution of $(\log 1.25)^2/\sigma_{W0}^2$ for IBC without an adjustment of the variance term approximately yields $\sigma_{W0} = 0.2$. It should be noted that although the FDA guidance recommends $\sigma_{WO} = 0.2$, the FDA uses (in a different context) $\sigma_{WO} = 0.25$.

2.3.3 Remarks

In practice, it is of particular interest to pharmaceutical scientists and researchers to determine whether similar ideas for assessing drug interchangeability for small-molecule drug products could be directly applied to biosimilar products if independent estimates of intra-subject variabilities, inter-subject variabilities, and the variability due to subject-by-drug interaction can be obtained under a valid study design.

2.4 Highly Variable Drugs

As indicated earlier, the assessment of ABE focuses on average bioavailability but ignores the variability associated with the PK responses. Thus, two drug products may fail the evaluation of ABE if the variability associated with the PK responses is large even though they have identical means. A drug with large variability is considered highly variable. It is generally accepted that a highly variable drug (HVD) is defined as one whose within-subject (or intra-subject) variation is larger than or equal to 30% (Shah et al., 1996). This definition based on intra-subject variation, however, is rather arbitrary. One of the problematic aspects of this definition is that the estimated within-subject variability depends on the metrics of PK responses such as AUC and C_{max}. In practice, the observed C_{max} is usually more variable than AUC. As indicated by Davit et al. (2008), among the 212 bioequivalence studies submitted to the FDA, 33 studies were considered highly variable. In 28 of the 33 studies, only the C_{max}, but not the AUC, had a variation higher than 30%. Among the 33 studies, no cases indicated that the AUC, but not the C_{max}, was highly variable. Tothfalusi et al. (2008) pointed out that HVDs show variable PKs as a result of their inherent properties (e.g., distribution, systemic metabolism, and elimination). A drug may have low variability if it is administered intravenously, whereas it can be highly variable after oral administration.

In practice, HVDs often fail to meet current regulatory acceptance criteria for ABE. In the past decade, the topic the evaluation of bioequivalence for HVDs has received much attention. This topic has been discussed several times at regulatory forums and international conferences. Academics, representatives of pharmaceutical industries and regulatory agencies have recently reached a consensus that the approach of scaled average bioequivalence (SABE), or an equivalent procedure, provides a reasonable means to deal with the problem. Tothfalusi et al. (2009) provided an excellent review for the evaluation of bioequivalence for HVDs with SABE. The approach of SABE, proposed by Tothfalusi et al. (2001) and implemented by the FDA (Haidar et al., 2008), is briefly described later.

2.4.1 Scaled Average Bioequivalence

To introduce SABE, we first consider the criterion for ABE. As indicated ear-lier, the PK response is a logarithmically transformed metric, e.g., log(AUC) or log(C_{max}). The two one-sided tests (TOST) procedure is usually applied to assess bioequivalence (Schuirmann, 1987). Accordingly, the average logarith-mic kinetic responses of the test (T) and reference (R) formulations, denoted by μ_T and μ_R, respectively, are compared. The acceptance of bioequivalence is claimed if the difference between the logarithmic means is between pre-specified regulatory limits. The limits (θ_A) are generally symmetrical on the logarithmic scale and usually equal $\pm\ln(1.25)$. Thus, the criterion for ABE can be expressed as follows:

$$-\theta_A \le \mu_T - \mu_R \le \theta_A. \tag{2.8}$$

In a bioequivalence study, the individual kinetic responses are evaluated from the measured concentrations. The means of the logarithmic responses of the two formulations are calculated. These sample averages estimate the true population means. A variance is also estimated for each kinetic response. It is a measure of the intra-subject variance, but not always identical to it. The FDA suggests the ABE mentioned previously could be scaled by a standard deviation as follows:

$$-\theta_S \le \frac{(\mu_T - \mu_R)}{\sigma_W} \le \theta_S, \tag{2.9}$$

where θ_S is the SABE regulatory cutoff. Here the standard deviation (σ_W) is the within-subject standard deviation. In applying a replicate design, σ_W is generally the within-subject standard deviation of the reference formulation (denoted by σ_{WR}). Thus, the scaling factor of SABE has similar features to the scaling factor of IBE.

2.4.2 Recent Considerations by Regulatory Agencies

Between the early 1990s and early 2000s, the FDA considered IBE and PBE as a possible solution for the problem of bioequivalence for HVDs. However, the development of this approach has been abandoned. In 2004, the FDA kicked off a *Critical Path Initiative* that focused on the challenges involved in the development of new drugs and generics. As part of this initiative, the FDA established a working group on the bioequivalence of HVDs for the development of a guidance dealing with HVDs. The group made pre-sentations to a meeting of its advisory committee in 2004 and at an AAPS symposium in 2005. The results and conclusions of the group's work were summarized recently by Haidar et al. (2008) and Davit et al. (2008). The sum-mary by Haidar et al. (2008) then serves as a basis for consideration by the

FDA of actual submissions. Consequently, SABE appears to have gained a measure of recognition and implementation.

For evaluation of bioequivalence of HVDs with SABE, as indicated in Equation 2.9, the bioequivalence limits for SABE can be expressed in the form of

$$\theta_S = \frac{\ln(1.25)}{\sigma_0},$$

where

σ_0 is a so-called regulatory standardized variation, which defines the proportionality factor between the logarithmic bioequivalence limits

σ_W in the highly variable region

The value of σ_0 must be defined by the regulators. The magnitude of σ_0 defines the bioequivalence limits (θ_S). For instance, when $\sigma_0 = 0.294$, then θ is 0.760.

EMA in the European Union applies a modified form of SABE (EMA, 2010c). Multiplying Equation 2.9 by σ_W:

$$-\theta_S \sigma_W \leq \mu_T - \mu_R \leq \theta_S \sigma_W.$$

This is average bioequivalence but with expanding limits (ABEL), a form that was recommended by Boddy et al. (1995).

2.4.3 Other Rules for Assessment of Bioequivalence

In addition to the SABE, several rules for the assessment of bioequivalence for highly variables are available in the literature. These possible rules include GMR-dependent bioequivalence limits (Karailis et al., 2004) and the reference-scaled approach by Liao and Heyse (2011). These rules are briefly summarized in the following.

The geometric mean ratio dependent (GMR-dependent) bioequivalence limits considered by Karalis et al. (2004) can be summarized as follows:

$$|\mu_T - \mu_R| \leq \log(1.25) + (5 - 4 \times GMR) \times 0.496 \sigma_{WR}$$

or

$$|\mu_T - \mu_R| \leq (\log(1.25) + 0.496 \sigma_{WR})(3 - 2 \times GMR),$$

where σ_{WR} is the within-subject standard deviation. Bioequivalence or similarity is claimed if the 90% confidence interval falls inside the limits. Liao and Heyse (2011) proposed the following reference scaled approach:

$$\left[(\mu_T - \mu_R)^2 + \sigma_D^2 \right] - 2\theta_L (GMR) \times \sigma_{WR}^2 \leq 0,$$

where

$$\theta_L(GMR) = \left(\frac{\log(1.25)}{\sqrt{2} \times (3.763 \times GMR - 2.763) \times 0.152} \right)^2.$$

Bioequivalence or similarity is claimed if the upper 95% confidence bound is negative or zero.

Liao and Heyse (2011) indicated that the SABE proposed by the FDA has too little power and is not sensitive to reference CV changes. The two GMR-dependent procedures are similar and are too sensitive to reference CV changes. Their method, on the other hand, has similar consumer's risk but has better power and reduces the producer's risk. In addition, their method is sensitive to the subject-by-product interaction and hence is preferred.

Both FDA and EMA require that a second regulatory criterion also be satisfied (Haidar et al., 2008; EMA, 2010c). Accordingly, the point estimate of GMR must be between 0.80 and 1.25. The two procedures presented in this section provide smooth, GMR-dependent transitions toward the constrained difference between the logarithmic means. The recent study of Zhang et al. (2013) achieves the same goal in a different way, see Chapter 10.

2.4.4 Remarks

For the evaluation of bioequivalence, the ABE approach has been criticized as follows: (1) generic companies are unable to obtain regulatory approval if the variability of the reference product is extremely large, and (2) it penalizes good products (with less variability). The SABE is an attempt to fix the problem. SABE is ABE adjusted for the standard deviation of the reference product, which is a special case of the IBE criterion. As a result, SABE also suffers from the disadvantages/limitations as described in Chow (1999).

In practice, it can be assumed that the test and reference formulations have the same within-subject variability although this assumption is not always true. For example, as indicated in Tothfalusi et al. (2009), a reference formulation of nadolol was found to have high within-subject variability ($CV = 50\%$ and 39% for the C_{max} and AUC, respectively). However, a test product showed much lower variability (26% and 19% for the C_{max} and AUC, respectively). In such cases, we are dealing with highly variable drug product (HVDP) rather than HVD. The most famous example of formulation-dependent (or drug product–dependent) within-subject variability is probably the case of cyclosporine when a change of the formulation leads to a marked decrease in within-subject variability. However, formulation-dependent variability can result in a paradoxical situation if the pooled variability (σ_W) is used for scaling. The paradox is that the chance of passing the SABE regulatory criterion increases with rising σ_W. It is bad enough that the test product has higher variability than the reference formulation, but it is really problematic if this behavior is rewarded and not punished as in the case of ABE. The only way to avoid this unfortunate situation is reference scaling.

But reference scaling also raises problems. First of these is that the symmetry of the equivalence relationship is broken. That is, by flipping the notation *T* and *R* we can come to a different conclusion. For instance, it is possible that *T* is equivalent to *R*, but *R* is not equivalent to *T*. This controversy was noted by Dragalin et al. (2003) who argued that for physicians and patients, bioequivalent drug formulations should not be used interchangeably to achieve a similar therapeutic effect. Therefore, in this sense, both formulations should be treated symmetrically from a theoretical point of view. However, from a practical point of view, the reference product has been shown to be safe and effective. Both effects depend on its within-subject variability which is, therefore, highly relevant. A new test product with a larger variability could possess a worse risk–benefit relationship. On the other hand, a test formulation with a lower variability than the reference product could indicate an improvement. Then, a switchback from a new test formulation with lower variability to the reference formulation with higher variability, but also with demonstrated safety and efficacy, is not seen as a clinical problem. Besides, it is not clear at present what kind of regulatory policy will be followed when several σ_{WR} estimates (i.e., results of previous submissions) are available to a drug regulatory agency. If regulators use all available data, then they can get an improved estimate for σ_{WR}, and possibly can draw a different conclusion from the sponsor. Finally, the term "reference" can be interpreted only in the context of approval of generics. It is questionable whether reference scaling is needed at all for other possible applications, such as the approval of new formulations of drugs under development.

2.5 Practical Issues

In this section, we shall focus on controversial issues related to the Fundamental Bioequivalence Assumption, the one size-fits-all criterion, and issues related to the log-transformation of PK data prior to analysis. These controversial issues are briefly described.

2.5.1 Fundamental Bioequivalence Assumption

As indicated earlier, the Fundamental Bioequivalence Assumption states that *if two drug products are shown to be bioequivalent, it is assumed that they will reach the same therapeutic effect or that they are therapeutically equivalent.* Under the Fundamental Bioequivalence Assumption, one of the controversial issues is that bioequivalence may not necessarily imply therapeutic equivalence and therapeutic equivalence does not guarantee bioequivalence either. The assessment of ABE for generic approval has been criticized to be based on legal/political deliberations rather than scientific considerations. In the past several decades, many sponsors/researchers have made an attempt to challenge this assumption with no success.

Note that the Fundamental Bioequivalence Assumption is also applied to drug products with local action such as nasal spray products via the assessment of in vitro bioequivalence testing. In either in vivo or in vitro bioequivalence testing, the verification of the Fundamental Bioequivalence Assumption is often difficult, if not impossible, without the conduct of clinical trials. It should be noted that the Fundamental Bioequivalence Assumption is for drug products with identical active ingredient(s). Note that for two products to be bioequivalent they must have, by general understanding, the same active ingredients.

In practice, the verification of the Fundamental Bioequivalence Assumption is often difficult, if not impossible, without the conduct of clinical trials. In practice, there are the following four possible scenarios:

1. Drug absorption profiles are similar and they are therapeutic equivalent.

2. Drug absorption profiles are not similar but they are therapeutic equivalent.

3. Drug absorption profiles are similar but they are not therapeutic equivalent.

4. Drug absorption profiles are not similar and they are not therapeutic equivalent.

The Fundamental Bioequivalence Assumption is nothing but scenario (1). Scenario (1) works if the drug absorption (in terms of the rate and extent of absorption) is predictive of the clinical outcome. In this case, PK responses such as AUC (area under the blood or plasma concentration–time curve for the measurement of the extent of drug absorption) and C_{max} (maximum concentration for the measurement of the rate of drug absorption) serve as surrogate endpoints for clinical endpoints for the assessment of efficacy and safety of the test product under investigation. Scenario (2) is the case which generic companies use to argue for generic approval of their drug products, especially when their products fail to meet the regulatory requirements for bioequivalence. In this case, it is doubtful that there is a relationship between PK responses and clinical endpoints. The innovator companies usually argue with the regulatory agency against the generic approval with scenario (3). However, more studies are necessarily conducted in order to verify scenario (3). There are no arguments with respect to scenario (4).

In practice, the Fundamental Bioequivalence Assumption is applied to all drug products across therapeutic areas without convincing scientific justification. In the past several decades, however, no significant safety incidences were reported for the generic drug products approved under the Fundamental Bioequivalence Assumption. One of the convincing explanations is that the Fundamental Bioequivalence Assumption is for drug products with *identical* active ingredient(s). Whether the Fundamental Bioequivalence Assumption is applicable to drug products with similar but different active ingredient(s) as in the case of follow-on products becomes an interesting but controversial question.

2.5.2 One-Size-Fits-All Criterion

For the assessment of ABE, FDA adopted a one size-fits-all criterion. That is, as noted earlier, a test drug product is said to be bioequivalent to a reference drug product if the estimated 90% confidence interval for the ratio of geometric means of the primary PK parameters (AUC and C_{max}) is (in %) totally within the bioequivalence limits of 80%–125%. The one size-fits-all criterion does not take into consideration the therapeutic window (TW) and ISV of a drug which have been identified to have nonnegligible impact on the safety and efficacy of generic drug products as compared to the innovative drug products.

In the past several decades, this one size-fits-all criterion has been challenged and criticized by many researchers. It was suggested that flexible criteria in terms of safety (upper bioequivalence limit) and efficacy (lower bioequivalence limit) should be developed based on the characteristics of the drug, its TW, and ISV (Table 2.1).

The approach of one size-fits-all has begun to dissipate in recent years. For instance, in some jurisdictions such as Europe and Canada, narrower BE limits have been proposed for drugs with narrow TWs (Health Canada, 2006; EMA, 2010c). However, FDA has maintained its usual requirement for these drugs with BE limits between 80% and 125%.

On the other hand, for orally administered drugs with high within-subject variability and wide TW (Class D, HVDs, see Table 2.1), the regulatory expectation has become, in some cases, more relaxed. For these drugs, the approach of SABE has been proposed (Haidar et al., 2008; Tothfalusi et al., 2009).

TABLE 2.1

Classification of Drugs

Class	TW	ISV	Example
A	Narrow	High	Cyclosporine
B	Narrow	Low	Theophylline
C	Wide	Low to moderate	Most drugs
D	Wide	High	Chlorpromazine or topical corticosteroids

Source: Chen, M.L. (1995). Dusseldorf, Germany, October 19–20, 1995.
Key: TW, therapeutic window; ISV, intra-subject variability.

This method is closely related to, and is a simplification of, the procedure recommended earlier for individual BE when the within-subject variation is high ($\sigma_{WR}^2 > \sigma_{W0}^2$). While the current FDA guidance does not contain special provisions for this class of drugs, the agency actually entertains submissions based on the criteria described in an "informal" publication (Haidar et al., 2008), which recommends the approach of SABE. Europe has recently also suggested the application of a variant of this procedure (EMA, 2010). However, some other agencies still apply the one size-fits-all approach and require the usual BE limits of 80%–125% also for this class of drugs.

2.5.3 Log-Transformation

In the past, bioequivalence could be assessed either based on raw data or log-transformed data depending upon which model followed normal distribution. This raised a controversial issue regarding which model should be used for the assessment of bioequivalence. The sponsors could choose the model which would serve their purposes (e.g., the demonstration of bioequivalence). In some cases, the raw data model could reach a different conclusion regarding bioequivalence than the log-transformation model. This controversial issue was discussed a great deal until a general understanding was reached on the use of log-transformed parameters.

The 2001 FDA guidance provides a rationale for the use of logarithmic transformation of exposure measures. The guidance emphasizes that the limited sample size in a typical BE study precludes a reliable determination of the distribution of the data. For this reason, the guidance does not encourage the sponsors to test for the normality of the error distribution after log-transformation, nor to use the normality of the error distribution as a reason for carrying out the statistical analysis on the original scale.

With respect to the (PK) rationale, deterministic multiplicative PK models are used to justify the routine use of logarithmic transformation for AUC($0-\infty$) and C_{max}. However, the deterministic PK models are theoretical derivations of AUC($0-\infty$) and C_{max} for a single object. The guidance suggests that AUC($0-\infty$) be calculated from the observed plasma/blood concentration–time curve using the trapezoidal rule, and that C_{max} be obtained directly from the curve, without interpolation. It is uncertain to what extent the observed AUC($0-\infty$) and C_{max} can provide good approximations to those under the theoretical models if the models are correct.

The use of the logarithmic transformation of PK parameters was questioned in the statistical literature (e.g., Liu and Weng, 1992, 1994, 1995; Patel, 1994). It was stated that the log-transformed AUC($0-\infty$) and C_{max} do not generally follow a normal distribution even when either the plasma concentrations or the log-plasma concentrations are normally distributed (Liu and Weng, 1994). It was suggested that performing a routine log-transformation of data and then applying normal, theory-based methods is not appropriate (Patel, 1994). It was suggested that normal probability plots for the studentized inter-subject and intra-subject residuals be examined and that the Shapiro–Wilk method be applied to test for normality of the inter-subject and intra-subject variabilities. However, the sample size of a typical bioequivalence study is generally too small to allow an adequate large-sample normal approximation and to enable clear discrimination between the normal and log-normal distributions of the estimated PK parameters.

In addition, the use of logarithmic PK (and generally kinetic) parameters has a strong basis in their multiplicative, rather than additive, sense. We typically think of doubling or halving a dose or concentration and not adding or taking away some units. Similarly, in tables of kinetic parameters, whether they are rate constants (including half-lives), equilibrium constants, or many other kinetic measures, we compare their orders of magnitudes and ask if one is, say, 10 times higher or lower than the other. Consequently, analyses involving kinetic parameters generally apply a multiplicative and not an additive model. An implementation of this sense is that the parameters are analyzed following their logarithmic transformation.

To achieve the objective of exchangeability among bioequivalent pharmaceutical products, the criteria for the assessment of bioequivalence must possess certain important properties. Chen (1995, 1997) outlined the desirable characteristics of bioequivalence criteria proposed by the FDA (Table 2.2). In addition, to address the issues of ISV and subject-by-formulation interaction and to ensure drug switchability, valid statistical procedures, both estimation and hypothesis testing, should be developed from the criteria to control the consumer's risk at the pre-specified nominal level (e.g., 5%). Furthermore, the statistical methods developed from the criteria should be able to provide sample size determination; to take into consideration the nuisance design parameters, such as period or sequence effects; and to develop user-friendly computer software. The most critical characteristics for the proposed criteria will be their interpretation to scientists and clinicians and the cost of conducting bioequivalence studies to provide inference for the criteria.

TABLE 2.2

Desirable Features of Bioequivalence Criteria

Comparison of both averages and variances

Assurance of switchability

Encouragement or reward of pharmaceutical companies to manufacture a better formulation

Control of type I error rate (consumer's risk) at 5%

Allowance for the determination of sample size

Admission of the possibility of sequence and period effects as well as missing values

User-friendly software application for statistical methods

Provision of easy interpretation for scientists and clinicians

Minimization of increased cost for conducting bioequivalence studies

---

Source: Chen, M.L., *J. Biopharm. Stat.*, 7, 5–11, 1997.

2.6 Frequently Asked Questions

Although the concepts of PBE and IBE for addressing drug prescribability and drug switchability were discussed tremendously especially during the 1990s, until 2002, the current position of FDA regarding the assessment of bioequivalence is that *ABE is required and individual/PBE may be considered.* FDA does not encourage the application of IBE. In any case, FDA suggests that a medical/statistical reviewer be consulted if individual/PBE is to be used. For the assessment of bioequivalence, some questions are frequently asked during regulatory submissions and reviews. In what follows, frequently asked questions in bioequivalence assessment are briefly described.

2.6.1 What if We Pass the Raw Data Model but Fail the Log-Transformed Data Model?

Most regulatory agencies, including FDA, EMA, and WHO, recommend that a log-transformation of PK parameters of AUC(0–t), AUC(0–∞), and C_{max} be performed before analysis. No assumption checking or verification of the log-transformed data is encouraged. However, sponsors often conduct analyses based on both raw data and log-transformed data and check which would pass bioequivalence testing. A sponsor would take a great risk of questioning and rejection by the regulators if it would submit results based on raw data just because they would pass within the BE limits. Some additional justification would be needed. If the sponsor passes BE testing under the log-transformed data model, then there is no problem because it meets the regulatory requirement.

It is possible, however, that a sponsor may fail BE testing under the log-transformed data model but pass under the raw data model. In this case, the sponsor can provide scientific/statistical justification for the use of raw data model. One of the most commonly seen scientific/statistical justifications is that the raw data model is a more appropriate statistical model than that of the log-transformed data model because all of the assumptions for the raw data model are met. However, for the raw data model, the bioequivalence limits are often expressed in terms of the ratio of the population means between the test and reference formulations. The equivalence limits are then expressed as a percentage of the population reference average, which has to be estimated from the data. Therefore, the variability of the estimated reference average is not considered in the equivalence limit. Hence, the false positive rate for claiming ABE for the two one-sided tests procedure can be inflated to 50%. As a result, one should apply the modified two one-sided tests procedure using the raw data proposed by Liu and Weng (1995) to control the size at the nominal level. In any case, it is advisable to consult the regulatory agency before submitting a clinical study report when the use of a calculational procedure is contemplated, which differs from that recommended in a guidance.

2.6.2 What if We Pass AUC but Fail C_{max}?

Based on log-transformed data, FDA requires that both AUC and C_{max} meet the bioequivalence limits of 80%–125% in order to establish ABE. In practice, however, it is not uncommon to pass AUC (the extent of absorption) but fail C_{max} (the rate of absorption). In this case, ABE cannot be claimed according to the FDA guidance.

If we pass AUC but fail C_{max}, Endrenyi et al. (1991) suggested considering C_{max}/AUC as an alternative bioequivalence measure for the rate of absorption. However, C_{max}/AUC is not currently selected as a required PK response for the approval of generic drug products by regulatory authorities. The condition of passing the regulatory requirement for AUC and not for C_{max} is less likely to arise in Canada where only the point estimate of the ratio of geometric means of C_{max} but not the 90% confidence interval must be (in%) between 80% and 125% (Health Canada, 1992, 2012).

It is possible that we would pass the regulatory requirement for C_{max} but not for AUC. It was suggested that we could look at partial AUC as an additional measure of bioequivalence (see, e.g., Chen et al., 2001).

2.6.3 What if We Fail by a Small Margin?

In practice, it is possible that we fail BE testing for either AUC or C_{max} by only a small margin. For example, suppose that the estimated 90% confidence interval for AUC is from 79.5% to 121.3%, which is slightly outside the lower limit of the regulatory range of 80.0%–125.0%. In this case, the FDA's position is very clear: *A rule is a rule and you fail.* In regulatory reviews and approvals, the FDA is very strict about this rule as described in the 2003 FDA guidance.

However, a sponsor may perform either an outlier detection analysis or a sensitivity analysis in order to resolve the issue. If a subject is found to be an outlier statistically, the data may be excluded from the analysis but only with appropriate clinical justification. Once the identified outlier is excluded from the analysis, the recalculated 90% confidence interval could be totally within the bioequivalence limits of 80%–125%, and the sponsor may present an argument for claiming bioequivalence.

Major regulatory agencies have recently encouraged additional design features which permit the later addition of subjects. Notably, they include group sequential extensions of the usual bioequivalence testing procedure (Gould, 1995). The results of a study would first be evaluated by the customary procedures. However, in order to maintain the overall type I error, the results would be assessed with adjusted significance levels which would yield confidence intervals higher than 90% (Pocock, 1983). If the analysis indicates that the calculated 90% confidence intervals of the PK parameters are moderately outside the regulatory BE interval of 80%–125%, then a second group of subjects could be investigated. A combined analysis of the two groups could be performed; these would apply a modified structure of the statistical computations and, again, adjusted significance levels.

Health Canada accepts also a simple add-on of at least 12 subjects (Health Canada, 1992, 2012). The structure of the statistical analysis should be modified and the level of significance should be 0.025 instead of 0.05. In all cases, the intention of applying either a group sequential or an add-on design as well as the details of the procedure should be specified in the protocol of the study.

2.6.4 Can We Still Assess Bioequivalence if There Is a Significant Sequence Effect?

As indicated in Chow and Liu (2008), under a standard two-sequence, two-period (2 × 2) crossover design, a significant sequence effect is an indication of the possible

1. Failure of randomization
2. A true sequence effect
3. A true carryover effect
4. A true formulation-by-period effect

Under the standard 2 × 2 crossover design, the sequence effect is confounded with the carryover effect. Therefore, if a significant sequence effect is found, the treatment effect and its corresponding 90% confidence interval cannot be estimated unbiasedly due to the possibly unequal carryover effects. However, in the 2001 FDA guidance, the following list of conditions is provided to rule out the possibility of unequal carryover effects:

1. It is a single-dose study.
2. The drug is not an endogenous entity.
3. More than an adequate washout period has been allowed between periods of the study, and in the subsequent periods the pre-dose biological matrix samples do not exhibit a detectable drug level in any of the subjects.
4. The study meets all scientific criteria (e.g., it is based on an acceptable study protocol and it contains a validated assay methodology).

The 2001 FDA guidance also recommends that sponsors conduct a bioequivalence study with parallel designs if unequal carryover effects become an issue.

2.6.5 What Should We Do When We Have Almost Identical Means but Still Fail to Meet the Bioequivalence Criterion?

It is not uncommon to run into the situation that we have almost identical means but still fail to meet the bioequivalence criterion. This may indicate that (1) the variation of the reference product is too large to establish bioequivalence between the test product and the reference product, (2) the bioequivalence study was poorly conducted, and (3) the analytical assay methodology is inadequate and not fully validated. The concept of IBE and/or PBE was an attempt to overcome this problem. More recently, the application of scaled average BE (Haidar et al., 2008; Tothfalusi et al., 2009; Liao and Heyse, 2011), or its variant (Boddy et al., 1995), is proving useful to deal with the problem of BE for highly variable drugs and drug products. The approach is favored by major regulatory agencies in the United States and Europe (Haidar et al., 2009; EMA, 2010c). It should be noted that these authorities impose also a secondary expectation which requires that the estimated ratio of test/reference geometric means be between 0.80 and 1.25.

2.6.6 Power and Sample Size Calculations Based on Raw-Data Model and Log-Transformed Model Are Different

The calculations of the statistical power and of the sample size are different when they are based on the raw data model and on the log-transformed model. Under different models, means, standard deviations, and coefficients of variation also differ. As mentioned earlier, for the assessment of bioequivalence, all regulatory authorities including the FDA, EMA, WHO, and Japan require that log-transformation of the parameters $AUC(0-t)$, $AUC(0-\infty)$, and C_{max} be performed before the analysis and evaluation of bioequivalence. As a result, one should use differences between logarithmic means and the corresponding standard deviations or the coefficients of variation for the power analysis and sample size calculation based on the method for the log-transformed model (see, e.g., chapter 5 of Chow and Liu, 2008).

Note that sponsors should make a decision as to which model (the raw data model or the log-transformed data model) will be used for bioequivalence assessment. Once the model is chosen, appropriate formulas can be used to determine the sample size. Fishing around for obtaining the smallest sample size is not a good clinical practice.

2.6.7 Multiplicity and Transitivity

The 2003 FDA guidance for general considerations requires that for $AUC(0-t)$, $AUC(0-\infty)$, and C_{max}, the following information be provided:

1. Geometric means
2. Arithmetic means
3. Ratio of means
4. 90% Confidence interval

In addition, as already noted, the 2003 FDA guidance recommends that logarithmic transformation be provided for each measure of $AUC(0-t)$, $AUC(0-\infty)$, and C_{max}, and that, for the demonstration of ABE, each of their 90% confidence intervals must fall within the bioequivalence limits of 80%–125%. It follows that according to the intersection-union principle (Berger, 1982), the type I error rate of ABE is still controlled under the nominal level of 5%. Therefore, there is no need for adjustment due to multiple PK measures.

Another issue involves the multiplicity of generic products of a drug. The bioequivalence of each generic formulation is determined against the reference, generally brand-name product. It is not obvious to what extent the generics could be equivalent with each other. This is particularly important when a patient is switched from one generic product to another. Anderson and Hauck (1990) examined the transitivity of bioequivalence, i.e., to what extent is there a potential of drift about the declaration of bioequivalence when a number of generics are tested against an innovator's product, With two or three generic formulations, the confidence of transitive bioequivalence is fairly high. With six generic products, this confidence is low.

2.7 Concluding Remarks

Current methods for the assessment of bioequivalence for drug products with identical active ingredients are not applicable to biosimilar products due to fundamental differences as described in Chapter 1. The assessment of biosimilarity between biosimilar products and the innovative biological product in terms of surrogate endpoints (e.g., PK parameters and/or pharmacodynamic responses) or biomarkers (e.g., genomic markers) requires the establishment of the Fundamental Biosimilarity Assumption in order to bridge the surrogate endpoints and/or biomarker data to clinical safety and efficacy.

Unlike small-molecule drug products, biosimilar products are very sensitive to small changes in variation during the manufacturing process, which have been shown to have an impact on the clinical outcome. Thus, it is a concern whether current criteria and regulatory requirements for the assessment of bioequivalence for drugs with small-molecules can be applied directly to the assessment of biosimilarity of biosimilar products. It is suggested that current, existing criteria for the evaluation of bioequivalence, similarity, and biosimilarity be scientifically/statistically evaluated in order to choose the most appropriate approach for assessing biosimilarity. It is recommended that the selected biosimilarity criteria should be able to address (1) sensitivity due to small variations in both location (bias) and scale (variability) parameters, and (2) the degree of similarity, which can reflect the assurance for drug interchangeability.

To assist the sponsors for the development of biosimilar products, several product-specific guidelines/guidances have been published by the EU EMA.

These guidelines/guidances, however, have been criticized for not having standards for the assessment of biosimilar products. Although product-specific guidelines/guidances do not help to establish standards for the assessment of biosimilarity, they do provide the opportunity for accumulating valuable experience/information for establishing standards in the future. Thus, it is recommended that numerical studies including simulations, meta-analysis, and/or sensitivity analysis be conducted, in order to (1) provide a better understanding of these product-specific guidelines/guidances, and (2) check the validity of the stated Fundamental Biosimilarity Assumption. This Assumption may constitute the legal basis for assessing biosimilarity if the process for bioequivalence assessment for small-molecule drug products is to be applied to the assessment of biosimilarity.

Note that recently the FDA circulated three draft guidances on the assessment of biosimilarity for public comments (on February 9, 2012) and conducted a public hearing on the discussion of the three guidances for public opinions and input (held on May 11, 2012). In one of the guidances, on scientific considerations in demonstrating biosimilarity, the FDA proposed the concept of the totality-of-the-evidence for similarity in all aspects related to clinical outcomes and the use of stepwise approach for providing the totality-of-the-evidence for a valid and reliable assessment of biosimilarity. These FDA draft guidances will be reviewed in Chapter 3.

3

Regulatory Requirements for Assessing Follow-on Biologics

3.1 Background

Biological drugs make up one of the fastest-growing sectors of the pharmaceutical and biotechnology industry in the past decade. For example, in 2005, worldwide spending on drug therapy grew by 7% and topped $600 billion. However, sales of biologics have grown even more rapidly, with an increase of about 17% in 2005 and annual expenditures worldwide of more than $50 billion. By 2010, spending on biologics roared to over $100 billion, with biologics making up nearly half of all newly approved medicines. Due to the high costs involved in the research, development, and production of many medicines, regulatory regimes have been created to balance the intellectual property interests and investments made by originator companies with the need for wider patient access through generic forms of the drugs. In the traditional chemical drug market, such a regime was created by the *Hatch–Waxman Act*. The Hatch–Waxman Act added Section 505(j) to the *Federal Food, Drug, and Cosmetic (FD&C) Act*. This section and its accompanying regulations created the Abbreviated New Drug Application (ANDA) process, which was designed to provide independent generic firms with a strong incentive to develop and introduce lower-cost and affordable generic drugs to majority of patient population. By virtually all accounts, the *Hatch–Waxman Act* has been extremely successful in bringing cheaper and affordable generic products to the market while maintaining incentives for the development and discovery of new drugs.

Because of the effectiveness of the *Hatch–Waxman Act* in the context of traditional small-molecule chemical drugs, some have called for applying a similar regime for biologics, given the high cost of this class of drugs. In particular, Rep. Henry Waxman (D-Cal.), one of the original authors of the *Hatch–Waxman Act* sponsored the *Access to Life-Saving Medicine Act* to determine whether such a legal infrastructure is appropriate for regulating the follow-on biologics (FOBs), a thorough policy assessment is necessary (see also, Liang, 2007). This effort has led to the passage of the *Biologics Price*

Competition and Innovation (BPCI) Act, which has given the FDA the authority to review and approve biosimilar products (biosimilars or FOBs). Following the passage of the BPCI Act, the FDA hosted a public hearing between November 2 and 3, 2010, to obtain public input regarding scientific factors for assessing biosimilarity and drug interchangeability of biosimilar products. After extensive discussions, the FDA developed and circulated three draft guidances on biosimilars on February 9, 2012, and hosted another public hearing to obtain public input and comments on the draft guidances on May 11, 2012. At this public hearing, special attention was directed to the discussion of drug interchangeability in terms of the concepts of switching and alternating as described in the BPCI Act.

On the other hand, the European Union (EU) has a well-established and well-documented legal and regulatory pathway for the review and approval of biosimilars. Other countries and organizations around the world, including Australia, Canada, Japan, and Switzerland and the World Health Organization (WHO), are also following the same scientific principles for establishing an abbreviated approval pathway for biosimilars. In contrast, the United States is at the very beginning of the process, with a legal pathway being discussed by Congress for a number of years. The FDA views and/or current position on biosimilars can be found from an excellent publication by Woodcock et al. (2007), from communications from the FDA to Congress (Torti, 2008), and from a number of internal User Fees Stakeholders meetings held within the FDA between 2010 and 2011. These discussions and/or documents indicate the FDA is contemplating similar but more stringent scientific principles and/or requirement to those established by the EMA.

The purpose of this chapter is to review regulatory requirements for the approval pathway of FOBs worldwide including WHO and various regions, such as the EU, United States, Canada, and the Asian Pacific Region (e.g., Japan and South Korea). Comparisons of these regulatory requirements, and some recommendations regarding global harmonization, will be made. In the next section, definitions and interpretations of biosimilar products from different regions are given. Regulatory requirements from different regions are briefly summarized in Section 3.3. Recommendations on global harmonization of the regulatory approval pathway are offered in Section 3.5. Section 3.6 provides some concluding remarks.

3.2 Definitions and Interpretations of Biosimilar Products

As indicated earlier, the similar biologic drug products (SBDP) are usually referred to as similar biotherapeutic products (SBPs) by WHO, biosimilars by the European Medicines Agency (EMA) of the EU, FOBs by the U.S. FDA, and subsequent-entered biologics (SEBs) by Health Canada. In some cases,

TABLE 3.1

Definitions of Biosimilar Products

Term	By	Definition
Biosimilar	EU EMA	A biological product claiming to be similar to another one already marketed
SBP	WHO	A biotherapeutic product similar to an already licensed reference biotherapeutic product in terms of quality, safety, and efficacy
FOB	U.S. FDA	A product highly similar to the reference product without clinically meaningful differences in safety, purity, and potency
SEB	Canada	A biologic drug that enters the market subsequent to a version previously authorized in Canada with demonstrated similarity to a reference biologic drug
Biosimilar	KFDA	A biological product which demonstrated its equivalence to an already approved reference product with regard to quality, safety, and efficacy

the term biosimilar has been used in an inappropriate way, and therefore it is important to review differences in definitions of biosimilar products in different regions (Table 3.1).

WHO defines an SBP as a product that is similar in terms of quality, safety, and efficacy to an already licensed reference biotherapeutic product (WHO, 2009). Health Canada defines biosimilar to be a biologic drug that enters the market subsequent to a version previously authorized in Canada, and with demonstrated similarity to a reference biologic drug (Health Canada, 2010). As indicated in the BPCI Act passed by the U.S. Congress and was written into law on March 23, 2010, a biosimilar product is defined as a product that is *highly similar* to the reference product, notwithstanding *minor* differences in clinically *inactive components*, and for which there are *no clinically meaningful differences in terms of safety, purity, and potency* from the reference product. EMA did not provide the definition of biosimilars in the original guidelines. However, a recently published concept paper on the revision of the guidelines on similar biological medicinal product indicated that it might be prudent to discuss if a definition of "biosimilar," in extension of what is in the legislation and relevant Committee for Medicinal Products for Human Use (CHMP) guidance, is necessary (EMA, 2011a).

Based on these different but similar definitions, we would interpret that there are three determinants in the definition of a biosimilar product: (1) it should be a biological products; (2) the reference product should be an already licensed biological products; (3) the demonstration of high similarity in safety, quality, and efficacy is necessary. Besides, it is well recognized that the similarity should be demonstrated using a set of comprehensive comparability exercises at the quality, nonclinical and clinical level. Products not authorized by this comparability regulatory pathway cannot be called biosimilars.

3.3 Regulatory Requirements

As indicated by Chow et al. (2011), standard methods for the assessment of bioequivalence for generic drug products with identical active ingredients are not appropriate for the assessment of biosimilarity due to the fundamental differences between small-molecule drug products and biological products. For the assessment of FOBs, regulatory requirements from the WHO and different regions such as the EU, the United States, and the Asian Pacific Region are similar and yet slightly different (Wang and Chow, 2012). In what follows, these regulatory requirements are briefly described.

3.3.1 World Health Organization

As an increasingly wide range of SBPs are under development or are already licensed in many countries, WHO formally recognized the need for the guidance for their evaluation and overall regulation in 2007. "Guidelines on Evaluation of Similar Biotherapeutic Products (SBPs)" were developed and adopted by the 60th meeting of the WHO Expert Committee on Biological Standardization in 2009. The intention of the guidelines is to provide globally acceptable principles for licensing biotherapeutic products that are claimed to be similar to the reference products that have been licensed based on a full licensing dossier (WHO, 2009). The scope of the guidelines includes well-established and well-characterized biotherapeutic products that have been marketed for a suitable period of time with a proven quality, efficacy, and safety, such as recombinant DNA-derived therapeutic proteins.

3.3.1.1 Key Principles and Basic Concepts

Key principles and basic concepts for licensing SBPs have been explained in WHO's guidelines. One of the most important principles of developing SBPs is the stepwise approach starting with the characterization of quality attributes of the product and followed by nonclinical and clinical evaluations. Manufactures should submit a full quality dossier that includes a complete characterization of the product, the demonstration of consistent and robust manufacture of their product, and the comparability exercise between the SBP and RBP in the quality part, which together serve as the basis for the possible reduction in data requirement in the nonclinical and clinical development. This principle indicates that the data reduction is only possible for the nonclinical and clinical parts of the development program, and significant differences between the SBP and the chosen RBP detected during the comparability exercise would result in a requirement for more extensive nonclinical and clinical data. In addition, the amount of nonclinical and clinical data considered necessary also depends on the class of products, which calls for a case-by-case approach for different classes of products.

3.3.1.2 Reference Biotherapeutic Product

The choice of the reference biotherapeutic product is another important issue covered in the WHO guidelines. Traditionally, National Regulatory Authorities (NRA) have required the use of a nationally licensed reference product for the licensing of generic medicines, but this may not be feasible for countries lacking nationally licensed RBPs. Thus additional criteria to guide the acceptability of using an RBP licensed in other jurisdiction may be needed. Considering the choice of the RBP, WHO requires that it should have been marketed for a suitable duration, have a volume of marketed use, and should be licensed based on full quality, safety, and efficacy data. Besides, the same RBP should be used throughout the development of the SBP, and the drug substance, dosage form, and route of administration of SBP should be the same as those of the RBP.

3.3.1.3 Quality

As mentioned in an earlier section, the comprehensive comparison showing quality similarity between SBP and RBP is a prerequisite for applying the clinical safety and efficacy profile of the RBP to SBP, thus a full quality dossier for both the drug substance and drug product is always required. To evaluate comparability, WHO recommends the manufacturer to conduct a comprehensive physicochemical and biological characterization of the SBP in head-to-head comparisons with the RBP. The following aspects of product quality and heterogeneity should be assessed.

3.3.1.3.1 Manufacturing Process

The manufacturing process should meet the same standards as required by NRA for originator products, and implement good manufacturing practices, modern quality control and assurance procedures, in-process controls, and process validation. The SBP manufacturer should assemble all available knowledge of the RBP with regard to the type of host cell, formulation, and container closure system, and submit a complete description and data package delineating the whole manufacturing process including obtaining target genes and their expression, the optimization and fermentation of gene engineering cells, the clarification and purification of the products, the formulation and testing, aseptic filling and packaging.

3.3.1.3.2 Characterization

Thorough characterization and comparability exercise are required, and details should be provided on primary and higher-order structures, post-translational modifications, biological activity, process- and product-related impurities, the relevant immunochemical properties, and results from accelerated degradation studies, and studies under various stress conditions.

3.3.1.4 Nonclinical and Clinical Studies

After demonstrating the similarity of SBP and RBP in quality, the proving the safety and efficacy of an SBP usually requires further nonclinical and clinical data. Nonclinical evaluations should be undertaken both in vitro (e.g., receptor-binding studies, cell-proliferation, cytotoxicity assays) and in vivo (e.g., biological/pharmacodynamic [PD] activity, repeat dose toxicity study, toxicokinetic measurements, anti-product antibody titers, cross-reactivity with homologous endogenous proteins, product neutralizing capacity).

In terms of the clinical evaluation, the comparability exercise should begin with pharmacokinetics (PK) and PD studies followed by the pivotal clinical trials. PK studies should be designed to enable the detection of potential differences between SBP and RBP. Single-dose, cross-over PK studies in a homogenous population are recommended by WHO. The manufacturer should justify the choice of single-dose studies, steady-state studies, or repeated determination of PK parameters, and the study population. Due to the lack of established acceptance criteria for the demonstration of similar PK between SBP and RBP, the traditional 80%–125% equivalence range is often used. Besides, PD studies and confirmatory PK/PD studies may be appropriate if there are clinically relevant PD markers. In addition, similar efficacy of SBP and RBP has to be demonstrated in randomized and well-controlled clinical trials, which should preferably be double-blind or at least observer-blind. In principle, equivalence designs (requiring lower and upper comparability margins) are clearly preferred for the comparison of efficacy and safety of SBP with RBP. Non-inferiority designs (requiring only one margin) may be considered if appropriately justified. WHO also suggests the pre-licensing safety data and the immunogenicity data should be obtained from the comparative efficacy trials.

In addition to the nonclinical and clinical data, applicants also need to present an ongoing risk management and pharmacovigilance plan, since data from pre-authorized clinical studies are usually too limited to identify all potential side effects of the SBP. The safety specifications should describe important identified or potential safety issues for the RBP, and any that are specific for the SBP.

In summary, the WHO guidelines on evaluating SBPs represent an important step forward in the global harmonization of evaluation and regulation of biosimilar products, and provide clear guidance for both regulatory bodies and the pharmaceutical industry.

3.3.2 European Union

The EU has pioneered the development of a regulatory system for biosimilar products. The EMA began formal consideration of scientific issues presented by biosimilar products at least as early as January 2001, when an ad hoc working group discussed the comparability of medicinal products containing biotechnology-derived proteins as active substances (CPMP, 2001). In 2003, the European Commission amended the provisions of the EU secondary legislation governing requirements for marketing authorization applications for medicinal products and established a new category of applications for "similar biological medicinal products" (CD, 2003). In 2005, the EMA issued a general guideline on similar biological medicinal products in order to introduce the concept of similar biological medicinal products, to outline the basic principles to be applied, and to provide applicants with a "user guide," showing where to find relevant scientific information (EMA, 2006). Since then, 14 biosimilar products have been approved by the EMA under the pathway (see Table 3.3). One of the rejected biosimilars is Alpheon (interferon alpha-2a). It was developed by BioPartners GmbH, and designed to become a biosimilar of the reference product Roferon-A for the treatment of adult patients with chronic hepatitis C. The EMA refused the marketing authorization for Alpheon due to the difference identified between Alpheon and the reference product, such as impurities, stability, and side effects.

3.3.2.1 Key Principles and Basic Concepts

Unlike WHO's guideline which seems to focus more on recombinant DNA–derived therapeutic proteins, the EMA guidelines clearly indicate that the concept of a "similar biological medicinal product" is applicable to a broad spectrum of products ranging from biotechnology-derived therapeutic proteins to vaccines, blood-derived products, monoclonal antibodies, gene and cell therapy, etc. However, comparability exercises to demonstrate similarity are more likely to be applied to highly purified products, which can be thoroughly characterized, such as biotechnology-derived medicinal products. Considering the amount of data submitted, EMA also requires a full quality dossier, while the comparability exercise at the quality level may allow a reduction of the nonclinical and clinical data requirement compared to a full dossier. In 2011, a concept paper on the revision of the guideline on similar biological medicinal product was published by EMA (EMA, 2011a), which emphasizes another main concept that clinical benefit has already been established by the reference medicinal product, and that the aim of a biosimilar development program is to demonstrate similarity to the reference product, and not clinical benefit. Besides, a clear definition of "biosimilar" is recommended as well as the feasibility to follow the generic legal basis for some biological products, and the refinement based on experience.

3.3.2.2 Reference Biotherapeutic Product

Similarly to the WHO, the EMA requires that the active substance, the pharmaceutical form, strength, and route of administration of the biosimilar should be the same as that of the reference product. The same chosen reference medicinal product should be used throughout the comparability program for quality, safety, and efficacy studies during the development of the biosimilar product. One of the major differences between WHO and EMA in terms of the choice of the reference product is that EMA requires the chosen medicinal reference product be authorized in the community. Data generated from comparability studies with medicinal products authorized outside the community may provide only supportive information.

3.3.2.3 Quality

In 2006, the "Guideline on Similar Biological Medicinal Products Containing Biotechnology-derived Proteins as Active Substance: Quality Issues" was adopted by the CHMP (EMA, 2006), which addresses the requirements regarding manufacturing processes, the comparability exercises for quality, analytical methods, physicochemical characterization, biological activity, purity, and specifications of the similar biological medicinal product. In 2011, the EMA issued a concept paper on the revision of this guideline (EMA, 2011b). This concept paper proposes that the guideline published in 2006 needs refinements taking into account the evolution of quality profile during the product lifecycle, since in the context of a biotherapeutic product claiming or claimed to be similar to another already marketed, the conclusion of a comparability exercise performed with a reference product at a given time may not hold true from the initial development of the biosimilar, through marketing authorization, until the product's discontinuation.

3.3.2.4 Nonclinical and Clinical Evaluation

The "Guideline on Similar Biological Medicinal Products Containing Biotechnology-derived Proteins as Active Substance: Non-clinical and Clinical Issues," published in 2006, lays down the nonclinical and clinical requirements for a biological medicinal product claiming to be similar to another already marketed product (EMA, 2006a–h). The nonclinical section of the guideline addresses the pharmaco-toxicological assessment, and the clinical section addresses the requirements for PK, PD, and efficacy studies. Clinical safety studies as well as the risk management plan with special emphasis on studying the immunogenicity of the biosimilar products are also required. In 2011, the EMA published a concept paper on the revision of this guideline (EMA, 2011c), which indicates several issues that need discussion for a potential revision. Firstly, the EMA emphasizes the need to follow the 3R principles (replacement, reduction, and refinement) with regard to the use of animal experiments. Secondly, a revised version of the guideline will consider a risk-based approach for the design of an appropriate nonclinical study program. Thirdly, the guideline should be clearer, considering the need and acceptance of PD markers, and what measures should be taken in case relevant markers are not available. Note that a draft guideline has been issued on May 24, 2012.

3.3.2.5 Product Class–Specific Guidelines

The principles of biosimilar drug development discussed in the earlier sections apply in general to all biological drug products. However, there are no standard data sets that can be applied to the approval of all classes of biosimilars. Each class of biologic varies in its benefit/risk profile, the nature and frequency of adverse events, the breadth of clinical indications, and whether surrogate markers for efficacy are available and validated. Accordingly, the EMA has developed product-class-specific guidelines that define the nature of comparative studies. So far, guidances for the development of biosimilar products have been developed for six different product classes, including erythropoietins, insulins, growth hormones, alpha interferons, granulocyte-colony-stimulating factors, and low-molecular-weight heparins (LMWH), with three more (beta interferons, follicle stimulation hormone, monoclonal antibodies) currently being drafted (EMA, 2006a–d, 2009a,b, 2010a,b, 2011d).

3.3.2.6 European Experience

As indicated earlier, the EU EMA has issued scientific guidelines on the quality, nonclinical, and clinical standards for the approval of biosimilars. A summary of EMA product-class-specific guidelines (including EPO, G-CSF, insulin, growth hormone, LMW heparin, and interferon-alpha) is given in Table 3.2. According to these product-class-specific guidelines, as of December 31, 2010, 14 biosimilar drugs have been approved in Europe. A list of these 14 biosimilars is provided in Table 3.3. As compared to other regions in the world, Europe holds the highest number of biosimilar approvals. This number is expected to increase as many biologic patents will soon expire in the near future, which will help to increase market size and competition among market participants.

3.3.2.7 Remarks

In summary, the EU has taken a thoughtful and evidence-based approach, and has established a well-documented legal and regulatory pathway for the approval of biosimilar products distinct from the generic pathway. In order to approve a biosimilar product, the EMA requires comprehensive and justified comparability studies between the biosimilar and the reference in the quality, nonclinical, and clinical level, which are explained in detail in the EMA guidelines. The approval pathway of biosimilar products in the EU is based on case-by-case reviews, owing to the complexity and diversity of the biological products. Therefore, besides the three general guidelines, the EMA also developed additional product-class-specific guidelines on non-clinical and clinical studies. This approval pathway is now held up as one of the gold standards for authorizing biosimilar products.

TABLE 3.2

Summary of EMA Product-Class-Specific Guidelines

Parameter	Method to demonstrate similar clinical characteristics in comparative study (studies).
Pharmacokinetics	Acceptance range should be based on clinical judgment.
	Standard bioequivalence criteria (i.e., 90% confidence interval within 80%–125% for select PK parameters) developed for orally administered products may not be appropriate.
Pharmacodynamics	PD markers should be selected on their relevance to therapeutic efficacy. Examples: reticulocyte count for erythropoietin, absolute neutrophil count for G-CSF, euglycemic clamp for insulin.
Efficacy	Demonstrate similar efficacy in at least one indication of the reference product. Indication chosen should be sensitive to differences in efficacy, should they exist. Demonstration of the clinical similarity in one indication may allow the extrapolation of the results to the other indications of the innovator biologic.
Safety	Demonstrate similar safety in at least one indication of the reference product.
Immunogenicity	Antibody testing should be part of all clinical studies.
Post-approval	Data from pre-authorization in clinical studies normally are insufficient to identify all potential differences.
	Clinical safety of biosimilars must be monitored on an ongoing basis post-approval, including continued benefit–risk assessment.

3.3.3 North America (the United States and Canada)

3.3.3.1 United States (FDA)

For the approval of FOBs in the United States, current regulations depend on whether the biological products is approved under the U.S. Food, Drug, and Cosmetic Act (U.S. FD&C) or it is licensed under the U.S. Public Health Service Act (U.S. PHS). For the biologic drugs marketed under the PHS Act, the BPCI Act passed by the U.S. Congress on March 23, 2010, amends the PHS Act to establish an abbreviated approval pathway for biological products that are highly similar or interchangeable with an FDA-authorized biologic drug, and gives the FDA the authority to approve FOBs under new Section 351(k) of the PHS Act. Some early biologic drugs such as somatropin and insulin were approved under the FD&C Act. In this case, biosimilar versions can receive approval for New Drug Applications (NDAs) under Section 505(b)(2) of the FD&C Act.

Following the passage of the BPCI Act, in order to obtain input on specific issues and challenges associated with the implementation of the BPCI Act from a broad group of stakeholders, the U.S. FDA conducted a 2 day public hearing on the Approval Pathway for Biosimilar and Interchangeability Biological Product held on November 2–3, 2010, at the FDA in Silver Spring, Maryland. The scientific issues included, but were not limited to, criteria and

TABLE 3.3

List of Approved Biosimilars in Europe Up to December 31, 2010

Product	Common Name (INN)	Company	Reference Product	Year of Approval
Omnitrope	Somatropin	Sandoz International Limited	Genotropin	2006
Valtropin	Somatropin	Biopartners GmbH	Humatrope	2006
Binocrit	Epoetin Alfa	Sandoz International Limited	Eprex	2007
Epoetin Alfa Hexal	Epoetin Alfa	HEXAL AG	Eprex	2007
Abseamed	Epoetin Alfa	Medice Arzneimittel Putter GmbH and Co. KG	Eprex	2007
Retacrit	Epoetin Zeta	Hospira, Inc.	Eprex	2007
Silapo	Epoetin Zeta	SAADA Arzneimittel AG	Eprex	2007
Biograstim	Filgrastim	CT Arzneimittel GmbH	Neupogen	2008
Filgrastim[a] Ratiopham	Filgrastim	Ratiopham GmbH	Neupogen	2008
Ratiograstim	Filgrastim	Ratiopham GmbH	Neupogen	2008
Tevagrastim	Filgrastim	Teva Generics GmbH	Neupogen	2008
Zarzio	Filgrastim	Sandoz International Limited	Neupogen	2009
Filgrastim Hexal	Filgrastim	HEXAL AG	Neupogen	2009
Nivestim	Filgrastim	Hospira, Inc.	Neupogen	2010

[a] Note that Filgrastim Ratiopharm was withdrawn on April 20, 2011, at the request of the sponsor.

design for establishing biosimilarity and interchangeability, comparability between manufacturing processes, patient safety and pharmacovigilance, exclusivity, and user fees.

In practice, there is a strong industrial interest and desire for the regulatory agencies to develop review standards and an approval process for biosimilars rather than an ad hoc case-by-case review of individual biosimilar applications. For this purpose, the FDA has established three committees to ensure consistency in the FDA's regulatory approach of FOBs. The three committees are the CDER/CBER Biosimilar Implementation Committee (BIC), the CDER Biosimilar Review Committee (BRC), and the CBER BRC. The CDER/CBER BRC will focus on the cross-center policy issues related to the implementation of the BPCI Act. The CDER BRC and CBER BRC are responsible for considering requests of applicants for advice about proposed development programs for biosimilar products, reviewing Biologic License Applications (BLAs) that are submitted under Section 351(k) of the PHS Act, and managing related issues. Thus, the review process steps of CDER BRC and CBER BRC include (1) the applicant submits request for advice, (2) internal review team meeting, (3) internal CDER BRC (CBER BRC) meeting, (4) internal post-BRC meeting, and (5) applicant meeting with CDER (CBER).

Another important issue discussed in the BPCI Act is the interchangeability of biosimilars. Once approved, standard generic drugs can be automatically substituted for the reference product without the intervention of the health-care provider in many states. However, the automatic interchangeability cannot be applied to all biosimilars. In order to meet the higher standard of interchangeability, a sponsor must demonstrate that the biosimilar products can be expected to produce the same clinical result as the reference product in any given patient.

On February 9, 2012, the FDA announced the publication of three draft guidance documents to assist industry in developing FOB products, including "Scientific Considerations in Demonstrating Biosimilarity to a Reference Product," "Quality Considerations in Demonstrating Biosimilarity to a Reference Protein Product," "Biosimilars: Questions and Answers Regarding Implementation of the BPCI Act of 2009" (FDA, 2012a–c). Similar to the require-ments of the WHO and EMA, a number of factors are considered to be important by the FDA when assessing applications for biosimilars, including the robust-ness of the manufacturing process; the demonstrated structural similarity, the extent to which the mechanism of action was understood; the existence of valid, mechanistically related PD assays; comparative PK and immunogenicity; and the amount of clinical data and experience available with the original products. The FDA was seeking public comments on the guidance within 60 days of the notice of publication in the Federal Register. Even though the guidances do not provide clear standards for assessing biosimilar products, they are the first step toward removing the uncertainties surrounding the biosimilar approval path-way in the United States.

3.3.3.2 Canada (Health Canada)

Health Canada, the federal regulatory authority that evaluates the safety, efficacy, and quality of drugs available in Canada, also recognizes that with the expiration of patents for biologic drugs, manufacturers may be interested in pursuing subsequent entry versions of these biologic drugs, which are called subsequent entry biologics (SEB) in Canada. In 2010, Health Canada issued a "Guidance for Sponsors: Information and Submission Requirements for Subsequent Entry Biologics (SEBs)," whose objective was to provide guid-ance on how to satisfy the data and regulatory requirements under the Food and Drugs Act and Regulations for the authorization of SEBs in Canada (Health Canada, 2010).

The concept of an SEB applies to all biologic drug products; however, there are additional criteria to determine whether the product will be eli-gible to be authorized as an SEB: (1) a suitable reference biologic drug exists that was originally authorized based on a complete data package, and has significant safety and efficacy data accumulated; (2) the product can be well characterized by state-of-the-art analytical methods; (3) the SEB can be judged similar to the reference biologic drug by meeting an appropriate set of pre-determined criteria. With regard to the similarity of products, Health Canada requires the manufacturer to evaluate the following factors: (1) relevant physicochemical and biological characterization data; (2) analysis of the relevant samples from the appropriate stages of the manufacturing process; (3) stability data and impurities data; (4) data obtained from multiple batches of the SEB and the reference product to understand the ranges in variability; (5) nonclinical and clinical data and safety studies. In addition, Health Canada also has stringent post-market requirements including the adverse drug reaction report, periodic safety update reports, suspension or revocation of notice of compliance (NOC).

The guidance of Canada shares similar concepts and principles as indicated in the WHO guidelines, since it is clearly mentioned in the guidance that Health Canada has the intention to harmonize as much as possible with other competent regulators and international organizations.

3.3.4 Asian Pacific Region (Japan and South Korea)

3.3.4.1 Japan (MHLW)

The Japanese Ministry of Health, Labor and Welfare (MHLW) has also been confronted with the new challenge of regulating biosimilar/FOB products. Based on the similarity concept outlined by the EMA, Japan has published a guideline for quality, safety, and efficacy of biosimilar products in 2009 (MHLW, 2009). The scope of the guideline includes recombinant plasma proteins, recombinant vaccines, PEGylated recombinant proteins, and non-recombinant proteins that are highly purified and characterized. Unlike the EU, polyglycans such as LMWH have been excluded from the guideline. Another class of product excluded is synthetic peptides, since the desired synthetic peptides can be easily defined by structural analyses and can be defined as generic drugs. Similar to the requirements by the EU, the original biologic should be already approved in Japan. However, there are some differences in the requirements of the stability test and toxicology studies for impurities in a biosimilar between the EU and Japan. A comparison of the stability of a biosimilar with the reference innovator products as a strategy for the development of a biosimilar is not always necessary in Japan. In addition, it is not required to evaluate the safety of impurities in the biosimilar product through nonclinical studies without a comparison to the original product. According to this guideline, two FOBs, "Somatropin" and "Epoetin alfa BS" have been recently approved in Japan.

3.3.4.2 South Korea (KFDA)

In Korea, the *Pharmaceutical Affairs Act* is a high-level regulation to license all medicines including biological products. The notifications by the Korean Food and Drug Administration (KFDA) serve as a lower-level regulation.

Biological products and biosimilars are subject to the *Notification of the Regulation on Review and Authorization of Biological Products*. The KFDA takes active participation in promoting a public dialog on the biosimilar issues. In 2008 and 2009, the KFDA held two public meetings and co-sponsored a workshop to gather input on scientific and technical issues. The regulatory framework of biosimilar products in Korea is a three-tiered system: (1) the Pharmaceutical Affairs Act; (2) the Notification of the Regulation on Review and Authorization of Biological Products; (3) the Guideline on Evaluation of Biosimilar Products (KFDA, 2011; Suh and Park, 2011). As the Korean guideline for biosimilar products was developed along with that of the WHO (WHO, 2009), most of the requirements are similar except for that of the clinical evaluation to demonstrate similarity. The KFDA requires that equivalent rather than noninferior efficacy should be shown in order to open the possibility of extrapolation of efficacy data to other indications of the reference product. Equivalence margins need to be pre-defined and justified, and should be established within the range which is judged not to be clinically different from reference products in clinical aspects.

3.4 Review of the FDA Draft Guidances

On February 9, 2012, the U.S. FDA released three draft guidances about the demonstration of biosimilarity. These draft guidances are (1) Scientific Considerations in Demonstrating Biosimilarity to a Reference Product, (2) Quality Considerations in Demonstrating Biosimilarity to a Reference Protein Product, (3) Biosimilars: Questions and Answers Regarding Implementation of the BPCI Act of 2009. As stated, these guidances are intended not only (1) to assist sponsors to demonstrate that a proposed therapeutic protein product is biosimilar to a reference product for the purpose of submitting a marketing application under Section 351(k) of the PHS Act, but also (2) to describe the FDA's current thinking on factors to consider when demonstrating that a proposed protein product is highly similar to a reference product which was licensed under Section 351(a) of the PHS Act. In addition, the guidances provide answers to common questions from sponsors interested in developing proposed biosimilar products, BLA holders, and other interested parties regarding FDA's interpretation of the BPCI Act of 2009.

3.4.1 Statistical Scientific Advisory Board

The Statistical Scientific Advisory Board (SSAB) focusing on *Statistical Considerations of Regulatory Approval for Biosimilars* consists of Dr. Shein-Chung Chow, a professor at Duke University School of Medicine; Dr. Laszlo Endrenyi, a professor at the University of Toronto; and Dr. Peter A. Lachenbruch, a professor at the Oregon State University. It was established and sponsored by Amgen, Inc. as an independent Board in 2009. The primary objectives of SSAB are (1) to identify statistical research topics that are critical to informing any future standards for the assessment of biosimilars, and (2) to discuss and obtain feedback on these identified statistical topics from regulatory agencies such as the FDA. The SSAB is very active in (1) statistical methodology development for the assessment of biosimilarity and interchangeability, and (2) communication and collaboration with regulatory agencies such as the FDA since established in 2009. SSAB also provided comments on one of the guidances entitled *Scientific Considerations in Demonstrating Biosimilarity to a Reference Product* for the Agency's consideration when preparing a revision of the draft guidance. In this section, we will focus on the comments from SSAB especially on the stepwise approach and the totality-of-the-evidence for assessment of biosimilarity.

3.4.2 FDA Draft Guidance on Scientific Considerations

The FDA draft guidance discusses important approaches for assessing biosimilarity, including (1) a stepwise approach to demonstrating biosimilarity, and (2) the concept of totality-of-the-evidence for the regulatory review and approval of biosimilar applications. The draft guidance covers various topics such as (1) complexities of protein products, (2) U.S.-licensed reference products and other comparators, (3) studies required for demonstrating biosimilarity, e.g., structural analysis, functional assays, animal data, and clinical studies, and (4) post-marketing safety monitoring considerations. Many important scientific factors and issues are discussed. They include (1) the use of human pharmacology data, (2) the assessment of clinical immunogenicity, (3) the use of clinical safety and effectiveness data, (4) the clinical study design issues, and (5) the extrapolation of clinical data across indications.

3.4.3 Comments on the FDA Draft Guidance

The draft guidances provide general concepts and principles for the assessment of biosimilarity although they do not present detailed information regarding the scientific factors or issues raised at the FDA *Public Hearing* and the FDA *Public Meeting for User Fees* held on November 2–3, 2010, and December 16, 2011, respectively, within the FDA in Silver Spring, Maryland. In addition, the current draft guidances did not mention the assessment of drug interchangeability, which was one of the major topics discussed at the 2010 FDA Public Hearing. In what follows, comments will be offered on some scientific factors or issues that still remain unanswered or unsolved.

3.4.3.1 Definition of Biosimilarity

As indicated in the section of *Background* of the draft guidance for *Scientific Considerations*, BPCI Act is part of the Affordable Care Act (the Healthcare Act) passed by the U.S. Congress on March 23, 2010. It adds new sections to the PHS Act. Section 351(i) defines biosimilarity, while Section 351(k) sets the procedures in a submission for biosimilarity. Note that a 351(k) application is to be distinguished from a 505(j) application for bioequivalence (generic drug products). Section 351(i) defines biosimilarity: a biological product is expected to be highly similar to the reference product notwithstanding minor differences in clinically inactive components. There should be no clinically meaningful differences between the biological product and the reference product in terms of safety, purity, and potency.

One of the major comments regarding the definition of biosimilarity is the question: "How similar is considered highly similar?" (see, e.g., Chow and Liu, 2008; Chow, 2011; Chow et al., 2011). There is little or no information regarding the definition of *highly similar*. In addition, no information is available regarding the degree of similarity such as *similar, generally similar*, and/or *highly similar*. Also: "What are the variables for which similarity should be demonstrated?" Presumably, variables used for the reference product should be studied.

The draft guidance introduces the concept of totality-of-the-evidence across different domains (such as PK/PD, immunogenicity, and clinical outcomes). The totality-of-the-evidence can be interpreted as expecting *global similarity* across different domains. *Local similarity* can be defined as similarity in some domains rather than in all domains. It is not clear that the demonstration of local similarity in some important domains would be sufficient for regulatory approval of biosimilar products.

Another comment is related to the demonstration of biosimilarity in terms of safety, purity, and potency, which are considered important, good drug characteristics as described in the FDA draft guidance. As indicated by USP/NF XXI (2000), important good characteristics, however, should include identity, strength (potency), quality, purity, safety, and stability.

3.4.3.2 Criteria of Biosimilarity

For the assessment of bioequivalence for generic (small-molecule) drug products, a one size-fits-all criterion is considered by most regulatory agencies such as the U.S. FDA and EMA of the EU. For PK studies, the one size-fits-all criterion has been directly applied for the assessment of biosimilar products regardless that there are fundamental differences between small-molecule drug products and biological products (Chow and Liu, 2010; Chow, 2011). The one size-fits-all criterion is for the assessment of average bioequivalence which does not take variabilities (inter-subject variability, intra-subject variability, and variability due to subject-by-drug interaction) into consideration. Thus, it has been criticized for penalizing drug products with smaller variability.

In the current draft guidance, however, there is little or no information regarding the criteria of biosimilarity in different domains (e.g., functional structures, PK/PD, clinical outcomes, manufacturing process). Criteria for the assessment of biosimilarity could include, but are not limited to, (1) average versus variability, (2) moment-based versus probability-based assessments, (3) aggregated versus disaggregated models, (4) scaled versus unscaled evaluations, (5) weighted versus nonweighted assessments, (6) fixed versus flexible criteria (Chow and Liu, 2010; Chow et al., 2010, Hsieh et al., 2010). At the 2010 FDA Public Hearing, it was pointed out by several presenters that the one size-fits-all criterion for the assessment of bioequivalence of generic drug products may not be appropriate for the assessment of biosimilarity of FOBs due to their fundamental differences (see also Chow and Liu, 2010). It is then suggested that a flexible, probability-based, disaggregated, scaled, weighted criterion which can account for variability should be considered (see also Chow et al., 2010).

3.4.3.3 Biosimilar Studies

For the assessment of biosimilarity by the concept of the totality-of-the-evidence, it is not clear what studies will be actually required. As stated in the draft guidance, the sponsor is required to show that there are no clinically meaningful differences between the biological product and the reference product in terms of safety, purity, and potency. This can be interpreted as the types of biosimilar studies required (e.g., PK/PD studies or clinical trials) for the demonstration of biosimilarity would depend upon the good (important) drug characteristics required by the regulatory agency. For example, if safety is of great concern, then demonstration of biosimilarity in safety, animal studies for toxicity, and immunogenicity for safety may be required.

3.4.3.4 Study Design

For human PK and PD studies, FDA recommends the use of a cross-over design for products with a short half-life (e.g., shorter than 5 days) and low incidence of immunogenicity. For products with a longer half-life (e.g., more than 5 days), a parallel-group design will usually be needed. In addition, FDA requires that scientific justification for the selection of study subjects, study dose, route of administration, and sample size be provided.

It can be suggested that in addition to the half-life and incidence rate of immunogenicity, the selection of study design should also be made based on the relative magnitude of the inter-subject and intra-subject variabilities of the test and reference drug products. It should be noted that Chow et al. (2010) proposed two useful study designs for the assessment of biosimilarity. In addition, an adaptive sequential design may be useful that (1) combines both cross-over design and parallel design and (2) links these in a bridging study.

3.4.3.5 Statistical Methods

In the current draft guidance, no specific (detailed) statistical methods for the assessment of biosimilarity were mentioned. For the assessment of generic, small-molecule drug products, under a valid study design (a cross-over design or a parallel design) and criteria for bioequivalence, standard statistical methods for the assessment of average bioequivalence such as a confidence interval approach and Schuirmann's two one-sided tests procedure are available (Chow and Liu, 2008). The FDA draft guidance may assume that these methods can be directly applied to the assessment of biosimilarity. As detailed in the following chapters, these methods may not be appropriate for the assessment of biosimilarity of FOBs due to some fundamental differences between small-molecule drug products and biological (large-molecule) drug products (Chow and Liu, 2010; Hsieh et al., 2010).

As indicated in the draft guidance, FDA recommends that sponsors use a stepwise approach to develop the evidence needed to demonstrate biosimilarity. FDA intends to consider the totality-of-the-evidence provided by a sponsor when the agency evaluates the sponsor's demonstration of biosimilarity, consistent with the longstanding approach of the agency to evaluating scientific evidence.

3.4.3.6 Stepwise Approach

The concept of the stepwise procedure is easy to comprehend. However, the term "stepwise approach" can be easily mistaken for "stepwise regression" in statistics. Thus, it is suggested that the term "stepwise approach" be changed to "step-by-step approach" in order to clarify the confusion.

A concern regarding the step-by-step approach proposed for the demonstration of evidence of biosimilarity is the control of the overall type I error rate for achieving the totality-of-the-evidence. In practice, the evidence obtained at different steps could carry different weights of clinical importance, which may or may not achieve statistical significance. In addition, the order of the step-by-step testing procedures may have an impact on the final test results. Also, the possible multiplicity of the variables could affect the type I error rate; this calls for clarification.

At each step of the approach, the "residual uncertainty" is to be evaluated which is still needed to demonstrate biosimilarity satisfactorily. At the end of the series of steps, the Draft Guidance presents clinical studies and thereby appears to leave the impression that the clinical program and its data are needed only if there is still "residual uncertainty" after evaluating the preceding steps (including structural analysis, functional assays, and studies in animals). On the other hand, the BPCI Act requires, not in a sequential manner, "a clinical study or studies (including the assessment of immunogenicity and PK or PD) that are sufficient to demonstrate safety, purity, and potency." It would be important to clarify the differing interpretations.

3.4.3.7 Totality-of-the-Evidence

The concept of totality-of-the-evidence is, in fact, global biosimilarity across different domains. The FDA seems to suggest that similarity should be demonstrated across different domains. The degree of biosimilarity in different domains, however, may have different degrees of impact on the clinical outcomes (i.e., safety and effectiveness). As a result, it is suggested that different criteria for biosimilarity in different domains should be considered. Thus, the criteria and degrees of biosimilarity in different domains will have an impact on the totality of evidence for global similarity. Chow (2011) proposed a biosimilarity index based on reproducibility probability, which may be helpful in achieving the totality of evidence for the assessment of biosimilarity. Details regarding Chow's proposed biosimilarity index and totality biosimilarity index are given in Chapters 5 and 7.

As indicated by Chow et al. (2011), the proposed biosimilarity index has the advantages that (1) it is robust with respect to the selected study endpoint, biosimilarity criteria, and study design; (2) it takes variability into consideration (one of the major criticisms in the assessment of average bioequivalence); (3) it allows the definition and assessment of the degree of similarity (in other words, it provides a partial answer to the question "how similar is considered similar?"); and (4) the use of the biosimilarity index will reflect the sensitivity of heterogeneity in variance.

Most importantly, the biosimilarity index proposed by Chow (2011) can be applied to different functional areas (domains) of biological products such as the good drug characteristics of safety (e.g., immunogenicity), purity, and potency (as described in the BPCI Act), PK, PD, biological activities, biomarkers (e.g., genomic markers), the manufacturing process, etc., used for the assessment of *global* biosimilarity.

3.4.3.8 Manufacturing Process Validation and Tests for Comparability

As the biological and reference products are very sensitive to small changes (variations) in environmental factors such as light and temperature, it is suggested that criteria for the assessment of biosimilarity based on *variability* should be developed. In addition, since different manufacturing processes could affect safety and effectiveness, the manufacturing process must be validated. *Sampling plan, acceptance criteria*, and *testing procedure* at critical stages of the manufacturing process must be described in detail in the protocol for process validation. In addition, tests for comparability between raw-material, in-process material, and the end product of manufacturing processes should be conducted based on some pre-specified *criteria for comparability*.

3.4.3.9 U.S.-Licensed Reference Product versus Other Comparators

In practice, a single reference product is less problematic. Different reference products may be problematic. Possibly, a U.S.-licensed reference product could be compared with another non-U.S.-licensed reference product. Alternatively, two different products licensed in the United States could be contrasted.

But, for example, what if the two reference products are not biosimilar under similar conditions of patient populations, study designs, and experiments?

Recently, Kang and Chow (2013) proposed a methodology for the assessment of biosimilarity with two reference products (say one from Europe and one from the United States) based on the concept of relative distance under a three-arm study design (T, R_1, and R_2). The criterion for biosimilarity is based on the relative distance between (T, R_1), (T, R_2), and (R_1, R_2). If there is no significant difference, R_1 and R_2 can be combined in order to increase the power for the assessment of biosimilarity. Conceivably, Bayesian analysis of the data could be helpful here.

3.4.3.10 Non-inferiority versus Similarity

Since non-inferiority is regarded as one-sided equivalence, we may consider establishing *non-inferiority* first and then test for *nonsuperiority* for the assessment of biosimilarity by utilizing the concept of *asymmetric* equivalence limits. This proposal deals with distinct values of α_1 and α_2 rather than $\alpha_1 = \alpha_2$. This enables us to adopt flexible biosimilarity criteria. However, the selection of the non-inferiority margin and the choices of α_1 and α_2 are controversial issues. Consideration of spending functions could be helpful. In any case, consensus among the regulatory agency, pharmaceutical/biotechnology industry, and academia should be reached based on appropriate and valid scientific/statistical justification.

3.4.3.11 Consultation with FDA

As pointed out in the draft guidance, many product-specific factors can influence the components of a product development program which intends to establish that a proposed product is biosimilar to a reference product. Therefore, FDA will provide feedback on a *case-by-case* basis on the components of a development program for a proposed product. Although the FDA's intention is good, one of the major criticisms is that case-by-case, product-specific regulatory requirements indicate that there are *no standards* for the assessment of biosimilarity. In addition, internal consistency among medical/statistical reviewers at the FDA with respect to regulatory requirements of similar drug products is another concern, especially when the decision is made subjectively and without valid and/or convincing scientific or statistical justification.

3.4.3.12 Remarks

In summary, many scientific factors still remain unresolved. These scientific factors and issues include, but are not limited to, (1) how similar is considered to be highly similar, (2) criteria for biosimilarity (average versus variability; one size-fits-all criterion or a more flexible criterion), (3) degree of biosimilarity (local similarity versus global similarity), (4) study design (potential use of adaptive designs in biosimilar studies) and sample size requirement, (5) statistical methods for achieving totality-of-the-evidence of biosimilarity, and (6) drug interchangeability (alternating versus switchability), even though it was not mentioned in the current draft guidance. More details for addressing these scientific factors and issues ought to be provided in the revised draft guidance.

The draft guidance suggests a step-by-step ("stepwise") approach for demonstrating evidence of biosimilarity. At each step the residual uncertainty of the still needed evidence can be evaluated. The sequence of structural analysis, functional analysis, animal studies, and clinical studies appears to be proposed in which, for instance, clinical investigations could be needed only in the light of the residual uncertainty. This is in contrast with the nonsequential approach of the BPCI Act according to which a clinical study or studies are required in submissions. The differing approaches ought to be clarified.

Under the step-by-step approach, it is not clear how the assessment of biosimilarity would be undertaken for different biosimilar studies in terms of criteria for biosimilarity, study designs (sample size requirement), and statistical methods. The guidance suggests consulting with FDA medical/statistical reviewers before biosimilar studies are conducted. Internal consistency at the FDA with respect to regulatory requirements of similar drug products is a concern, especially when the decision is made without valid and/or convincing scientific or statistical justifications.

3.5 Global Harmonization

According to the regulatory requirements of different regions described in the previous section, there seems to be no significant difference in the general concept and basic principles in these guidelines. There are five well-recognized principles with regard to the assessment of biosimilar products: (1) the generic approach is not appropriate for biosimilars; (2) biosimilar products should be similar to the reference in terms of quality, safety, efficacy; (3) a stepwise comparability approach, required to indicate the similarity of the SBP to RBP in terms of quality, is a prerequisite for the reduction of the submitted nonclinical and clinical data; (4) the assessment of biosimilarity is based on a case-by-case approach for different classes of products; (5) the importance of pharmacovigilance is stressed.

However, differences have been noted in the scope of the guidelines, the choice of the reference product, and the data required for product approval. The concept of a "similar biological medicinal product" in the EU is applicable to a broad spectrum of products ranging from biotechnology-derived therapeutic proteins to vaccines, blood-derived products, monoclonal antibodies, gene and cell-therapy, etc. However, the scopes of other organizations or countries are limited to recombinant protein drug products.

Concerning the choice of the reference product, the EU and Japan require that the reference product should be previously licensed in their own jurisdiction, while other countries do not have this requirement. A detailed comparison of the guidelines of the WHO, the EU, Canada, Korea, and Japan for the biosimilar products is summarized in Table 3.4.

TABLE 3.4

Comparison of Requirements among Different Regions

	WHO	Canada	Korea	EU	Japan
Term	SBPs	SEBs	Biosimilars	Biosimilars	Follow-on Biologics
Scope	Recombinant protein drugs			Mainly recombinant protein drugs	Recombinant protein drugs
Efficacy	Double-blind or observer-blind; equivalence or non-inferiority design		Equivalence design	Comparability margins should be pre-specified and justified	
Reference product	Authorized in a jurisdiction with well-established regulatory framework			Authorized in the EU	Authorized in Japan
Stability	• Accelerated degradation studies • Studies under various stress conditions				Not necessary
Purity	Process-related and product-related impurities				
Manufacture	• Same standards required by the NRA for originator products • Full chemistry and manufacture data package				
Physicochemical	• Primary and higher-order structure • Post-translational modifications				
Biological activity	• Qualitative measure of the function • Quantitative measure (e.g., enzyme assays or binding assays)				
Non-clinical studies	• In vitro (e.g., receptor-binding, cell-based assays) • In vivo (PD activity, at least one repeat dose toxicity study, antibody measurements, local tolerance)				
PK study design and criteria	• Single dose, steady-state studies, or repeated determination of PK • Cross-over or parallel • Include absorption and elimination characteristics • Traditional 80%–125% equivalence range is used				
PD	PD markers should be selected and comparative PK/PD studies may be appropriate				
Safety	Pre-licensing safety data and risk management plan				
Principles	• Generic approach is not appropriate for FOB • Follow-on biologic should be similar to the reference in terms of quality, safety, efficacy • Stepwise comparability approach: similarity of the SBP to RBP in terms of quality is a prerequisite for reduction of non-clinical and clinical data required for approval • Case-by-case approach for different classes of products • Pharmacovigilance is stressed				

Note: See also Wang and Chow (2012).

In order to facilitate the global harmonization of evaluation of the FOBs, the first workshop on implementing "WHO Guidelines on Evaluating Similar Biotherapeutic Products" into the regulatory and manufacturing practice at the global level was held on August 24–26, 2010, in Seoul, Republic of Korea. The workshop featured speakers from regulatory agencies from various countries, clinical and scientific experts, representatives from the biopharmaceutical industry and WHO.

It was recognized in the workshop that some progress toward implementation and development of guidance documents in various countries had been made. For instance, the biosimilar guidances of Singapore and Malaysia are amended mainly based on the EU's biosimilar guidelines, while Brazil and Cuba chose the WHO and Canadian guidelines as the basis for developing regulations. However, there are also many challenges which need to be addressed for global harmonization of the regulatory framework for licensure of biotherapeutics. For example, the manufacturing of SBPs in the Arab region is not well controlled due to the lack of expertise in the assessment of biotechnology products and inexperience with regulatory processes. Besides, large emerging economies such as China and India are currently lagging behind in terms of their regulations and need to act rapidly in developing appropriate regulations for biosimilar product approval.

In summary, the status of SBPs and the implementation of the WHO guidelines are highly diverse worldwide, and a harmonized approach for SBPs worldwide is unlikely to occur rapidly. While some countries have developed guidelines or are developing guidelines, other countries are taking a relaxed view and are not committed to the approach to adopt for the approval of SBPs. Accordingly, in order to promote the global harmonization, NRA should take an active role in building capacity for the regulatory evaluation of biotherapeutics; the existing guidelines should be revised as considerable experience is being gained through scientific advice, marketing authorization, applications, and workshops; WHO should continue monitoring progress with the implementation of the guidelines on the evaluation of SBPs into regulatory and manufacturers' practices.

3.6 Concluding Remarks

For the assessment of bioequivalence of generic drug products, with identified active ingredient(s) to the innovative drug products, the regulatory approval pathway through the conduct of bioequivalence studies is possible under the Fundamental Bioequivalence Assumption. For the assessment of biosimilar products, a similar Fundamental Biosimilarity Assumption is established. Biosimilar products are not identical, but merely similar to the innovative products.

As described in Section 3.3, most regulatory requirements for the approval of biosimilar products are similar but slightly different in the definitions of biosimilarity, the scope of the guidelines, the choice of the reference product, and the data required for product approval. Only few or no discussions regarding the criteria and/or the degree of biosimilarity and/or interchangeability have been pursued. In practice, it is an unresolved question, "how similar is considered highly similar?," and it is of particular interest to the sponsors to establish "how many studies are required for the regulatory approval of biosimilar products?" Besides, the degree of similarity may have an impact on the interchangeability of biosimilar products. As indicated in the BPCI Act, biosimilar products are considered interchangeable provided that they can produce the same therapeutic effect in any given patient. This, however, is not possible to achieve. Alternatively, we would suggest that biosimilar products are considered interchangeable provided that they can produce the same therapeutic effect in any given patient with certain statistical assurance.

In summary, there are still many unsolved scientific issues regarding criteria, design, and analysis for the assessment of biosimilarity and/or interchangeability of FOBs. Detailed regulatory guidances for global harmonization are needed whenever possible.

4

Criteria for Similarity

4.1 Introduction

For comparisons between drug products, some criteria for testing similarity are available in either regulatory guidelines/guidances and/or the literature. These criteria include (1) criteria for the assessment of in vivo bioequivalence testing and in vitro bioequivalence testing (FDA, 1992, 1999, 2003; Chow and Liu, 2008), (2) similarity factors for dissolution profiles comparison (Moore and Flanner, 1996; Chow and Ki, 1997; FDA, 1997), and (3) tests for consistency in raw materials, in-process materials, and end-products for quality control/assurance (Tse et al., 2006). These criteria are useful for assessing biosimilarity. However, these criteria do not discuss the issue regarding the degree of similarity. In general, these criteria can be classified into (1) absolute change versus relative change, (2) aggregated versus disaggregated, (3) scaled (weighted) versus unscaled (unweighted), or (4) moment-based (MB) versus probability-based (PB) criteria.

In clinical research and development, for a given study endpoint, post-treatment absolute change from baseline or post-treatment relative change from baseline is usually considered for comparisons between treatment groups. In practice, it is not clear whether absolute change or relative change should be selected for the assessment of similarity. As a result, several controversial issues are raised (see, e.g., Chow, 2011). First, which endpoint (i.e., absolute change or relative change from baseline) is telling the truth? Second, it is not clear whether a clinically meaningful difference in absolute change from baseline can be similarly translated to a clinically meaningful difference in relative change from baseline. Third, sample size calculations based on power analysis in terms of absolute change from baseline or relative change from baseline could lead to a very different result. It should be noted that current regulation for the assessment of bioequivalence between drug products is based on relative change.

In the development of aggregated criteria, individual criteria for the assessment of differences in average, intra-subject variability, and variance due to subject-by-product interaction between drug products are often adjusted for (or scaled with respect to) the variability associated with the reference product. The intention of the scaled criteria is not to penalize (good) products with less variability during the bioequivalence review. The scaled criteria for the assessment of bioequivalence for highly variable drug products have been in practice since introduced by the U.S. Food and Drug Administration (FDA) (Haidar et al., 2008).

For the evaluation of similarity, one can develop either an MB criterion or a PB criterion. An MB criterion assures that the difference (in terms of either absolute change or relative change) is within some pre-specified similarity limits with certain statistical assurance. For example, a 90% confidence interval of the ratio of means is totally within the similarity limits of (δ_L, δ_U). On the other hand, a PB criterion assures that there is a desired probability that the true difference (in terms of either absolute change or relative change) is within some pre-specified similarity limits. That is, for example, the probability that μ_T/μ_R is within the limits of δ_L and δ_U is higher than or equal to some pre-specified value p_0. Current requirements for the assessment of bioequivalence focus on relative change using an MB criterion.

To address the degree of similarity, similarity can be assessed by evaluating differences in average, intra-subject variability, and variance due to subject-by-product interaction between drug products *separately*. Individual criteria for the assessment of differences in average, intra-subject variability, and variance due to subject-by-product interaction between drug products are referred to as disaggregated criteria. If the criterion is a single summary measure composed of these individual criteria, it is called an aggregated criterion. Between early 1990s and early 2000s, aggregated criteria for the assessment of population bioequivalence (PBE) and individual bioequivalence (IBE) were considered for addressing drug prescribability and drug switchability (Chow and Liu, 2008).

In the next section, criteria for the assessment of average bioequivalence (ABE), PBE, IBE, and in vitro bioequivalence testing are briefly described. Similarity factors used for the comparison of dissolution profiles are given in Section 4.3. Section 4.4 provides a criterion for testing consistency in the process of quality control/assurance. Section 4.5 compares the relative performances between MB criterion and PB criterion for the assessment of bioequivalence or similarity by means of extensive simulation studies. Other alternative criteria for the assessment of similarity such as PB relative distance and a biosimilarity index based on reproducibility probability are discussed in Section 4.6. Section 4.7 provides some concluding remarks.

4.2 Criteria for Bioequivalence

As indicated in Chapter 2, bioequivalence assessment is possible under the Fundamental Bioequivalence Assumption. Accordingly, if two drug products are shown to be bioequivalent in their drug absorption profiles (which are measured in terms of the extent and rate of absorption), it is generally assumed that they will reach the same therapeutic effect or that they are therapeutically equivalent and hence can be used interchangeably. The extent and rate of drug absorption are usually measured by pharmacokinetic parameters such as the area under the blood or plasma concentration–time curve (AUC) and the maximum concentration (C_{max}). The Fundamental Bioequivalence Assumption assumes that there is an association between pharmacokinetic responses and clinical outcomes. The association between bioequivalence limits and clinical difference, however, is difficult to assess in practice.

4.2.1 Average Bioequivalence

For the assessment of ABE, the following criteria were considered by the FDA since 1977 (Chow and Liu, 2008):

75/75 Rule: Bioequivalence is claimed if at least 75% of individual subject ratios (relative individual bioavailability of the test product to the reference product) are within (75%, 125%). This criterion has the advantages that (1) it is easy to apply, (2) it compares the relative bioavailability within subjects, and (3) it removes the effect of heterogeneity from the comparison between products. However, this criterion is not viewed favorably by the FDA due to some undesirable statistical properties (see, e.g., Chow and Liu, 2008).

80/20 Rule: Bioequivalence is concluded if the average measure of the test product is not statistically significantly different from that of the reference product, and if there is at least 80% power for the detection of a 20% difference of the reference product average. This criterion has been criticized because it is based on hypothesis testing for *equality*, not for *equivalence* (*similarity*).

±20 Rule: Bioequivalence is concluded if the average bioavailability of the test product is within ±20% of that of the reference product with a certain statistical assurance. This criterion allows a test product to exhibit up to a 20% variation in average bioavailability in comparison with a reference product. The ±20 rule has been widely used for the assessment of bioequivalence for most drug products. Levy (1986), however, indicated that the ±20 rule does not accommodate the effect that the 20% variation could have on the safety and efficacy of the drug product under investigation.

80/125 Rule: Bioequivalence is concluded if the geometric means ratio between the test product and the reference product is within (80%, 125%), with a certain statistical assurance. This criterion is not symmetric about 1 on the original scale. However, on the logarithmic scale, the criterion is symmetric about 0, that is, it has a range of –0.2231 to 0.2231.

Note that according to current regulations, the 75/75 rule is not required for the assessment of bioequivalence because it is not based on rigorous statistical tests. It appears that the ±20 rule was acceptable to the FDA for the evaluation of ABE in the early 1980s. The 80/20 rule was recommended as a secondary analysis, which is often used as a supplement to the ±20 rule. However, frequently, the ±20 rule and the 80/20 rule may result in inconsistent conclusions. The 80/125 rule is the current regulation for the assessment of ABE (FDA, 2003).

4.2.2 Population/Individual Bioequivalence

In the early 1990s, as more generic drug products became available, it was a concern whether the use of generic drug products was safe, and whether the approved generic drug products could be used interchangeably. The FDA indicates that an approved generic drug product can be used as a substitution of the innovative (brand-name) drug product. However, the FDA does not indicate that generic drug products can be used interchangeably. Since generic drug products are approved based on the criterion of the 80/125 rule, there may be a drastic change in blood concentration if one shall switch from one generic drug to another. For example, if one switches from a drug which was approved on the lower end of the 80/125 rule (say 80%) to another drug which was approved on the higher end of the 80/125 rule (say 120%), then there would be a sudden 50% increase in blood concentration, which may cause a potential safety concern. In order to address the issue of drug interchangeability in terms of drug prescribability and switchability, between early 1990s and early 2000s, the FDA suggested using the concepts of PBE for addressing drug prescribability and IBE for addressing drug switchability.

Let y_T be the PK response from the test product, and y_R and $y_{R'}$ be two identically distributed PK responses from the reference product. Now consider a measure of the relative difference between the mean squared errors of $y_T - y_R$ and $y_R - y_{R'}$. Thus,

$$\theta = \begin{cases} \dfrac{E(y_T - y_R)^2 - E(y_R - y_{R'})^2}{E(y_R - y_{R'})^2/2} & \text{if } E(y_R - y_{R'})^2/2 \geq \sigma_0^2 \\[4mm] \dfrac{E(y_T - y_R)^2 - E(y_R - y_{R'})^2}{\sigma_0^2} & \text{if } E(y_R - y_{R'})^2/2 < \sigma_0^2 \end{cases},$$

where σ_0^2 is a given constant. If y_T, y_R, and $y_{R'}$ are independent observations from different subjects, then the two drug products show PBE when $\theta < \theta_P$. On the other hand, if y_T, y_R, and $y_{R'}$ are independent observations from the same subject, then the two drug products exhibit IBE when $\theta < \theta_I$. Thus, as indicated in Section 2.3, for the assessment of IBE the criterion proposed in the FDA guidance (FDA, 2001) can be expressed as

$$\theta_I = \frac{\delta^2 + \sigma_D^2 + \sigma_{WT}^2 - \sigma_{WR}^2}{\max\{\sigma_{W0}^2, \sigma_{WR}^2\}}, \tag{4.1}$$

where $\delta = \mu_T - \mu_R$, $\sigma_{WT}^2, \sigma_{WR}^2, \sigma_D^2$ are the true difference in means, intra-subject variabilities of the test product and the reference product, and the variance component due to subject-by-formulation interaction between the drug products, respectively. σ^2_{W0} is the scale parameter specified by the user. Similarly, the criterion for the assessment of PBE suggested in the FDA guidance (FDA, 2001) is given by

$$\theta_P = \frac{\delta^2 + \sigma^2_{TT} - \sigma^2_{TR}}{\max\{\sigma^2_{T0}, \sigma^2_{TR}\}}, \tag{4.2}$$

where

$\sigma^2_{TT}, \sigma^2_{TR}$ are the total variances for the test product and the reference product, respectively

σ^2_{T0} is the scale parameter specified by the user

A typical approach is to construct a one-sided 95% confidence interval for $\theta_I(\theta_P)$ for the assessment of individual (population) bioequivalence. If the one-sided 95% upper confidence limit is less than the bioequivalence limit of $\theta_I(\theta_P)$, we then conclude that the test product is bioequivalent to that of the reference product in terms of individual (population) bioequivalence. More details regarding individual and PBE can be found in Chow and Liu (2008).

4.2.3 Profile Analysis for In Vitro Bioequivalence Testing

As indicated in the FDA draft guidance for in vitro bioequivalence testing, profile analysis using a confidence interval approach should be applied to studies with a cascade impactor or multistage liquid impinger for particle size distribution. Equivalence may be assessed based on chi-square differences. The idea is to compare the profile difference between test product and reference product samples to the profile variation between reference product samples. More specifically, let y_{ijk} denote the observation from the *j*th subject's *i*th stage of the *k*th treatment. Given a sample (j_0) from the test product and two samples (j_0, j_1) from the reference products and assuming that there are a total of S stages, the profile distance between the test and reference products is given by

$$d_{TR} = \sum_{i=1}^{S} \frac{(y_{ij_0T} - 0.5(y_{ij_1R} + y_{ij_2R}))^2}{(y_{ij_0T} + 0.5(y_{ij_1R} + y_{ij_2R}))}.$$

Similarly, the profile variability within the reference formulation is defined as

$$d_{RR} = \sum_{i=1}^{S} \frac{(y_{ij_1R} - y_{ij_2R})^2}{0.5(y_{ij_1R} + y_{ij_2R})}.$$

For a given triplet sample of (Test, Reference 1, Reference 2), the ratio of d_{TR} and d_{RR}, that is,

$$rd = \frac{d_{TR}}{d_{RR}},$$

can then be used as a bioequivalence measure for the triplet samples between the two drug products. For a selected sample, the 95% upper confidence bound of $E(rd) = E(d_{TR}/d_{RR})$ is then used as a measure for the determination of bioequivalence. In other words, if the 95% upper confidence bound is less than the bioequivalence limit, then we claim that the two products are bioequivalent. The 1999 FDA draft guidance recommends a bootstrap procedure to construct the 95% upper bound for $E(rd)$. The procedure is described later.

Assume that the samples are obtained in a two-stage sampling manner. In other words, for each treatment (test or reference), three lots are randomly sampled. Within each lot, 10 samples (e.g., bottles or canisters) are sampled. The following is quoted from the 1999 FDA draft guidance regarding the bootstrap procedure to establish profile bioequivalence.

For an experiment consisting of three lots each of the test and reference products, and with 10 canisters per lot, the lots can be matched into six different combinations of triplets with two different reference lots in each triplet. The 10 canisters of a test lot can be paired with the 10 canisters of each of the two reference lots in $(10 \text{ factorial})^2 = (3{,}628{,}800)^2$ combinations in each of the lot triplets. Hence a random sample of the N canister pairings of the six Test-Reference 1-Reference 2 lot triplets is needed. rd is estimated by the sample mean of the rds calculated for the triplets in 10 selected samples of N. Note that the FDA recommends that $N = 500$ be considered.

4.3 Similarity Factor for Dissolution Profile Comparison

In vivo bioequivalence studies are surrogate trials for assessing equivalence between test and reference formulations based on the rate and extent of drug absorption in humans to establish similar effectiveness and safety under the Fundamental Bioequivalence Assumption. However, drug absorption depends on the dissolved state of a drug product, and dissolution testing provides a rapid in vitro assessment of the rate and extent of drug release. Leeson (1995), therefore, suggested that in vitro dissolution testing be used as a surrogate for in vivo bioequivalence studies to assess equivalence between the test and the reference formulations for post-approval changes. For the comparison of dissolution profiles, the

FDA guidance suggests considering the assessment of (1) the overall profile similarity and (2) the similarity at each sampling time point (FDA,
1997). Since dissolution profiles are curves over time, Chow and Ki (1997)
introduced the concepts of local similarity and global similarity. Two dissolution profiles are said to be locally similar at a given time point if their
difference or ratio at the given time point is within some equivalence
(similarity) limits, denoted by (δ_L, δ_U). Two dissolution profiles are considered globally similar if their differences or ratios are within (δ_L, δ_U) across
all time points. Note that global similarity is also known as *uniformly
similar*. Chow and Ki (1997) suggested the following similarity limits for
comparing dissolution profiles:

$$\delta_L = \frac{Q-\delta}{Q+\delta} \quad \text{and} \quad \delta_U = \frac{Q+\delta}{Q-\delta},$$

where
> Q is the desired mean dissolution rate of a drug product as specified in the
> USP/NF individual monograph
> δ is a meaningful difference of scientific importance in mean dissolution
> profiles of two drug products under consideration

In practice, δ is usually determined by a pharmaceutical scientist.

In order to achieve these two objectives, based on Moore and Flanner
(1996), both the FDA SUPAC guidance (SUPAC, 1995) and guidance on dissolution testing (FDA, 1997) suggest the similarity and difference factor for the
assessment of similarity. The similarity factor is then defined as the logarithmic reciprocal square root transformation of 1 plus the mean-squared (the
average sum of squares) difference in mean cumulative percentage dissolved
between the test and the reference formulations (μ_T and μ_R, respectively) over
all sampling time points. That is,

$$f_2 = 50 \log \left\{ \left[1 + \frac{Q}{n} \right]^{-0.5} 100 \right\}, \tag{4.3}$$

where

$$Q = \sum_{t=1}^{n} (\mu_{Rt} - \mu_{Tt})^2,$$

where log denotes the logarithm based on 10.

On the other hand, the difference factor is the sum of the absolute differences in mean cumulative percentage dissolved between the test and

reference formulations divided by the sum of the mean cumulative dissolved amounts of the reference formulation:

$$f_1 = \frac{\sum_{t=1}^{n} |\mu_{Ri} - \mu_{Ti}|}{\sum_{t=1}^{n} \mu_{Ri}}. \qquad (4.4)$$

It should be noted that the definitions of f_1 and f_2 provided by Moore and Flanner (1996), and in the SUPAC and guidance on dissolution testing, are not clear whether they are defined based on the population means or the sample averages. However, following the traditional statistical inference with ability for the evaluation of error probability, we define both f_1 and f_2 based on the population mean dissolution rates. It follows that f_1 and f_2 are population parameters for the assessment of similarity of dissolution profiles between the test and reference formulations.

The use of the f_2 similarity factor has been discussed and criticized by many researchers (e.g., Liu et al., 1997; Shah et al., 1998; Ma et al., 1999). Chow and Shao (2002) pointed out two main problems in using the f_2 similarity factor for assessing similarity between the dissolution profiles of two drug products. The first problem is its lack of statistical justification. Since f_2 is a statistic and, thus, a random variable, $P(f_2 > 50)$ may be quite large when the two dissolution profiles are not similar. However, $P(f_2 > 50)$ can be very small when the two dissolution profiles are similar. Suppose the expected value $E(f_2)$ exists and that we can find a 95% lower confidence bound for $E(f_2)$. Then, a reasonable modification to the f_2 similarity factor approach is to replace f_2 with the 95% lower confidence bound for $E(f_2)$. The second problem with using the f_2 similarity factor is that the f_2 similarity factor assesses neither local similarity nor global similarity, owing to the use of the average of the dissolution data.

4.4 Measures of Consistency

4.4.1 Moment-Based Method

Consider that a parallel design of the study is employed for evaluating the ABE of the test product with the reference product. Let T and R be the parameters of interest (e.g., a pharmacokinetic response) with means of μ_T and μ_R, respectively. Thus, the interval hypothesis for testing the ABE of two products can be expressed as

$$H_0 : \theta_L \geq \frac{\mu_T}{\mu_R} \quad \text{or} \quad \theta_U \leq \frac{\mu_T}{\mu_R} \quad \text{vs.} \quad H_a : \theta_L < \frac{\mu_T}{\mu_R} < \theta_U, \qquad (4.5)$$

where (θ_L, θ_U) is the ABE limit. Furthermore, if X and Y are the log-transformed values of T and R, respectively, then the Hypothesis 4.5 can be expressed as

$$H_0 : \theta'_L \geq \mu_X - \mu_Y \quad \text{or} \quad \theta'_U \leq \mu_X - \mu_Y \quad \text{vs.} \quad H_a : \theta'_L < \mu_X - \mu_Y < \theta'_U, \quad (4.6)$$

where
μ_X and μ_Y are the means of X and Y which are equal to the log-transformed values of μ_T and μ_R
(θ'_L, θ'_U) is $(-0.2231, 0.2231)$ which is equal to the log-transformed values of (80%, 125%)

Let X_i and Y_j be the log-transformed values of the observations of T and R obtained in the study following the normal distribution with means of μ_X, μ_Y, variances of V_X, V_Y, and numbers of the observations of n_X and n_Y, respectively. The $100(1 - 2\alpha)\%$ confidence interval (L, U) based on the parallel design for $\mu_X - \mu_Y$ can be obtained as

$$\left((\overline{X} - \overline{Y}) - t_{\alpha, df} \sqrt{\frac{S_X^2}{n_X} + \frac{S_Y^2}{n_Y}}, (\overline{X} - \overline{Y}) + t_{\alpha, df} \sqrt{\frac{S_X^2}{n_X} + \frac{S_Y^2}{n_Y}} \right), \quad (4.7)$$

where $\overline{X}$, $\overline{Y}$, S_X^2, and S_Y^2 are the unbiased estimators of μ_X, μ_Y, V_X, and V_Y, respectively. Under the assumption that $V_X \neq V_Y$, the df which is the degrees of freedom for the t-distribution mentioned earlier can be obtained by

$$df = \frac{\left(S_X^2/n_X + S_Y^2/n_Y \right)^2}{\left(S_X^2/n_X \right)^2 / (n_X - 1) + \left(S_Y^2/n_Y \right)^2 / (n_Y - 1)}.$$

The ABE of the test and reference products will be concluded if (L, U) lies within (θ'_L, θ'_U).

4.4.2 Probability-Based Approach

Tse et al. (2006) proposed a PB index for measuring consistency between raw materials, in-process materials, and end products between two traditional Chinese medicines in the process of quality control/assurance. The idea of testing consistency is described later.

Let T and R be the parameters of interest with means μ_T and μ_R, respectively. Also, let X and Y be the log-transformed values of T and R, respectively. Tse et al. (2006) proposed to test for consistency between T and R by the following probability:

$$p_C = P\left(1 - \delta < \frac{T}{R} < 1 + \delta \right) = P(\log(1 - \delta) < X - Y < \log(1 + \delta)), \quad (4.8)$$

where $0 < \delta < 1$ is an acceptance limit for consistency. Note that this idea can be applied to assess bioequivalence (biosimilarity) between drug products. In this case, we will refer to this PB index p_C as the ABE index or average biosimilarity index (denoted by p_{PB}), that is, $p_C = p_{PB}$. Let X_i and Y_j be the log-transformed values of the observations of T and R obtained in the study following the normal distribution with means μ_X, μ_Y, variances V_X, V_Y, and numbers of the observations n_X and n_Y, respectively.

From the second expression of $p_{PB} = p_C$ in Equation 4.8 by the invariance principle, the maximum likelihood estimator (MLE) of p_{PB} can be obtained as

$$\hat{p}_{PB} = \Phi\left(\frac{\log(1+\delta) - (\overline{X} - \overline{Y})}{\sqrt{\hat{V}_X + \hat{V}_Y}}\right) - \Phi\left(\frac{\log(1-\delta) - (\overline{X} - \overline{Y})}{\sqrt{\hat{V}_X + \hat{V}_Y}}\right), \qquad (4.9)$$

where

$\Phi(z_0) = P(Z < z_0)$ with Z being a standard normal random variable
$\hat{V}_X$ and $\hat{V}_Y$ are the MLE of V_X and V_Y, respectively

Moreover, the asymptotic distribution can be obtained as $\hat{p}_{PB}$:

$$\frac{\hat{p}_{PB} - p_{PB} - B(\hat{p}_{PB})}{\sqrt{C(\hat{p}_{PB})}} \rightarrow N(0,1),$$

where $B(\hat{p}_{PB})$ and $C(\hat{p}_{PB})$ are the MLEs of $B(p_{PB})$ and $C(p_{PB})$, respectively, and $B(p_{PB})$ and $C(p_{PB})$ are defined as follows:

$$B(p_{PB}) = -\frac{\partial p_{PB}}{\partial V_X}\frac{V_X}{n_X} - \frac{\partial p_{PB}}{\partial V_Y}\frac{V_Y}{n_Y}$$

$$+ \frac{1}{2}\left[\frac{\partial^2 p_{PB}}{\partial \mu_X^2}\frac{V_X}{n_X} + \frac{\partial^2 p_{PB}}{\partial \mu_Y^2}\frac{V_Y}{n_Y} + \frac{\partial^2 \hat{p}_{PB}}{\partial V_X^2}\left(\frac{2V_X^2}{n_X}\right) + \frac{\partial^2 \hat{p}_{PB}}{\partial V_Y^2}\left(\frac{2V_Y^2}{n_Y}\right)\right],$$

$$C(p_{PB}) = \left[\left(\frac{\partial p_{PB}}{\partial \mu_X}\right)^2\frac{V_X}{n_X} + \left(\frac{\partial p_{PB}}{\partial \mu_Y}\right)^2\frac{V_Y}{n_Y} + \left(\frac{\partial p_{PB}}{\partial V_X}\right)^2\left(\frac{2V_X^2}{n_X}\right) + \left(\frac{\partial \hat{p}_{PB}}{\partial V_Y}\right)^2\left(\frac{2V_Y^2}{n_Y}\right)\right],$$

$$\frac{\partial \hat{p}_{PB}}{\partial \mu_X} = -\frac{\partial \hat{p}_{PB}}{\partial \mu_Y} = \left(\frac{-1}{\sqrt{V_X + V_Y}}\right)\left[\phi(Z_2) - \phi(Z_1)\right]\overline{X},$$

$$\frac{\partial \hat{p}_{PB}}{\partial V_X} = \frac{\partial \hat{p}_{PB}}{\partial V_Y} = \left(\frac{-1}{2(V_X + V_Y)}\right)\left[Z_2\phi(Z_2) - Z_1\phi(Z_1)\right],$$

$$\frac{\partial^2 \hat{p}_{PB}}{\partial \mu_X^2} = \frac{\partial^2 \hat{p}_{PB}}{\partial \mu_Y^2} = \left(\frac{-1}{V_X + V_Y}\right)\left[Z_2 \phi(Z_2) - Z_1 \phi(Z_1)\right],$$

$$\frac{\partial^2 \hat{p}_{PB}}{\partial V_X^2} = \frac{\partial^2 \hat{p}_{PB}}{\partial V_Y^2} = \frac{1}{4(V_X + V_Y)^2}\left[(3Z_2 - Z_2^3)\phi(Z_2) - (3Z_1 - Z_1^3)\phi(Z_1)\right],$$

where

$$Z_1 = \frac{\log(1-\delta) - (\overline{X} - \overline{Y})}{\sqrt{\hat{V}_X + \hat{V}_Y}}, \quad Z_2 = \frac{\log(1+\delta) - (\overline{X} - \overline{Y})}{\sqrt{\hat{V}_X + \hat{V}_Y}},$$

and

$$\phi(Z) = \frac{1}{\sqrt{2\pi}}\exp\left(-\frac{z^2}{2}\right).$$

The PB method for hypothesis testing of ABE or average biosimilarity can be conducted based on the index of p_{PB} by considering the following hypotheses:

$$H_0 : p_{PB} \le p_0 \quad \text{vs.} \quad H_a : p_{PB} > p_0,$$

where p_0 is the lower limit of p_{PB} for concluding the ABE or average biosimilarity. We then reject the null hypothesis and conclude the alternative hypothesis if

$$\hat{p}_{PB} > p_0 + B(\hat{p}_{PB}) + Z_\alpha \sqrt{C(\hat{p}_{PB})},$$

where $B(\hat{p}_{PB})$ and $C(\hat{p}_{PB})$ can be obtained by substituting $\hat{V}_X$ and $\hat{V}_Y$ for V_X and V_Y into $B(p_{PB})$ and $C(p_{PB})$, respectively.

4.5 Comparison of Moment-Based and Probability-Based Criteria

To study the feasibility and applicability of the MB and the PB criteria described earlier for the assessment of biosimilarity between biological products, the following hypotheses and probabilities of correctly concluding biosimilarity are considered. Let T_i be the ith test statistic for the assessment of similarity based on the ith criterion, where $i = $ MB is the moment-based criterion and $i = $ PB is the probability-based criterion. Consider the following hypotheses for testing biosimilarity between a follow-on biologics and an innovator:

$$H_{0i} : \text{Dis-similarity} \quad \text{vs.} \quad H_{ai} : \text{Similarity},$$

where the ith null hypothesis of dissimilarity is tested by means of T_i based on the ith method. Thus,

$$\alpha_i = P(\text{reject } H_{0i}|H_{0i})$$

is the probability of rejecting the null hypothesis of H_{0i} when H_{0i} is true. Also,

$$p_i = 1 - \beta_i = 1 - P(\text{reject } H_{ai}|H_{ai}) = P(\text{reject } H_{0i}|H_{ai})$$

is the power of concluding biosimilarity when the follow-on biologic is indeed biosimilar to the innovator. Thus, (p_{PB}) is the probability of correctly concluding biosimilarity when applying the MB (or PB) criterion.

To compare the relative performance of the MB criterion and the PB criterion for the assessment of biosimilarity, we consider examining the following probabilities of consistency (see also Table 4.1):

P_{11}: The probability by which both the MB and PB methods conclude ABE

P_{12}: The probability by which the MB method does not conclude ABE but the PB method does

P_{21}: The probability by which the MB method concludes ABE but the PB method does not

P_{22}: The probability by which both the MB and PB methods do not conclude ABE

Let $P_{PB} = p$ and $P_{MB} = q$. Then, we have

$$P_{11} = pq$$

$$P_{12} = p(1-q)$$

$$P_{21} = (1-p)q$$

$$P_{22} = (1-p)(1-q)$$

TABLE 4.1

Probabilities of Consistency

Probability-Based Method	Moment-Based Method	
	Similar q	Not Similar $(1 - q)$
Similar p	$P_{11} = pq$	$P_{12} = p(1 - q)$
Not similar $(1 - p)$	$P_{21} = (1 - p)q$	$P_{22} = (1 - p)(1 - q)$

As a result, $P_{11} + P_{22}$ is considered the probability of consistency, while $P_{12} + P_{21}$ is a measure of inconsistency for the assessment of biosimilarity. A small value of P_{12} suggests that the conclusion of biosimilarity based on the PB criterion could imply the conclusion of biosimilarity based on the MB criterion. On the other hand, a large value of P_{21} indicates that meeting the MB criterion for biosimilarity does not guarantee the data would also meet the PB criterion for biosimilarity.

A simulation study was conducted to evaluate the performance of the MB criterion and PB criterion by observing the relationship of P_{12}, P_{21} under the following parameter settings for the simulation:

According to the parameter settings, 10,000 random samples were generated for each of a total 27 combinations of $\left(n, \mu_T, \mu_R, \sqrt{V_T}, \sqrt{V_R}\right)$, where the numbers of samples were assumed to be equal to n for test and reference products, respectively. The generated random samples were evaluated for ABE by the MB and PB methods simultaneously based on each of a total eight combinations of ABE criteria $((\theta_L, \theta_U), \delta, p_0)$. Empirical values of P_{11}, P_{12}, P_{21}, and P_{22} were calculated for each of a total 216 combinations of parameters listed in Table 4.2. In addition, for the purpose of investigating the impact of the biosimilarity limit δ and the variability V_T and V_R on the consistency and inconsistency between the two methods, separate simulations based on the combinations of parameters listed in Tables 4.3 and 4.4 were also conducted.

Results of the simulations for the parameter specifications in Table 4.2 are summarized in Tables 4.5 and 4.6. We have the following findings from these tables:

TABLE 4.2

Parameter Specifications for Simulation Study

Population Parameters for T and R			ABE Criteria for Moment-Based Method	ABE Criteria for Probability-Based Method	
n	(μ_T, μ_R)	$\left(\sqrt{V_T}, \sqrt{V_R}\right)$	(θ_L, θ_U)	δ	p_0
12	(100, 95)	(10, 5)	(80%, 125%)	0.10	0.70
	(100, 100)	(10, 10)	(90%, 111%)	0.20	0.90
	(100, 105)	(10, 15)			
		(20, 15)			
		(20, 20)			
		(20, 25)			
		(30, 25)			
		(30, 30)			
		(30, 35)			

TABLE 4.3

Parameter Specifications for Simulation Study to Investigate the Impact of δ

	Population Parameters for T and R		ABE Criteria for Moment-Based Method	ABE Criteria for Probability-Based Method	
n	(μ_T, μ_R)	$\left(\sqrt{V_T}, \sqrt{V_R}\right)$	(θ_L, θ_U)	Δ	p_0
12	(100, 100)	(10, 10)	(80%, 125%)	0.10	0.7
		(20, 20)	(90%, 111%)	0.15	0.9
				0.20	
				0.25	
				0.30	
				0.35	
				0.40	

TABLE 4.4

Parameter Specifications for Simulation Study to Investigate the Impact of the Variability

	Population Parameters for T and R		ABE Criteria for Moment-Based Method	ABE Criteria for Probability-Based Method	
n	(μ_T, μ_R)	$\left(\sqrt{V_T}, \sqrt{V_R}\right)$	(θ_L, θ_U)	δ	p_0
12	(100, 100)	(5, 5)	(80%, 125%)	0.10	0.7
		(10, 10)	(90%, 111%)	0.20	0.9
		(15, 15)			
		(20, 20)			
		(25, 25)			
		(30, 30)			
		(35, 35)			
		(40, 40)			

1. p_{MB} is uniformly higher than p_{PB} for all combinations of the parameters under study. The difference is very significant and more stringent than the MB criterion. However, if we reset especially for large variability, this indicates that the PB criterion is much the bioequivalence limits from (80%, 125%) to (90%, 111%), the rejection rate of the MB criterion would increase and p_{MB} would move close to p_{PB}.

2. Studies that pass the bioequivalence or biosimilarity testing based on the MB criterion have relatively low probability of passing the testing based on the PB criterion. From Table 4.5, when $n = 24$ (i.e., 12 subjects per treatment arm), the probabilities of inconsistencies (i.e., P_{12} and P_{21}) are 0.0000 and 0.7179, respectively, for the case of $(\mu_T, \mu_R, V_T, V_R, \delta, p_0) = (100, 100, 20, 20, 0.2, 0.7)$ with $(\theta_L, \theta_U) = (80\%, 125\%)$. This suggests that the PB criterion is much more stringent compared to the MB criterion.

TABLE 4.5

Empirical P_{11}, P_{12}, P_{21}, and P_{22} with the Moment-Based Equivalence Limits of (80%, 125%) and $n = 12$ (per Group)

μ_R	σ_T	σ_R	$p_0 = 0.7$				$p_0 = 0.9$			
			P_{11}	P_{12}	P_{21}	P_{22}	P_{11}	P_{12}	P_{21}	P_{22}
$\delta = 0.10$										
95	1	5	0.005	0.0000	0.9938	0.0004	0.0000	0.0000	0.9996	0.0004
		10	0.000	0.0000	0.9916	0.0084	0.0000	0.0000	0.9916	0.0084
		15	0.000	0.0000	0.9239	0.0761	0.0000	0.0000	0.9239	0.0761
	2	15	0.000	0.0000	0.7192	0.2808	0.0000	0.0000	0.7192	0.2808
		20	0.000	0.0000	0.6095	0.3905	0.0000	0.0000	0.6095	0.3905
		25	0.000	0.0000	0.4588	0.5412	0.0000	0.0000	0.4588	0.5412
	30	25	0.000	0.0000	0.2495	0.7505	0.0000	0.0000	0.2495	0.7505
		30	0.000	0.0000	0.1597	0.8403	0.0000	0.0000	0.1597	0.8403
		35	0.0000	0.0000	0.0963	0.9037	0.0000	0.0000	0.0963	0.9037
100	10	5	0.024	0.0000	0.9753	0.0000	0.0001	0.0000	0.9999	0.0000
		10	0.000	0.0000	0.9992	0.0003	0.0000	0.0000	0.9997	0.0003
		15	0.000	0.0000	0.9912	0.0088	0.0000	0.0000	0.9912	0.0088
	20	15	0.000	0.0000	0.8412	0.1588	0.0000	0.0000	0.8412	0.1588
		20	0.000	0.0000	0.7185	0.2815	0.0000	0.0000	0.7185	0.2815
		25	0.000	0.0000	0.5551	0.4449	0.0000	0.0000	0.5551	0.4449
	30	25	0.000	0.0000	0.2962	0.7038	0.0000	0.0000	0.2962	0.7038
		30	0.000	0.0000	0.1928	0.8072	0.0000	0.0000	0.1928	0.8072
		35	0.000	0.0000	0.1248	0.8752	0.0000	0.0000	0.1248	0.8752
105	10	5	0.011	0.0000	0.9880	0.0001	0.0001	0.0000	0.9998	0.0001
		10	0.000	0.0000	0.9947	0.0049	0.0000	0.0000	0.9951	0.0049
		15	0.000	0.0000	0.9568	0.0432	0.0000	0.0000	0.9568	0.0432
	20	15	0.000	0.0000	0.7762	0.2238	0.0000	0.0000	0.7762	0.2238
		20	0.000	0.0000	0.6597	0.3403	0.0000	0.0000	0.6597	0.3403
		25	0.000	0.0000	0.5391	0.4609	0.0000	0.0000	0.5391	0.4609
	30	25	0.000	0.0000	0.2921	0.7079	0.0000	0.0000	0.2921	0.7079
		30	0.000	0.0000	0.2093	0.7907	0.0000	0.0000	0.2093	0.7907
		35	0.000	0.0000	0.1422	0.8578	0.0000	0.0000	0.1422	0.8578
$\delta = 0.20$										
95	10	5	0.7314	0.0000	0.2682	0.0004	0.0976	0.0000	0.9020	0.0004
		10	0.3712	0.0000	0.6204	0.0084	0.0088	0.0000	0.9828	0.0084
		15	0.0786	0.0000	0.8453	0.0761	0.0005	0.0000	0.9234	0.0761
	20	15	0.0023	0.0000	0.7169	0.2808	0.0000	0.0000	0.7192	0.2808
		20	0.0004	0.0000	0.6091	0.3905	0.0000	0.0000	0.6095	0.3905
		25	0.0000	0.0000	0.4588	0.5412	0.0000	0.0000	0.4588	0.5412
	30	25	0.0000	0.0000	0.2495	0.7505	0.0000	0.0000	0.2495	0.7505
		30	0.0000	0.0000	0.1597	0.8403	0.0000	0.0000	0.1597	0.8403
		35	0.0000	0.0000	0.0963	0.9037	0.0000	0.0000	0.0963	0.9037

(continued)

TABLE 4.5 (continued)

Empirical P_{11}, P_{12}, P_{21}, and P_{22} with the Moment-Based Equivalence Limits of (80%, 125%) and $n = 12$ (per Group)

			$p_0 = 0.7$				$p_0 = 0.9$			
μ_R	σ_T	σ_R	P_{11}	P_{12}	P_{21}	P_{22}	P_{11}	P_{12}	P_{21}	P_{22}
100	10	5	0.9536	0.0000	0.0464	0.0000	0.3081	0.0000	0.6919	0.0000
		10	0.7049	0.0000	0.2948	0.0003	0.0330	0.0000	0.9667	0.0003
		15	0.1869	0.0000	0.8043	0.0088	0.0010	0.0000	0.9902	0.0088
	20	15	0.0037	0.0000	0.8375	0.1588	0.0000	0.0000	0.8412	0.1588
		20	0.0006	0.0000	0.7179	0.2815	0.0000	0.0000	0.7185	0.2815
		25	0.0002	0.0000	0.5549	0.4449	0.0000	0.0000	0.5551	0.4449
	30	25	0.0000	0.0000	0.2962	0.7038	0.0000	0.0000	0.2962	0.7038
		30	0.0000	0.0000	0.1928	0.8072	0.0000	0.0000	0.1928	0.8072
		35	0.0000	0.0000	0.1248	0.8752	0.0000	0.0000	0.1248	0.8752
105	10	5	0.9439	0.0000	0.0560	0.0001	0.2910	0.0000	0.7089	0.0001
		10	0.7203	0.0000	0.2748	0.0049	0.0342	0.0000	0.9609	0.0049
		15	0.2126	0.0000	0.7442	0.0432	0.0022	0.0000	0.9546	0.0432
	20	15	0.0058	0.0000	0.7704	0.2238	0.0000	0.0000	0.7762	0.2238
		20	0.0005	0.0000	0.6592	0.3403	0.0000	0.0000	0.6597	0.3403
		25	0.0002	0.0000	0.5389	0.4609	0.0000	0.0000	0.5391	0.4609
	30	25	0.0000	0.0000	0.2921	0.7079	0.0000	0.0000	0.2921	0.7079
		30	0.0000	0.0000	0.2093	0.7907	0.0000	0.0000	0.2093	0.7907
		35	0.0000	0.0000	0.1422	0.8578	0.0000	0.0000	0.1422	0.8578

3. In the interest of achieving the same level of precision and reliability for detecting bioequivalence or biosimilarity based on the MB criterion as suggested by the FDA, we may loosen the specification limits of δ or P_0 with the PB criterion. For example, for the case of $(\mu_T, \mu_R, V_T, V_R) = (100, 100, 10, 5)$ with $(\theta_L, \theta_U) = (90\%, 111\%)$, the choice of $P_0 = 0.9$ and $\delta = 0.1$ with the PB criterion cannot reach the same probability (p = 0.0001 vs. q = 0.8628) of concluding bioequivalence or biosimilarity as with the MB criterion. However, with $\delta = 0.2$ and $p_0 = 0.7$, similar probabilities can be reached (p = 0.8628 vs. q = 0.9536) of concluding bioequivalence or biosimilarity. On the other hand, when the variability is large, it is almost impossible for the MB criterion to reach the same level of precision and reliability for detecting bioequivalence or biosimilar based on the proposed PB criterion regardless of how tight the bioequivalence or biosimilarity limit would be.

TABLE 4.6

Empirical P_{11}, P_{12}, P_{21}, and P_{22} with the Moment-Based Equivalence Limits of (90%, 111%) and $n = 12$ (per Group)

μ_R	σ_T	σ_R	P_{11}	P_{12}	P_{21}	P_{22}	P_{11}	P_{12}	P_{21}	P_{22}
				$p_0 = 0.7$				$p_0 = 0.9$		
$\delta = 0.10$										
95	10	5	0.0058	0.0000	0.4626	0.5316	0.0000	0.0000	0.4684	0.5316
		10	0.0000	0.0000	0.3153	0.6847	0.0000	0.0000	0.3153	0.6847
		15	0.0000	0.0000	0.1438	0.8562	0.0000	0.0000	0.1438	0.8562
	20	15	0.0000	0.0000	0.0138	0.9862	0.0000	0.0000	0.0138	0.9862
		20	0.0000	0.0000	0.0033	0.9967	0.0000	0.0000	0.0033	0.9967
		25	0.0000	0.0000	0.0009	0.9991	0.0000	0.0000	0.0009	0.9991
	30	25	0.0000	0.0000	0.0002	0.9998	0.0000	0.0000	0.0002	0.9998
		30	0.0000	0.0000	0.0000	1.0000	0.0000	0.0000	0.0000	1.0000
		35	0.0000	0.0000	0.0000	1.0000	0.0000	0.0000	0.0000	1.0000
100	10	5	0.0247	0.0000	0.8381	0.1372	0.0001	0.0000	0.8627	0.1372
		10	0.0005	0.0000	0.6061	0.3934	0.0000	0.0000	0.6066	0.3934
		15	0.0000	0.0000	0.2684	0.7316	0.0000	0.0000	0.2684	0.7316
	20	15	0.0000	0.0000	0.0225	0.9775	0.0000	0.0000	0.0225	0.9775
		20	0.0000	0.0000	0.0047	0.9953	0.0000	0.0000	0.0047	0.9953
		25	0.0000	0.0000	0.0011	0.9989	0.0000	0.0000	0.0011	0.9989
	30	25	0.0000	0.0000	0.0000	1.0000	0.0000	0.0000	0.0000	1.0000
		30	0.0000	0.0000	0.0001	0.9999	0.0000	0.0000	0.0001	0.9999
		35	0.0000	0.0000	0.0000	1.0000	0.0000	0.0000	0.0000	1.0000
105	10	5	0.0119	0.0000	0.5052	0.4829	0.0001	0.0000	0.5170	0.4829
		10	0.0004	0.0000	0.3746	0.6250	0.0000	0.0000	0.3750	0.6250
		15	0.0000	0.0000	0.1986	0.8014	0.0000	0.0000	0.1986	0.8014
	20	15	0.0000	0.0000	0.0218	0.9782	0.0000	0.0000	0.0218	0.9782
		20	0.0000	0.0000	0.0061	0.9939	0.0000	0.0000	0.0061	0.9939
		25	0.0000	0.0000	0.0020	0.9980	0.0000	0.0000	0.0020	0.9980
	30	25	0.0000	0.0000	0.0001	0.9999	0.0000	0.0000	0.0001	0.9999
		30	0.0000	0.0000	0.0000	1.0000	0.0000	0.0000	0.0000	1.0000
		35	0.0000	0.0000	0.0000	1.0000	0.0000	0.0000	0.0000	1.0000
$\delta = 0.20$										
95	10	5	0.4616	0.2698	0.0068	0.2618	0.0973	0.0003	0.3711	0.5313
		10	0.2621	0.1091	0.0532	0.5756	0.0088	0.0000	0.3065	0.6847
		15	0.0579	0.0207	0.0859	0.8355	0.0005	0.0000	0.1433	0.8562
	20	15	0.0015	0.0008	0.0123	0.9854	0.0000	0.0000	0.0138	0.9862
		20	0.0002	0.0002	0.0031	0.9965	0.0000	0.0000	0.0033	0.9967
		25	0.0000	0.0000	0.0009	0.9991	0.0000	0.0000	0.0009	0.9991
	30	25	0.0000	0.0000	0.0002	0.9998	0.0000	0.0000	0.0002	0.9998
		30	0.0000	0.0000	0.0000	1.0000	0.0000	0.0000	0.0000	1.0000
		35	0.0000	0.0000	0.0000	1.0000	0.0000	0.0000	0.0000	1.0000

(continued)

TABLE 4.6 (continued)

Empirical P_{11}, P_{12}, P_{21}, and P_{22} with the Moment-Based Equivalence Limits of (90%, 111%) and $n = 12$ (per Group)

μ_R	σ_T	σ_R	P_{11}	P_{12}	P_{21}	P_{22}	P_{11}	P_{12}	P_{21}	P_{22}
					$p_0 = 0.7$				$p_0 = 0.9$	
100	10	5	0.8504	0.1032	0.0124	0.0340	0.3029	0.0052	0.5599	0.1320
		10	0.5326	0.1723	0.0740	0.2211	0.0325	0.0005	0.5741	0.3929
		15	0.1283	0.0586	0.1401	0.6730	0.0010	0.0000	0.2674	0.7316
	20	15	0.0026	0.0011	0.0199	0.9764	0.0000	0.0000	0.0225	0.9775
		20	0.0004	0.0002	0.0043	0.9951	0.0000	0.0000	0.0047	0.9953
		25	0.0002	0.0000	0.0009	0.9989	0.0000	0.0000	0.0011	0.9989
	30	25	0.0000	0.0000	0.0000	1.0000	0.0000	0.0000	0.0000	1.0000
		30	0.0000	0.0000	0.0001	0.9999	0.0000	0.0000	0.0001	0.9999
		35	0.0000	0.0000	0.0000	1.0000	0.0000	0.0000	0.0000	1.0000
105	10	5	0.5136	0.4303	0.0035	0.0526	0.2499	0.0411	0.2672	0.4418
		10	0.3457	0.3746	0.0293	0.2504	0.0314	0.0028	0.3436	0.6222
		15	0.1064	0.1062	0.0922	0.6952	0.0020	0.0002	0.1966	0.8012
	20	15	0.0035	0.0023	0.0183	0.9759	0.0000	0.0000	0.0218	0.9782
		20	0.0004	0.0001	0.0057	0.9938	0.0000	0.0000	0.0061	0.9939
		25	0.0002	0.0000	0.0018	0.9980	0.0000	0.0000	0.0020	0.9980
	30	25	0.0000	0.0000	0.0001	0.9999	0.0000	0.0000	0.0001	0.9999
		30	0.0000	0.0000	0.0000	1.0000	0.0000	0.0000	0.0000	1.0000
		35	0.0000	0.0000	0.0000	1.0000	0.0000	0.0000	0.0000	1.0000

Figure 4.1 presents the relationship of probabilities of consistency and inconsistency of MB and PB methods versus δ and σ based on the simulation results of parameters specified in Tables 4.3 and 4.4, respectively, where σ denotes the standard deviation of the population which is assumed to be the same for test and reference products. The findings are summarized as follows:

1. In Figure 4.1, $p = P_{11} + P_{12}$, that is, the probability concluding biosimilarity by the PB method increases when δ increases in both subfigures. On the other hand, the slope for the curve p becomes flatter when σ and p_0 increase. With respect to $q = P_{11} + P_{21}$ which stands for the probability concluding biosimilarity by the MB method, it remains as a horizontal line throughout the change of δ since δ is the ABE criterion for the PB method and has no impact on the performance of the MB method. However, q becomes smaller when (θ_L, θ_U) changes from (80%, 125%) to (90%, 111%) since the ABE limit of the MB method becomes tighter. On the other hand, P_{12} increases when δ increases while P_{21} decreases because the ABE limit for the PB method becomes looser. In addition, when $(\theta_L, \theta_U) = (80\%, 125\%)$, the probability for concluding the biosimilarity by both methods, that is, $P_{11} + P_{22}$,

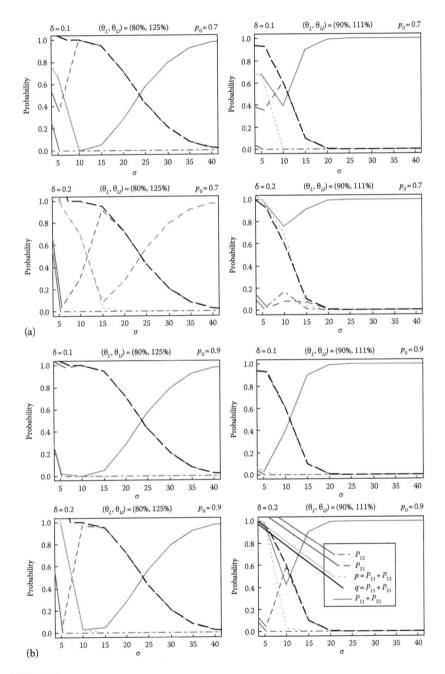

FIGURE 4.1
(a) Probabilities of consistency and inconsistency of the moment-based method and the probability-based method versus δ when $p_0 = 0.7$. (b) Probabilities of consistency and inconsistency of moment-based method and probability-based method versus δ when $p_0 = 0.9$.

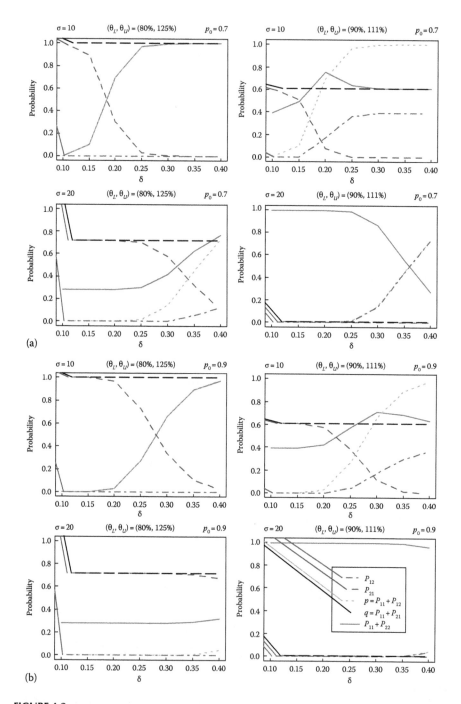

FIGURE 4.2
Probabilities of consistency and inconsistency of the moment-based method and the probability-based method versus the variability for (a) $p_0 = 0.7$ and (b) $p_0 = 0.9$.

remains the same at the smaller value of δ and increases, while $P_{11} + P_{22}$ increases at the smaller value of δ but decreases at the later value of δ when $(\theta_L, \theta_U) = (90\%, 111\%)$. It should be noticed that most of the decreases of $P_{11} + P_{22}$ result from the decrease of P_{22}. Therefore, when the ABE limit of the MB method becomes tighter from (80%, 125%) to (90%, 111%), $P_{11} + P_{22}$ decreases due to the decrease of P_{22}.

2. In Figure 4.2, both p and q decrease quickly when σ increases in all subfigures. The slopes become flatter if δ increases and (θ_L, θ_U) is looser. However, in most cases, p is more sensitive to the change of σ than q since it decreases faster. On the other hand, P_{21} varies a lot throughout with the change in σ while P_{12} maintains its value in most of the subfigures. The change in σ impacts the probability of concluding the biosimilarity by the PB method more than the MB method. Therefore, the simulation results of Figure 4.2 demonstrate that the PB method is more sensitive to the change of variability than the MB method.

4.6 Alternative Criteria

4.6.1 Probability-Based Relative Distance

In addition to the MB criterion relying on relative distance as described in Section 4.2.2, Schall and Luus (1993) also proposed PB measures for the expected discrepancy in pharmacokinetic responses between drug products. Their presentation involved the determination of bioequivalence. The arguments also apply to the evaluation of biosimilarity. The MB measure suggested by Schall and Luus (1993) is based on the following expected mean-squared differences:

$$d(Y_j; Y_{j'}) = \begin{cases} E(Y_T - Y_R)^2 & \text{if } j = T \text{ and } j' = R \\ E(Y_R - Y_R')^2 & \text{if } j = R \text{ and } j' = R. \end{cases} \quad (4.10)$$

For some pre-specified positive number r, one of the PB measures for the expected discrepancy is given as (Schall and Luus, 1993)

$$d(Y_j; Y_{j'}) = \begin{cases} P\{|Y_T - Y_R| < r\} & \text{if } j = T \text{ and } j' = R \\ P\{|Y_R - Y_R'| < r\} & \text{if } j = R \text{ and } j' = R. \end{cases} \quad (4.11)$$

$d(Y_T; Y_R)$ measures the expected discrepancy for some pharmacokinetic metric between test and reference formulations, and $d(Y_R; Y_R')$ provides the expected discrepancy between the repeated administrations of the reference formulation. The role of $d(Y_R; Y_R')$ in the formulation of bioequivalence criteria is to serve as a control. The rationale is that the reference formulation should be bioequivalent to itself. Therefore, for the MB measures, if the test formulation is indeed bioequivalent to the reference formulation, then $d(Y_T; Y_R)$ should be very close to $d(Y_R; Y_R')$. It follows that if the criteria are functions of the difference (or ratio) between $d(Y_T; Y_R)$ and $d(Y_R; Y_R')$, then bioequivalence is concluded if they are smaller than some pre-specified limit. On the other hand, for PB measures, if the test formulation is indeed bioequivalent to the reference formulation, as compared with $d(Y_R; Y_R')$, then $d(Y_T; Y_R)$ should be relatively large. As a result, bioequivalence is concluded if the criterion relying on the PB measure is larger than some pre-specified limit.

4.6.2 Reproducibility Probability

Most recently, Chow et al. (2011) proposed a biosimilarity index, based on the concept of reproducibility probability proposed by Shao and Chow (2002), for the assessment of biosimilarity for a given biosimilarity criterion. The idea is described later. Suppose that the null hypothesis H_0 is rejected if and only if $|T| > c$, where c is a positive known constant and T is a test statistic. Thus, the reproducibility probability of observing a significant clinical result when H_a is indeed true is given by

$$p = P\left(|T| > c \mid H_a\right) = P\left(|T| > c \mid \hat{\theta}\right), \qquad (4.12)$$

where $\hat{\theta}$ is an estimate of θ, which is an unknown parameter or vector of parameters. Following the similar idea, a reproducibility probability can also be used to evaluate biosimilarity between a test product and a reference product based on any pre-specified criteria for biosimilarity. As an example, the biosimilarity index proposed by Chow et al. (2011) is illustrated based on the well-established bioequivalence criterion by the following steps. First, assess the average biosimilarity between the test product and the reference product based on a given biosimilarity criterion. For illustration, consider the bioequivalence criterion as a biosimilarity criterion. That is, biosimilarity is claimed if the 90% confidence interval of the ratio of means of a given study endpoint falls within the biosimilarity limits of (80%, 125%) based on log-transformed data. Once the product passes the test for biosimilarity in Step 1, calculate the reproducibility probability based on the observed ratio (or observed mean difference) and *variability*. Chow et al. (2011) refer to the calculated reproducibility probability as the *biosimilarity index*. We then claim biosimilarity if the following null hypothesis is rejected:

$$H_0 : p \leq p_0 \quad \text{vs.} \quad H_a : p > p_0. \qquad (4.13)$$

A confidence interval approach can be similarly applied. In other words, we claim biosimilarity if the lower 95% confidence bound of the reproducibility probability is larger than a pre-specified number p_0. In practice, p_0 can be obtained based on an estimate of reproducibility probability for a study comparing a reference product to itself (the reference product). We will refer to such a study as an R–R study.

4.7 Concluding Remarks

Although several criteria for similarity are available in either regulatory guidelines/guidances or the literature, these criteria do not translate into one another. In other words, one may pass one criterion but fail to pass others. Besides, these criteria do not address the critical questions that (1) how similar is considered to be highly similar and (2) the impact of the degree or level of similarity on drug interchangeability.

EMA is not clear regarding what specific scientific requirements will be applied to biosimilar applications, or how innovator data from reference products will be treated. They do provide a summary of biosimilar legislations and previous publications in the European Union but do not address the question of scientific requirements. On the other hand, the FDA does not have clear regulatory requirements, currently, though guidelines are in preparation, and there does appear to be a preference for multiple testing and/or sequential testing procedures to establish biosimilarity.

In this chapter, we compare the MB criterion with the PB criterion for the assessment of bioequivalence and also of biosimilarity under a parallel-group design. The results indicate that the PB criterion is not only much more stringent but also sensitive to any small changes in variability. This justifies the use of the proposed PB criterion for the assessment of biosimilarity between follow-on biologics if a certain level of precision and reliability of biosimilarity is desired.

Moreover, since the comparison is made based on the concept of ABE (biosimilarity), the criterion does not take into consideration variability, which is known to have a significant impact on the clinical performance of follow-on biologics. Thus, it is suggested that a statistical methodology for comparing variabilities based on the PB criterion should be developed by following similar ideas described earlier. It should be noted that major sources of variabilities include intra-subject and inter-subject variabilities and variability due to possible subject-by-treatment interaction, which is known to have an impact on drug interchangeability.

In practice, we may consider to assess bioequivalence or biosimilarity by comparing average and variability separately or simultaneously. This leads to the so-called disaggregated criterion and aggregated criterion.

A disaggregate criterion will provide different levels of biosimilarity. For example, a study that passes both average and variability of biosimilarity provides stronger evidence of biosimilarity as compared to studies that pass only average biosimilarity. On the other hand, it is not clear whether an aggregated criterion would provide a stronger evidence of biosimilarity due to potential offset (or masked) effect between the average and variability in the aggregated criterion. Further research may be needed for establishing the appropriate statistical testing procedures based on the aggregate criterion and comparing its performance with the disaggregate criterion.

5

Statistical Methods for Assessing Average Biosimilarity

5.1 Introduction

In recent years, as more biological products are going off patent protection, the assessment of biosimilarity between biosimilar products (or follow-on biologics) and an innovative (reference) product has received considerable attention. For the approval of biosimilar products, the European Medicines Agency (EMA) has published several product-specific concept papers as regulatory guidelines for the approval pathway of biosimilar products (EMA, 2006a–g). In the United States, the *Biologics Price Competition and Innovation* (BPCI) Act (as part of the *Affordable Care* Act) has given FDA the authority to approve biosimilar drug products. As indicated in the BPCI Act, a biosimilar product is defined as a product that is *highly similar* to the reference product notwithstanding minor differences in clinically inactive components and there are no clinically meaningful differences in terms of safety, purity, and potency. However, no discussion regarding the criterion for similarity and how similar is considered highly similar is given in the BPCI Act.

For the assessment of biosimilarity, standard methods for the assessment of bioequivalence for small-molecule drug products are usually considered. They include the classical methods such as the confidence interval approach and interval hypotheses testing such as Schuirmann's two one-sided tests procedure, Bayesian methods, and non-parametric methods such as the Wilcoxon–Mann–Whitney two one-sided tests procedure. It should be noted that these methods were derived based on a raw data model under a crossover design although they can be easily applied to a parallel-group design based on log-transformed data. In practice, it is a concern whether these methods are appropriate for the assessment of biosimilarity due to fundamental differences between small-molecule drug products and large-molecule biological drug products as described in earlier chapters (see also Chow et al., 2011). As a result, the search for biosimilarity criteria, study endpoints (measures of biosimilarity), and statistical methods has become the center of attention for the assessment of biosimilarity.

In practice, one of the most widely used designs for assessing biosimilarity between biosimilar products and an innovator biological product is probably either a two-sequence, two-period (2×2) crossover design or a two-arm parallel-group design. Under a valid study design, biosimilarity can then be assessed by means of an equivalence test under the following interval hypotheses:

$$H_0 : \mu_T - \mu_R \leq \theta_L \quad \text{or} \quad \mu_T - \mu_R \geq \theta_U \quad \text{versus} \quad H_a : \theta_L < \mu_T - \mu_R < \theta_U, \quad (5.1)$$

where
   (θ_L, θ_U) are pre-specified equivalence limits (margins)
   μ_T and μ_R are the population means of a biological (test) product and an innovator biological (reference) product, respectively

That is, biosimilarity is assessed in terms of the *absolute* difference between the two population means. Alternatively, biosimilarity can be assessed in terms of the *relative* difference (i.e., ratio) between the population means. Note that for the assessment of similarity between small-molecule drug products, average bioequivalence, population bioequivalence, and individual bioequivalence are defined in terms of ratios of appropriate parameters under a crossover design. In practice, since many biological products have long half-lives, a crossover design may not be appropriate for the assessment of biosimilarity. Instead, a parallel-group design is considered to be more appropriate.

The purpose of this chapter is to provide a comprehensive summarization of standard statistical methods that are commonly used for the assessment of average bioequivalence for small-molecule drug products under a crossover design. In addition, we will focus on the discussion of statistical methods proposed by Kang and Chow (2013) under a newly proposed three-arm parallel design for the investigation of biosimilarity. The statistical analysis methods proposed by Kang and Chow (2013) consider the relative distance based on the absolute mean differences. Under the three-arm design, patients who are randomly assigned to the first group receive a biosimilar (test) product, while patients who are randomly assigned to the second and the third groups receive the innovator biological (reference) product from different batches. The distance between the test product and the reference product is defined by the absolute mean difference between the two products. Similarly, the distance is defined between the reference products from two different batches. The relative distance is defined as the ratio of the two distances whose denominator is the distance between the two reference products from different batches. Under the proposed design, Kang and Chow (2013) claim that the two products are biosimilar if the relative distance is less than a pre-specified margin.

In the next section, classic methods such as the shortest confidence interval approach and Schuirmann's two one-sided tests procedure are introduced.

The Bayesian method proposed by Rodda and Davis (1980) is given in Section 5.3. Section 5.4 outlines the non-parametric method of the Wilcoxon–Mann–Whitney two one-sided tests procedure. In Section 5.5, two statistical methods for assessing biosimilarity of biosimilar products in a three-arm design proposed by Kang and Chow (2013) are discussed. Also included in this section are the power functions of two statistical methods and a comparison of the powers of the two statistical methods. In Section 5.6, future studies are discussed.

5.2 Classic Methods for Assessing Biosimilarity

Under a $p \times q$ crossover design, consider the following statistical model for raw data:

$$Y_{ijk} = \mu + S_{ik} + P_j + F_{j,k} + C_{(j-1,k)} + e_{ijk}, \qquad (5.2)$$

where
  Y_{ijk} is the response (e.g., AUC) of the ith subject in the kth sequence at the jth period
  μ is the overall mean
  S_{ik} is the random effect of the ith subject in the kth sequence, where $i = 1, 2, ..., q$
  P_j is the fixed effect of the jth period, where $j = 1, ..., p$ and $\Sigma_j P_j = 0$
  $F_{(j,k)}$ is the direct fixed effect of the drug product in the kth sequence which is administered in the jth period, and $\Sigma F_{(j,k)} = 0$
  $C_{(j-1,k)}$ is the fixed first-order carryover effect of the drug product in the kth sequence which is administered in the $(j = 1)$th period, where $C_{(0,k)} = 0$; and $\Sigma C_{(j-1,k)} = 0$
  e_{ijk} is the (within-subject) random error in observing Y_{ijk}

It is assumed that $\{S_{ik}\}$ are independently and identically distributed (i.i.d.) with mean 0 and variance σ_s^2 and $\{e_{ijk}\}$ are independently distributed with mean 0 and variances σ_t^2, where $t = 1, 2, ..., L$ (the number of formulations to be compared). $\{S_{ik}\}$ and $\{e_{ijk}\}$ are assumed mutually independent. The estimate of σ_s^2 is usually used to explain the inter-subject variability, and the estimates of σ_t^2 are used to assess the intra-subject variabilities for the tth drug product.

5.2.1 Confidence Interval Approach

For bioequivalence assessment of small-molecule drug products, the FDA adopts the 80/125 rule based on log-transformed data. The 80/125 rule states that bioequivalence is concluded if the geometric means ratio (GMR) between the test product and the reference product is within the bioequivalence limits of (80%, 125%), with a certain statistical assurance. Thus, a typical approach is to consider the method of classic (shortest) confidence interval.

Consider a standard two-sequence, two-period (i.e., $p=q=2$) crossover design, under Model 5.2, after the log-transformation of the data, let $\bar{Y}_T$ and $\bar{Y}_R$ be the respective least-squares means for the test and reference formulations, which can be obtained from the sequence-by-period means. The classic (or shortest) $(1-2\alpha) \times 100\%$ confidence interval can then be obtained based on the following t statistic:

$$T = \frac{(\bar{Y}_T - \bar{Y}_R) - (\mu_T - \mu_R)}{\hat{\sigma}_d \sqrt{(1/n_1) + (1/n_2)}}, \qquad (5.3)$$

where

n_1 and n_2 are the numbers of subjects in sequences 1 and 2, respectively

$\hat{\sigma}_d$ is an estimate of the variance of the period differences for each subject within each sequence, which is defined as follows:

$$d_{ik} = \frac{1}{2}(Y_{i2k} - Y_{i1k}), \quad i = 1, 2, \ldots, n_k; \quad k = 1, 2.$$

Thus, $V(d_{ik}) = \sigma_d^2 = \sigma_e^2/2$. Under normality assumptions, T follows a central Student t distribution with degrees of freedom $n_1 + n_2 - 2$. Thus, the classic $(1-2\alpha) \times 100\%$ confidence interval for $\mu_T - \mu_R$ can be obtained as follows:

$$L_1 = (\bar{Y}_T - \bar{Y}_R) - t(\alpha, n_1 + n_2 - 2)\hat{\sigma}_d \sqrt{(1/n_1) + (1/n_2)},$$

$$U_1 = (\bar{Y}_T - \bar{Y}_R) - t(\alpha, n_1 + n_2 - 2)\hat{\sigma}_d \sqrt{(1/n_1) + (1/n_2)}. \qquad (5.4)$$

The previously mentioned $(1-2\alpha) \times 100\%$ confidence interval for $\log(\mu_T) - \log(\mu_R) = \log(\mu_T/\mu_R)$ can be converted into a $(1 - 2\alpha) \times 100\%$ confidence interval for μ_T/μ_R by taking an anti-log transformation.

Note that under a parallel-group design, a $(1-2\alpha) \times 100\%$ confidence interval for μ_T/μ_R can be similarly obtained.

5.2.2 Schuirmann's Two One-Sided Tests Procedure

The assessment of average bioequivalence is based on the comparison of bioavailability profiles between drug products. However, in practice, it is recognized that no two drug products will have exactly the same bioavailability profiles. Therefore, if the profiles of two drug products differ by less than a (clinically) meaningful limit, the profiles of the two drug products may be considered equivalent. Following this concept, Schuirmann (1987) first introduced the use of interval Hypotheses 5.1 for assessing average bioequivalence. The concept of interval Hypotheses 5.1 is to show average bioequivalence by rejecting the null hypothesis of average bioinequivalence. In most bioavailability and bioequivalence studies, δ_L and δ_U are often chosen to be $-\theta_L = \theta_U = 20\%$ of the reference mean (μ_R). When the natural logarithmic transformation of the data is considered, the hypotheses corresponding to Hypotheses 5.1 can be stated as

$$H_0' : \frac{\mu_T}{\mu_R} \le \delta_L \quad \text{or} \quad \frac{\mu_T}{\mu_R} \ge \delta_U \quad \text{versus} \quad H_a' : \delta_L < \frac{\mu_T}{\mu_R} < \delta_U, \tag{5.5}$$

where
$$\delta_L = \exp(\theta_L)$$
$$\delta_U = \exp(\theta_U)$$

The FDA and other regulatory authorities recommend $(\delta_L, \delta_U) = (80\%, 125\%)$ for assessing average bioequivalence.

Note that the test for hypotheses in Equation 5.5, formulated on the log-scale, is equivalent to testing for Hypotheses 5.1 on the raw scale. The interval Hypotheses 5.1 can be decomposed into two sets of one-sided hypotheses

$$H_{01} : \mu_T - \mu_R \le \theta_L \quad \text{versus} \quad H_{a1} : \mu_T - \mu_R > \theta_L$$

and

$$H_{02} : \mu_T - \mu_R \ge \theta_U \quad \text{versus} \quad H_{a2} : \mu_T - \mu_R < \theta_U. \tag{5.6}$$

The first set of hypotheses is to verify that the average bioavailability of the test formulation is not too low, whereas the second set of hypotheses is to verify that the average bioavailability of the test formulation is not too high. A relatively low (or high) average bioavailability may refer to the concern of efficacy (or safety) of the test formulation. If one concludes that $\theta_L < \mu_T - \mu_R$ (i.e., rejects H_{01}) and $\mu_T - \mu_R < \theta_U$ (i.e., rejects H_{02}), then it has been concluded that

$$\theta_L < \mu_T - \mu_R < \theta_U.$$

Thus, μ_T and μ_R are equivalent. The rejection of H_{01} and H_{02}, which leads to the conclusion of average bioequivalence, is equivalent to rejecting H_0 in Equation 5.1.

Under Hypotheses 5.1, Schuirmann (1987) introduced the two one-sided tests procedure for assessing average bioequivalence between drug products. The proposed two one-sided tests procedure suggests the conclusion of the equivalence of μ_T and μ_R at the α level of significance if, and only if, H_{01} and H_{02} in Equation 5.6 are rejected at a pre-determined α-level of significance. Under the normality assumptions, the two sets of one-sided hypotheses can be tested with ordinary one-sided t tests. We conclude that μ_T and μ_R are average equivalent if

$$T_L = \frac{(\bar{Y}_T - \bar{Y}_R) - \theta_L}{\hat{\sigma}_d \sqrt{(1/n_1) + (1/n_2)}} > t(\alpha, n_1 + n_2 - 2)$$

and

$$T_U = \frac{(\bar{Y}_T - \bar{Y}_R) - \theta_U}{\hat{\sigma}_d \sqrt{(1/n_1) + (1/n_2)}} < -t(\alpha, n_1 + n_2 - 2). \tag{5.7}$$

The two one-sided t tests procedure is operationally equivalent to the classic (shortest) confidence interval approach; that is, both the classic confidence interval approach and Schuirmann's two one-sided tests procedure will lead to the same conclusion on bioequivalence.

Note that under a parallel-group design, Schuirmann's two one-sided tests procedure can be similarly derived with a slight modification from a paired-t test statistic to a two-sample t test statistic.

5.3 Bayesian Methods

In previous sections, statistical methods for the assessment of biosimilarity were derived based on the sampling distribution of the estimate of the parameter of interest, such as the direct drug effect (i.e., $\theta = \mu_T - \mu_R$), which is assumed to be fixed, but unknown. Although statistical inference (e.g., confidence interval and interval hypothesis testing) on the unknown direct drug effect can be drawn from the sampling distribution of the estimate, there is little information on the probability of the unknown direct drug effect being within the equivalent limits (θ_L, θ_U). To have a certain assurance on the probability of the direct drug effect being within (θ_L, θ_U), a Bayesian approach is useful (Box and Tiao, 1973), which assumes that the unknown direct drug effect is a random variable and follows a prior distribution.

In practice, before a biosimilar study is conducted, investigators may have some prior knowledge of the drug product under development. As an example, for a PK biosimilar study, according to past experiments, the investigator may have some information on (1) the inter-subject and the intra-subject variabilities, and (2) the ranges of AUC or C_{max} for the test and reference products.

This information can be used to choose an appropriate prior distribution of the unknown direct drug effect. An appropriate prior distribution can reflect the investigator's belief about the drug products under study. After the study is completed, the observed data can be used to adjust the prior distribution of the direct drug effect, which is called the posterior distribution. Given the posterior distribution, a probability statement on the direct drug effect being within the biosimilarity limits can be made.

A different prior distribution can lead to a different posterior distribution that has an influence on statistical inference on the direct drug effect. Thus, an important issue in a Bayesian approach is how to choose a prior distribution. Box and Tiao (1973) introduced the use of a locally uniform distribution over a possible range of AUC or C_{max} as a non-informative prior distribution. A non-informative prior distribution assumes that there is an equally likely chance for any two points within the possible range being the true state of the location of the direct drug effect. In this case, the resultant posterior distribution can be used to provide the true state of the location of a direct drug effect. In practice, however, it is also desirable to provide an interval showing a range in which most of the distribution of a direct drug effect will fall. We shall refer to such an interval as a highest posterior density (HPD) interval. The HPD interval is also known as a credible interval (Edwards et al., 1963) and a Bayesian confidence interval (Lindley, 1965). An HPD interval possesses the following properties (Box and Tiao, 1973): (1) the density for every point inside the interval is higher than that for every point outside the interval, and (2) for a given probability distribution, the interval is the shortest. It can be verified that the above two properties imply each other.

In what follows, for the sake of illustration, the Bayesian method proposed by Rodda and Davis (1980) is discussed under the following model, which assumes that there are no carryover effects because a washout period of sufficient length can be chosen to completely eliminate the residual effects form one dosing period to the next:

$$Y_{ijk} = \mu + S_{ik} + F_{(j,k)} + P_j + e_{ijk}, \tag{5.8}$$

where Y_{ijk}, μ, S_{ik}, $F_{(j,k)}$, P_j, and e_{ijk} were defined in Equation 5.2. Given the results of a bioequivalence/biosimilar study, Rodda and Davis (1980) proposed a Bayesian evaluation to estimate the probability of a clinically important difference (i.e., the probability that the true direct drug effect will fall within the bioequivalent limits is estimated). Under the assumption of normality and equal carryover effects, $\bar{d}_{.1}$, $\bar{d}_{.2}$, and $(n_1 + n_2 - 2)\sigma_d^2$ are independently distributed as $N(\theta_1, \sigma_d^2/n_1)$, $N(\theta_2, \sigma_d^2/n_2)$, and $\sigma_d^2 \chi^2(n_1 + n_2 - 2)$,

where

$$\bar{d}_{.k} = \frac{1}{n_k} \sum_{i=1}^{n_k} d_{ik}, \quad k = 1, 2.$$

$$\theta_1 = \frac{1}{2}[(P_2 - P_1) + (F_T - F_R)],$$

$$\theta_2 = \frac{1}{2}[(P_2 - P_1) + (F_R - F_T)].$$

Note that $F = \theta_1 - \theta_2 = (\mu + F_T) - (\mu + F_R)$

$$= \mu_T - \mu_R$$

Assuming that the non-informative prior distributions for θ_1, θ_2, and log (σ_d) are approximately independent and locally uniformly distributed, then the joint posterior distributions of θ_1, θ_2, and σ_d^2, given the data $Y = \{Y_{ijk}, i = 1, 2, ..., n_k;$ $j, k = 1, 2\}$, are

$$p(\theta_1, \theta_2, \sigma_d^2 \mid Y) = p(\theta_1 \mid \sigma_d^2, \bar{d}_{.1}) p(\theta_2 \mid \sigma_d^2, \bar{d}_{.2}) p(\sigma_d^2 \mid \hat{\sigma}_d^2), \qquad (5.9)$$

$$p(\theta_i \mid \sigma_d^2, \bar{d}_{.i}) = N(\bar{d}_{.i}, \hat{\sigma}_d^2 / n_i), \quad i = 1, 2.$$

$$p(\sigma_d^2 \mid \hat{\sigma}_d^2) = (n_1 + n_2) \hat{\sigma}_d^2 \chi^{-2}(n_1 + n_2 - 2),$$

where χ^{-2} $(n_1 + n_2 - 2)$ is the distribution of the inverse of χ^2 $(n_1 + n_2 - 2)$. Therefore, the joint distribution of $\mu_T - \mu_R$ $(=F)$ and σ_d^2 is given by

$$p(\mu_T - \mu_R, \sigma_d^2 \mid Y) = p(\mu_T - \mu_R \mid \sigma_d^2, \bar{d}_{.1} - \bar{d}_{.2}) p(\sigma_d^2 \mid \hat{\sigma}_d^2), \qquad (5.10)$$

where

$$p(\mu_T - \mu_R \mid \sigma_d^2, \bar{d}_{.1} - \bar{d}_{.2}) = N\left[\bar{d}_{.1} - \bar{d}_{.2}, \hat{\sigma}_d^2 \left(\frac{1}{n_1} + \frac{1}{n_2}\right)\right]$$

$$= N\left[\bar{Y}_T - \bar{Y}_R, \hat{\sigma}_d^2 \left(\frac{1}{n_1} + \frac{1}{n_2}\right)\right].$$

The marginal posterior distribution of F, given the data Y, is

$$p(\mu_T - \mu_R \mid Y) = \frac{(\hat{\sigma}_d^2 m)^{-1/2}}{B(1/2, v/2)\sqrt{n}} \left\{1 + \frac{[(\mu_T - \mu_R) - (\bar{Y}_T - \bar{Y}_R)]^2}{v \hat{\sigma}_d^2 m}\right\}^{-(v+1)/2}, \qquad (5.11)$$

where $m = 1/n_1 + 1/n_2$, $v = n_1 + n_2 - 2$ and $-\infty < \mu_T - \mu_R < \infty$.
Thus, we have

$$T_{RD} = \frac{(\mu_T - \mu_R) - (\bar{Y}_T - \bar{Y}_R)}{\hat{\sigma}_d \sqrt{(1/n_1) + (1/n_2)}}, \qquad (5.12)$$

which has a central Student t distribution with $n_1 + n_2 - 2$ degrees of freedom. From Equation 5.12, the probability of F being within the biosimilarity limits of (θ_L, θ_U) can be estimated by

$$P_{RD} = P\{\theta_L < \mu_T - \mu_R < \theta_U\}$$

$$= F_t(t_U) - F_t(t_L),\tag{5.13}$$

where F_t is the cumulative distribution function of a central t variable with $n_1 + n_2 - 2$ degrees of freedom, and

$$t_U = \frac{\theta_U - (\bar{Y}_T - \bar{Y}_R)}{\hat{\sigma}_d\sqrt{(1/n_1) + (1/n_2)}} \quad \text{and} \quad t_L = \frac{\theta_L - (\bar{Y}_T - \bar{Y}_R)}{\hat{\sigma}_d\sqrt{(1/n_1) + (1/n_2)}}.\tag{5.14}$$

The lower and upper limits of the $(1 - 2\alpha) \times 100\%$ HPD interval are given by

$$L_{RD} = (\bar{Y}_T - \bar{Y}_R) - t(\alpha, n_1 + n_2 - 2)\hat{\sigma}_d\sqrt{\frac{1}{n_1} + \frac{1}{n_2}},$$

$$\tag{5.15}$$

$$U_{RD} = (\bar{Y}_T - \bar{Y}_R) + t(\alpha, n_1 + n_2 - 2)\hat{\sigma}_d\sqrt{\frac{1}{n_1} + \frac{1}{n_2}}.$$

Hence, it is verified that the $(1 - 2\alpha) \times 100\%$ HPD interval in Equation 5.15 is numerically equivalent to the $(1 - 2\alpha) \times 100\%$ classic confidence interval obtained from the sampling theory. However, the interpretation of these two intervals is totally different. For example, a 90% classic confidence interval for F indicates that, in the long run, if the study is repeatedly carried out numerous times, 90% of the times the interval will contain the unknown direct drug effect $\mu_T - \mu_R$. On the other hand, based on the posterior distribution of $\mu_T - \mu_R$, the chance of $\mu_T - \mu_R$ being within the lower and upper limits of a 90% HPD interval is 90%.

5.4 Wilcoxon–Mann–Whitney Two One-Sided Tests Procedure

As described in the previous sections, statistical methods for assessing average biosimilarity between drug products were derived under the assumption that $\{S_{ik}\}$ and $\{e_{ijk}\}$ are mutually independent and normally distributed with mean 0 and variance σ_s^2 and σ_e^2. Under these normality assumptions, confidence intervals and tests for interval hypotheses were obtained based on either a two-sample t statistic or an F statistic. In practice, however, one of the difficulties commonly encountered in comparing drug products is whether the assumption of normality (for raw or untransformed data) or log-normality (for log-transformed data) is valid. If the normality (or log-normality) is seriously violated, the approach based on a two-sample t statistic or an F statistic is no longer justified. In this situation, a distribution-free (or non-parametric) method is useful. In this section, a non-parametric version of the two one-sided tests procedure for testing interval hypotheses, namely, the Wilcoxon–Mann–Whitney two one-sided tests procedure, is discussed. The Hodges–Lehmann estimator associated with the Wilcoxon rank sum test will be used to construct a $(1-2\alpha) \times 100\%$ confidence interval for $\mu_T - \mu_R$, the difference in average biosimilarity.

The standard 2×2 crossover design consists of a pair of dual sequences (i.e., RT and TR). A distribution-free rank sum test can then be applied directly to the two one-sided tests procedure (Cornell, 1990; Hauschke et al., 1990). We shall refer to this approach as the Wilcoxon–Mann–Whitney two one-sided tests procedure. Let $\theta = \mu_T - \mu_R$. The two sets of hypotheses in Equation 5.6 can then be rewritten as

$$H_{01} : \theta_L^* \leq 0 \quad \text{vs.} \quad H_{a1} : \theta_L^* > 0$$

and

$$H_{02} : \theta_U^* \geq 0 \quad \text{vs.} \quad H_{a2} : \theta_U^* < 0,$$

where
$$\theta_L^* = \theta - \theta_L$$
$$\theta_U^* = \theta - \theta_U$$

Thus, the estimates of θ_L^* and θ_U^* can be obtained as a linear function of period differences d_{ik}, $i = 1, 2, \ldots, n_k$, $k = 1, 2$. Let

$$b_{hik} = \begin{cases} d_{ik} - \theta_h & h = L, U, \text{ for subjects in sequence 1} \\ d_{ik} & \text{for subjects in sequence 2.} \end{cases} \qquad (5.16)$$

When there are no carryover effects, the expected value and variance of b_{hik}, where $h = L, U, i = 1, 2, \ldots, n_k$, and $k = 1, 2$, are given by

$$E(b_{hik}) = \begin{cases} \dfrac{1}{2}[(P_2 - P_1) + (\theta - 2\theta_h)] & \text{for } k = 1 \\ \dfrac{1}{2}[(P_2 - P_1) - \theta] & \text{for } k = 2, \end{cases} \qquad (5.17)$$

and

$$V(b_{hik}) = V(d_{ik}) = \sigma_d^2 = \frac{\sigma_e^2}{2}.$$

It can be seen that $E(b_{hi1}) - E(b_{hi2}) = (\theta - \theta_h) = \theta_h^*$.

Thus, for a fixed h, $\{b_{hi1}\}$ and $\{b_{hi2}\}$ have the same distribution except for the difference $(= \theta_h^*)$ in location of the true formulation effect. Here, the Wilcoxon–Mann–Whitney rank sum test (Wilcoxon, 1945; Mann and Whitney, 1947) for the unpaired two-sample location problem can be directly applied to test each of the two sets of hypotheses given earlier. Consider the first set of hypotheses that

$$H_{01} : \theta_L^* \le 0 \quad \text{versus} \quad H_{a1} : \theta_L^* > 0.$$

The Wilcoxon–Mann–Whitney test statistic can be derived based on $\{b_{Li1}\}$, $i = 1, 2, \ldots, n_1$ and $\{b_{Li2}\}$, $i = 1, 2, \ldots, n_2$. Let $R(b_{Lik})$ be the rank of b_{Lik} in the combined sample $\{b_{Lik}\}$, $i = 1, 2, \ldots, n_k$, $k = 1, 2$. Also, let R_L be the sum of the ranks of the responses for subjects in sequence 1; that is,

$$R_L = \sum_{i=1}^{n_1} R(b_{Li1}).$$

Thus, the Wilcoxon–Mann–Whitney test statistic for H_{01} is given by

$$W_L = R_L - \frac{n_1(n_1 + 1)}{2}.$$

We then reject H_{01} if

$$W_L > w(1 - \alpha), \tag{5.18}$$

where $w(1 - \alpha)$ is the $(1 - \alpha)$th quantile of the distribution of W_L. Similarly, for the second set of hypotheses that

$$H_{02} : \theta_U^* \ge 0 \quad \text{versus} \quad H_{a2} : \theta_U^* < 0,$$

we reject H_{02} if

$$W_U = R_U - \frac{n_1(n_1 + 1)}{2} < w(\alpha), \tag{5.19}$$

where R_u is the sum of the ranks of $\{b_{Uik}\}$ for subjects in the first sequence. Hence, average bioequivalence is concluded if both H_{01} and H_{02} are rejected; that is,

$$W_L > w(1-\alpha) \quad \text{and} \quad W_U < w(\alpha). \tag{5.20}$$

The expected values and variances for W_L and W_U under the null hypotheses H_{01} and H_{02}, when there are no ties, are given by

$$E(W_L) = E(W_U) = \frac{n_1 n_2}{2},$$

$$V(W_L) = V(W_U) = \frac{1}{12} n_1 n_2 (n_1 + n_2 + 1). \tag{5.21}$$

When there are ties among observations, average ranks can be assigned to compute W_L and W_U. In this case, however, the expected values and variances of W_L and W_U become

$$E(W_L) = E(W_U) = \frac{n_1 n_2}{2},$$

$$V(W_L) = V(W_U) = \frac{1}{12} n_1 n_2 (n_1 + n_2 + 1 - Q), \tag{5.22}$$

where

$$Q = \frac{1}{(n_1 + n_2)(n_1 + n_2 - 1)} \sum_{v=1}^{q} (r_v^3 - r_v),$$

where
  q is the number of tied groups
  r_v is the size of the tied group v

Note that if there are no tied observations, $q = n_1 + n_2$, $r_v = 1$ for $v = 1, 2, \ldots, n$, and $Q = 0$, then Equation 5.22 reduces to Equation 5.21. Since W_L and W_U are symmetric about their mean $(n_1 n_2)/2$, we have

$$w(1-\alpha) = n_1 n_2 - w(\alpha). \tag{5.23}$$

When $n_1 + n_2$, the total number of subjects, is large (say, $n_1 + n_2 > 40$) and the ratio of n_1 and n_2 is close to ½; the standard normal distribution can be used for a large-sample approximation of average biosimilarity testing; that is, we may conclude bioequivalence if

$$Z_L > z(\alpha) \quad \text{and} \quad Z_U < -z(\alpha),$$

where $z(\alpha)$ is the αth quantile of a standard normal distribution, and

$$Z_L = \frac{W_L - E(W_L)}{\sqrt{V(W_L)}} = \frac{R_L - \left[n_1(n_1 + n_2 + 1)/2\right]}{\sqrt{\frac{1}{12}n_1 n_2(n_1 + n_2 + 1)}},$$

$$Z_U = \frac{W_U - E(W_U)}{\sqrt{V(W_U)}} = \frac{R_U - \left[n_1(n_1 + n_2 + 1)/2\right]}{\sqrt{\frac{1}{12}n_1 n_2(n_1 + n_2 + 1)}}.$$

(5.24)

Note that the variances in Z_L and Z_U should be replaced with those given in Equation 5.21 if there are ties.

5.5 Three-Arm Parallel Design

Let T denote a biosimilar product, and R_1 and R_2 represent innovator biological products from different batches, respectively. Suppose that the N patients are randomized into the following three groups. The patients who are assigned to the first group receive the biosimilar product T and the number of patients is denoted by n_1. The patients who are assigned to the second and the third groups receive the innovator biological products R_1 and R_2, respectively, and the number of patients in both groups is denoted by n_2 for simplicity. The randomization ratio $2:1:1$ is employed. So $n_1 = 2n_2$ and the total sample size is $N = n_1 + 2n_2$. Suppose that we have only one primary continuous response variable Y. If this trial is a pharmacokinetic study, Y can be either AUC or C_{max}. If the trial is a pivotal trial, Y can be a clinical response.

5.5.1 Criteria for Biosimilarity

Let $d(T, R)$ represent the distance between the biosimilar product T and the innovator biological product R. Similarly, $d(R_1, R_2)$ denotes the distance between R_1 and R_2. There are many possible choices for specific forms of distance. For example,

$$d_1(T, R) = \left| \mu_T - \mu_R \right|$$

$$d_2(T, R) = \left| \frac{\mu_T}{\mu_R} \right|$$

$$d_3(T, R) = (\mu_T - \mu_R)^2$$

$$d_4(T,R) = E(\mu_T - \mu_R)^2$$

where

μ_T is the population mean of Y in patients with the biosimilar product T
μ_R is defined as $(\mu_{R_1} + \mu_{R_2})/2$ where μ_{R_1} and μ_{R_2} denote the population means of Y in patients who receive the reference product R_1 and R_2, respectively

In this chapter, we consider the following relative distance to assess biosimilarity between the biosimilar product and the innovator biological product

$$rd = \frac{d(T,R)}{d(R_1,R_2)}.$$

Since the distances take on only non-negative values, the relative distances are also non-negative numbers. If the relative distance rd is less than a pre-specified margin δ ($\delta > 0$) in the proposed design, we claim that the two products are biosimilar. Therefore, the hypotheses of interest are given by

$$H_0 : rd \geq \delta \quad \text{versus} \quad H_a : rd < \delta.$$

Kang and Chow (2013) consider the absolute mean difference $d_1(T,R) = |\mu_T - \mu_R|$ to evaluate biosimilarity between the two products. Then, assuming that $\mu_{R_1} \neq \mu_{R_2}$, the relative distance is given by

$$rd = \left| \frac{d(T,R)}{d(R_1,R_2)} \right| = \left| \frac{\mu_T - (\mu_{R_1} + \mu_{R_2})/2}{\mu_{R_1} - \mu_{R_2}} \right|.$$

Then the hypotheses in Equation 5.1 can be rewritten as

$$H_0 : \theta \leq -\delta \quad \text{or} \quad \theta \geq \delta \quad \text{versus} \quad H_a : -\delta < \theta < \delta, \tag{5.25}$$

where

$$\theta = \frac{\mu_T - (\mu_{R_1} + \mu_{R_2})/2}{\mu_{R_1} - \mu_{R_2}}. \tag{5.26}$$

It is well-known that the hypotheses in Equation 5.25 can be decomposed into two one-sided hypotheses as follows:

$$H_{01} : \theta \leq -\delta \quad \text{versus} \quad H_{a1} : -\delta < \theta, \tag{5.27}$$

and

$$H_{02} : \theta \geq \delta \quad \text{versus} \quad H_{a2} : \theta < \delta. \tag{5.28}$$

5.5.2 Statistical Tests for Biosimilarity

Let $Y_{T,i}$ $(i = 1, 2,..., n_1)$ and $Y_{R_k,i}$ $(k = 1, 2, i = 1, 2,..., n_2)$ denote the response variables from the biosimilar product in the first group and the innovator biological product in the second and the third groups, respectively, with $n_1 = 2n_2$. First, it is assumed that $Y_{T,i}$ and $Y_{R_k,i}$ $(k = 1, 2)$ follow independently the normal distribution with the means μ_T and μ_{R_k} $(k = 1, 2)$ and the common variance σ^2. When we need to derive an asymptotic distribution of a test statistic and the power functions, we assume that the sample size is large enough so that the central limit theorem can be employed. In the following two subsections, we propose two statistical tests in order to test the hypotheses in Equations 5.27 and 5.28.

5.5.2.1 Statistical Test Based on the Ratio Estimator

A natural estimator of θ in Equation 5.26 is to replace the population means with the corresponding sample means. It is given by

$$\hat{\theta} = \frac{\bar{V}}{\bar{U}} \equiv \frac{\bar{Y} - (\bar{Y}_{R_1} + \bar{Y}_{R_2})/2}{\bar{Y}_{R_1} - \bar{Y}_{R_2}},$$

where

$$\bar{Y}_T = \frac{1}{n_1} \sum_{i=1}^{n_1} Y_{T,i},$$

$$\bar{Y}_{R_k} = \frac{1}{n_2} \sum_{i=1}^{n_2} Y_{R_k,i} \quad \text{for } k = 1, 2.$$

Since the exact distribution of $\hat{\theta}$ is very complicated, Kang and Chow (2013) obtained the asymptotic normality of $\sqrt{n_1}(\hat{\theta} - \theta)$ as follows. First, note that

$$\frac{\bar{V}}{\bar{U}} - \frac{v}{\mu} = \frac{\bar{V}_\mu - \bar{U}_v}{\bar{U}_\mu} = \frac{\mu(\bar{V} - v) - v(\bar{U} - \mu)}{\bar{U}_\mu} = \frac{(\bar{V} - v)}{\bar{U}} - \frac{v}{\mu} \frac{(\bar{U} - \mu)}{\bar{U}},$$

where

$$\mu = \mu_{R_1} - \mu_{R_2} \quad \text{and} \quad v = \mu_T - \frac{\mu_{R_1} + \mu_{R_2}}{2}.$$

Therefore, we have

$$\sqrt{n_1}(\hat{\theta}-\theta) = \sqrt{n_1}\left(\frac{\bar{V}}{\bar{U}}-\frac{v}{\mu}\right)$$

$$= \sqrt{n_1}\frac{(\bar{V}-v)}{\bar{U}} - \frac{\sqrt{n_1}}{\sqrt{n_2}}\frac{v}{\mu}\sqrt{n_2}\frac{(\bar{U}-\mu)}{\bar{U}}.$$

Since $\bar{U} \xrightarrow{p} \mu$, we have

$$\sqrt{n_1}(\hat{\theta}-\theta) \sim \sqrt{n_1}\frac{(\bar{V}-v)}{\mu} - \sqrt{2}\frac{v}{\mu^2}\sqrt{n_2}(\bar{U}-\mu)$$

$$\xrightarrow{d} N\left(0, \frac{2\sigma^2}{\mu^2} + \frac{4v^2}{\mu^4}\sigma^2\right).$$

By using this asymptotic normality of $\sqrt{n_1}(\hat{\theta}-\theta)$, we can conduct hypothesis testing and establish an asymptotic confidence interval for θ. The null hypothesis H_{01} in Equation 5.27 is rejected if $Z_1 > z_\alpha$ where

$$Z_1 = \frac{\hat{\theta}+\delta}{(s/\sqrt{n_1})\sqrt{(2/(\bar{U})^2)+4((\bar{V})^2/(\bar{U})^4)}} = \frac{(\bar{V}/\bar{U})+\delta}{(s/\sqrt{n_1})\sqrt{(2/(\bar{U})^2)+4((\bar{V})^2/(\bar{U})^4)}},$$

and z_α is the upper α quantile of the standard normal distribution and

$$s^2 = \frac{1}{n_1+2n_2-3}\left[\sum_{i=1}^{n_1}(Y_{T,i}-\bar{Y}_T)^2 + \sum_{i=1}^{n_2}(Y_{R_1,i}-\bar{Y}_{R_1})^2 + \sum_{i=1}^{n_2}(Y_{R_2,i}-\bar{Y}_{R_2})^2\right].$$

$$(5.29)$$

Similarly, the null hypothesis H_{02} in Equation 5.28 is rejected if $Z_2 < -z_\alpha$, where

$$Z_1 = \frac{(\bar{V}/\bar{U})-\delta}{(s/\sqrt{n_1})\sqrt{(2/(\bar{U})^2)+4((\bar{V})^2/(\bar{U})^4)}}$$

If each null hypothesis in both Equations 5.27 and 5.28 is rejected at the significance level α, we claim that the two products are biosimilar.

An alternative method to assess biosimilarity between the two products is to use a two-sided asymptotic confidence interval for θ. Since an $(1-\alpha) \times 100\%$ asymptotic confidence interval for θ is given by

$$\left(\frac{\bar{V}}{\bar{U}} \pm z_{\alpha/2} \frac{s}{\sqrt{n_1}} \sqrt{\frac{2}{(\bar{U})^2} + 4\frac{(\bar{V})^2}{(\bar{U})^4}} \right), \tag{5.30}$$

we claim that the two products are biosimilar if the $(1-\alpha) \times 100\%$ asymptotic confidence interval for θ lies within the interval $(-\delta, \delta)$.

Although we have obtained the $(1-\alpha) \times 100\%$ asymptotic confidence interval for θ, actually we can obtain an exact $(1-\alpha) \times 100\%$ confidence interval for θ based on Fieller's theorem (Fieller, 1954, 1944), because we assume that $Y_{T,i}$ and $Y_{R_k,i}\,(k=1,2)$ follow the normal distribution. From the Fieller's theorem, since

$$\text{Var}(\bar{V}) = \left[\frac{1}{n_1} + \frac{1}{2n_2} \right] \sigma^2 \quad \text{Var}(\bar{U}) = \frac{1}{n_2}\sigma^2 \quad \text{Cov}(\bar{V},\bar{U}) = 0,$$

an exact $(1-\alpha) \times 100\%$ confidence interval for θ is given by

$$\frac{1}{1-g}\left\{ \frac{\bar{V}}{\bar{U}} \pm \frac{t_{\alpha,m}s}{\bar{U}}\left[\frac{1}{n_1} + \frac{1}{2n_2} + \left(\frac{\bar{V}}{\bar{U}}\right)^2 \frac{2}{n_2} - g\left(\frac{1}{n_1} + \frac{1}{2n_2}\right) \right]^{1/2} \right\}, \tag{5.31}$$

where

$$g = \frac{t_{1-\alpha,m}^2 s^2}{(\bar{U})^2}\left(\frac{2}{n_2}\right), \quad m = n_1 + 2n_2 - 3,$$

and $t_{\alpha,m}$ is the upper α quantile of the t distribution with m degrees of freedom.

5.5.2.2 Linearization Method

When we conduct a hypothesis testing for a parameter which is the ratio of parameters, a popular method of constructing a hypothesis testing is the linearization method (Howe, 1974; Hyslop et al., 2000). Both sides of the inequality in the hypothesis are multiplied by the parameter in the denominator of the ratio, and then the numerator of the ratio is moved to the opposite side of the inequality, so that the linearized parameter can be obtained.

The parameter of interest in this chapter is θ in Equation 5.8 and the denominator is $\mu_{R_1} - \mu_{R_2}$. First, we need to check the sign of the denominator, because the direction of inequalities in the hypotheses changes depending on the sign of the denominator. It is assumed that $\mu_{R_1} \neq \mu_{R_2}$. Otherwise, θ cannot be defined. In order to check the sign of the denominator $\mu_{R_1} - \mu_{R_2}$, we test the following preliminary hypotheses:

$$H_0 : \mu_{R_1} < \mu_{R_2} \quad \text{versus} \quad H_a : \mu_{R_1} > \mu_{R_2}. \tag{5.32}$$

The null hypothesis in Equation 5.32 is rejected if

$$T_R = \frac{\bar{Y}_{R_1} - \bar{Y}_{R_2}}{s_R \sqrt{2/n_2}} > t_{\alpha, 2n_2 - 2},$$

where

$$s_R^2 = \frac{1}{2n_2 - 2} \left[\sum_{i=1}^{n_2} (Y_{R_1,i} - \bar{Y}_{R_1})^2 + \sum_{i=1}^{n_2} (Y_{R_2,i} - \bar{Y}_{R_2})^2 \right].$$

When the null hypothesis in Equation 5.32 is rejected, the null hypothesis $H_{01} : \theta \leq -\delta$ in Equation 5.9 can be expressed as

$$H_{01} : \mu_T - \frac{1}{2}(\mu_{R_1} + \mu_{R_2}) + \delta(\mu_{R_1} - \mu_{R_2}) \leq 0.$$

Similarly, the null hypothesis $H_{02} : \theta \geq \delta$ in Equation 5.28 can be rewritten as

$$H_{02} : \mu_T - \frac{1}{2}(\mu_{R_1} + \mu_{R_2}) - \delta(\mu_{R_1} - \mu_{R_2}) \geq 0.$$

Therefore, the two products are claimed to be biosimilar if

$$T_1^L > t_{\alpha, n_1 + 2n_2 - 3} \quad \text{and} \quad T_2^L < -t_{\alpha, n_1 + 2n_2 - 3},$$

where

$$T_1^L \equiv \frac{\bar{Y}_T - ((1/2) - \delta)\bar{Y}_{R_1} - ((1/2) + \delta)\bar{Y}_{R_2}}{s\sqrt{(1/n_1) + ((1/2) - \delta)^2 (1/n_2) + ((1/2) + \delta)^2 (1/n_2)}},$$

$$T_2^L \equiv \frac{\bar{Y}_T - ((1/2) + \delta)\bar{Y}_{R_1} - ((1/2) - \delta)\bar{Y}_{R_2}}{s\sqrt{(1/n_1) + ((1/2) + \delta)^2 (1/n_2) + ((1/2) - \delta)^2 (1/n_2)}}.$$

In a similar fashion, when the null hypothesis is accepted, the null hypothesis $H_{01} : \theta \leq -\delta$ in Equation 5.27 can be expressed as

$$H_{01} : \mu_T - \frac{1}{2}(\mu_{R_1} + \mu_{R_2}) + \delta(\mu_{R_1} - \mu_{R_2}) \geq 0,$$

and the null hypothesis $H_{02} : \theta \geq \delta$ in Equation 5.28 can be rewritten as

$$H_{02} : \mu_T - \frac{1}{2}(\mu_{R_1} + \mu_{R_2}) - \delta(\mu_{R_1} - \mu_{R_2}) \leq 0.$$

Hence, biosimilarity between the two products is claimed if

$$T_1^L < -t_{\alpha, n_1 + 2n_2 - 3} \quad \text{and} \quad T_2^L > t_{\alpha, n_1 + 2n_2 - 3}.$$

5.5.2.3 Power Functions

In the previous section, we described two statistical tests proposed by Kang and Chow (2013) to test the hypotheses in Equation 5.25. In this section, following Kang and Chow (2013), the power functions of two statistical tests (in large samples) will be given. First, under the alternative hypothesis that $H_a : -\delta < \theta < \delta$, the power function of the statistical test based on the ratio estimator in large samples is given by

$$\text{Power} = P\left(Z_2 < -z_\alpha \quad \text{and} \quad Z_1 > z_\alpha \mid -\delta < \theta < \delta\right)$$

$$\sim P\left(\frac{(\bar{V}/\bar{U}) - \delta}{\sigma/\sqrt{n_1}\sqrt{(2/\mu^2) + 4(v^2/\mu^4)}} < -z_\alpha\right.$$

$$\text{and} \quad \frac{(\bar{V}/\bar{U}) + \delta}{\sigma/\sqrt{n_1}\sqrt{(2/\mu^2) + 4(v^2/\mu^4)}} > z_\alpha \left.\mid -\delta < \theta < \delta\right)$$

$$= P\left(Z < -z_\alpha + \frac{\delta - \theta}{\sigma/\sqrt{n_1}\sqrt{(2/\mu^2) + 4(v^2/\mu^4)}}\right.$$

$$\text{and} \quad Z > z_\alpha - \frac{\delta + \theta}{\sigma/\sqrt{n_1}\sqrt{(2/\mu^2) + 4(v^2/\mu^4)}}\right)$$

$$= \Phi\left(-z_\alpha + \frac{\delta - \theta}{\sigma/\sqrt{n_1}\sqrt{(2/\mu^2) + 4(v^2/\mu^4)}}\right) \qquad (5.33)$$

$$- \Phi\left(z_\alpha - \frac{\delta + \theta}{\sigma/\sqrt{n_1}\sqrt{(2/\mu^2) + 4(v^2/\mu^4)}}\right),$$

where

$$\theta = \frac{\mu_T - (\mu_{R_1} + \mu_{R_2})/2}{\mu_{R_1} - \mu_{R_2}}, \quad \mu = \mu_{R_1} - \mu_{R_2}, \quad v = \mu_T - \frac{\mu_{R_1} + \mu_{R_2}}{2}$$

and the random variable Z follows the standard normal distribution, and Φ represents the cumulative distribution function of the standard normal distribution. Since the following condition should be satisfied in order to have positive powers

$$-z_\alpha + \frac{\delta - \theta}{\sigma/\sqrt{n_1}\sqrt{(2/\mu^2) + 4(v^2/\mu^4)}} > z_\alpha - \frac{\delta + \theta}{\sigma/\sqrt{n_1}\sqrt{(2/\mu^2) + 4(v^2/\mu^4)}},$$

the margin δ should satisfy the following inequality:

$$\delta > z_\alpha \frac{\sigma}{\sqrt{n_1}} \sqrt{\frac{2}{\mu^2} + 4\frac{v^2}{\mu^4}}.$$

In order to investigate the power function of the linearization method, we need to note that, as the sample size increases, the random vector (T_1^L, T_2^L) converges to the random vector (Z_1^L, Z_2^L) which follows a bivariate normal distribution $N_2(\mu_{2\times1}, \Sigma_{2\times2})$ where the mean vector $\mu_{2\times1}$ is $(0,0)^t$ under H_{01} and H_{02} and

$$\mu_{2\times1} = (\mu_1, \mu_2)^t$$

$$= \left(\frac{\mu_T - ((1/2) - \delta)\mu_{R_1} - ((1/2) + \delta)\mu_{R_2}}{\sigma\sqrt{(1/n_1) + ((1/2) - \delta)^2 (1/n_2) + ((1/2) + \delta)^2 (1/n_2)}}, \right.$$

$$\left. \frac{\mu_T - ((1/2) + \delta)\mu_{R_1} - ((1/2) - \delta)\mu_{R_2}}{\sigma\sqrt{(1/n_1) + ((1/2) - \delta)^2 (1/n_2) + ((1/2) + \delta)^2 (1/n_2)}} \right)^t.$$

Under H_{a1} and H_{a2} and the variance-covariance matrix is

$$\Sigma_{2\times2} = \begin{pmatrix} 1 & \rho \\ \rho & 1 \end{pmatrix}$$

and

$$\rho = \frac{1 - 2\delta^2}{1 + 2\delta^2}. \tag{5.34}$$

Therefore, the power function of the linearization method in large sample is given by

$$\text{Power} = Pr(\mu_T, \mu_{R_1}, \mu_{R_2})$$

$$= P(\text{reject } H_0 \text{ in Equation 5.32}) + P(\text{accept } H_0 \text{ in Equation 5.32})$$

$$= P\left(T_1^L > t_{\alpha, n_1 + 2n_2 - 3} \quad \text{and} \quad T_2^L < -t_{\alpha, n_1 + 2n_2 - 3}\right)$$

$$+ P\left(T_1^L < -t_{\alpha, n_1 + 2n_2 - 3} \quad \text{and} \quad T_2^L > t_{\alpha, n_1 + 2n_2 - 3}\right)$$

$$\sim [1 - \Phi(w_1)]\left(P\left(Z_1^L < \infty, Z_2^L < -z_\alpha\right) - P\left(Z_1^L < z_\alpha, Z_2^L < -z_\alpha\right)\right) \qquad (5.35)$$

$$+ \Phi(w_1)\left(P\left(Z_1^L < -z_\alpha, Z_2^L < \infty\right) - P\left(Z_1^L < -z_\alpha, Z_2^L < z_\alpha\right)\right)$$

$$= [1 - \Phi(w_1)](\Phi_2(\infty, -z_\alpha - \mu_2, \rho) - \Phi_2(z_\alpha - \mu_1, -z_\alpha - \mu_2, \rho))$$

$$+ \Phi(w_1)(\Phi_2(-z_\alpha - \mu_1, \infty, \rho) - \Phi_2(-z_\alpha - \mu_1, z_\alpha - \mu_2, \rho)),$$

where Φ_2 is the cumulative distribution function of a standardized bivariate normal distribution with mean 0, variance 1, and a correlation coefficient ρ in Equation 5.34 and

$$w_1 = z_\alpha - \frac{\mu_{R_1} - \mu_{R_2}}{\sigma\sqrt{2/n_2}}.$$

5.5.2.4 Numerical Results

Kang and Chow (2013) compare the power of the statistical test based on the ratio estimator and the linearization method whose formulae are given in Equations 5.33 and 5.35, respectively. It seems that it may not be feasible to compare the two formulae in Equations 5.33 and 5.35 analytically. Therefore, numerical comparisons are conducted. Figures 5.1 through 5.3 show the powers of the two methods which are computed with the formulae in Equations 5.33 and 5.35. The power of the statistical test based on the ratio estimator is always higher than that of the linearization method over the investigated ranges of the parameters. Tables 5.1 and 5.2 present sample size calculations computed numerically with Formula 5.33.

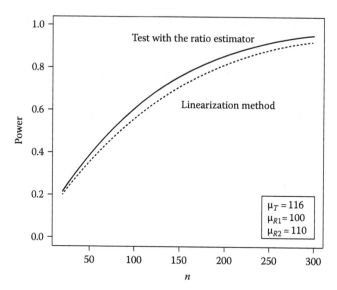

FIGURE 5.1
The power of two statistical tests ($\delta = 1.2$, $\sigma = 2$).

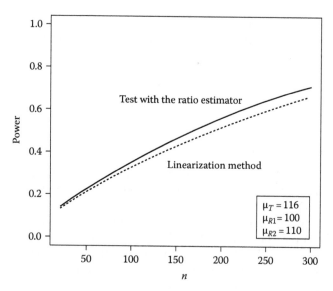

FIGURE 5.2
The power of two statistical tests ($\delta = 1.2$, $\sigma = 3$).

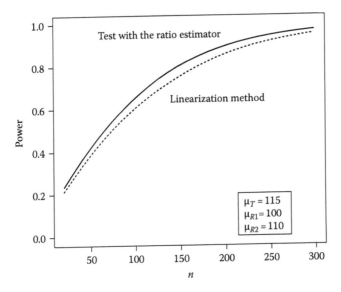

FIGURE 5.3
The power of two statistical tests ($\delta = 1.1$, $\sigma = 2$).

TABLE 5.1

Sample Size Calculations of the Statistical Test Based on the
Ratio Estimator with $\mu = 8$ and $\mu = 10$

μ	ν	Σ	n_1 (80%)	n_1 (90%)	μ	ν	σ	n_1 (80%)	n_1 (90%)
10	11.5	2	722	999	8	9.0	2	486	673
10	11.0	2	170	235	8	8.5	2	134	185
10	10.5	2	71	98	8	8.0	2	58	81
10	10.0	2	38	52	8	7.5	2	31	43
10	9.5	2	23	31	8	7.0	2	19	26
10	9.0	2	15	20	8	6.5	2	12	17
10	10.5	3	159	220	8	8.5	3	300	416
10	10.0	3	84	116	8	8.0	3	131	181
10	9.5	3	50	70	8	7.5	3	70	97
10	9.0	3	33	45	8	7.0	3	42	58
10	8.5	3	23	31	8	6.5	3	27	38
10	8.0	3	16	22	8	6.0	3	19	26
10	10.0	4	149	206	8	8.0	4	232	322
10	9.5	4	89	124	8	7.5	4	124	172
10	9.0	4	58	80	8	7.0	4	75	103
10	8.5	4	40	55	8	6.5	4	48	67
10	8.0	4	29	40	8	6.0	4	33	45
10	7.5	4	21	29	8	5.5	4	23	32

TABLE 5.2

Sample Size Calculations of the Statistical Test Based
on the Ratio Estimator with $\mu = 4$ and $\mu = 6$

μ	ν	σ	n_1 (80%)	n_1 (90%)	μ	ν	σ	n_1 (80%)	n_1 (90%)
6	6.5	2	338	469	4	4.2	2	441	610
6	6.3	2	196	272	4	4.0	2	232	322
6	6.0	2	104	143	4	3.8	2	139	193
6	5.5	2	46	64	4	3.5	2	75	103
6	5.0	2	25	34	4	3.0	2	33	45
6	4.5	2	15	20	4	2.5	2	17	24
6	6.3	3	441	610	4	4.0	3	522	723
6	6.0	3	232	322	4	3.8	3	313	433
6	5.5	3	104	143	4	3.5	3	167	231
6	5.0	3	55	77	4	3.0	3	73	102
6	4.5	3	33	45	4	2.5	3	38	52
6	4.0	3	21	29	4	2.0	3	22	30
6	6.0	4	413	571	4	3.2	4	177	245
6	5.5	4	184	255	4	3.0	4	130	180
6	5.0	4	98	136	4	2.7	4	86	119
6	4.5	4	58	80	4	2.5	4	67	93
6	4.0	4	37	51	4	2.0	4	38	53
6	3.5	4	25	34	4	1.4	4	24	33

Since the statistical test based on the ratio estimator employs large-sample theory, we need to investigate the performance in finite samples. We generate random samples of $X_{T,i}$ and $X_{Rk,i}$ ($k = 1, 2$) from normal distributions. Two test statistics, Z_1 and Z_2, are computed. If $Z_1 > z_{0.05}$ and $Z_2 < -z_{0.05}$, then the null hypothesis in Equation 5.25 is rejected. Kang and Chow (2013) generated 5000 simulation samples and the empirical type I error rate is calculated as the proportion of samples for which the null hypothesis in Equation 5.25 is rejected. The simulation results in Table 5.3 show that the statistical test based on the ratio estimator controls the empirical type I error rates under the nominal level.

5.6 Concluding Remarks

In this chapter, much discussion was given to the design and analysis methods proposed by Kang and Chow (2013) for the assessment of biosimilarity. Kang and Chow's methods were derived based on the relative distance of

TABLE 5.3

Empirical Type I Error Rates of the Statistical Test Based on the Ratio Estimator

δ	μ_T	μ_{R_1}	μ_{R_2}	σ	n_1	Type I Error	μ_T	μ_{R_1}	μ_{R_2}	σ	n_1	Type I Error
1.2	117	100	110	1	30	0.028	110.2	106	100	1	30	0.033
					50	0.031					50	0.027
					100	0.030					100	0.032
1.2	117	100	110	2	30	0.034	110.2	106	100	2	30	0.043
					50	0.033					50	0.036
					100	0.034					100	0.034
1.2	117	100	110	3	30	0.035	110.2	106	100	3	30	0.045
					50	0.038					50	0.045
					100	0.038					100	0.036
1.1	116	100	110	1	30	0.032	109.6	106	100	1	30	0.032
					50	0.029					50	0.033
					100	0.033					100	0.030
1.1	116	100	110	2	30	0.034	109.6	106	100	2	30	0.043
					50	0.033					50	0.037
					100	0.032					100	0.035
1.1	116	100	110	3	30	0.043	109.6	106	100	1	30	0.050
					50	0.035					50	0.049
					100	0.034					100	0.035

means observed from the test and reference products. The proposed design consists of three arms: one arm is for the test product and the other two arms are for the reference products from different batches. This design will allow us to assess the relative distance in terms of the ratio of the difference between T and R and the difference between R_1 and R_2. Under the design, the performances of the derived statistical tests were evaluated both theoretically and through the simulation study. Since the statistical test based on the ratio estimator is more powerful than the linearization method, Kang and Chow (2013) recommend the statistical test based on the ratio estimator.

In practice, one of the most commonly used designs for assessing biosimilarity between a biosimilar product and an innovative biological product is probably a two-arm balanced design, and biosimilarity is assessed by using the difference between two population means. A disadvantage of this approach is that the variability of a reference product among different batches cannot be incorporated. Hence, when an equivalence/similarity margin is larger than the variability of a reference product, this approach may tend to conclude that two products are biosimilar, although there could exist a considerable difference between the two products. This problem can be fixed if the equivalence/similarity margin can be determined by incorporating variability of a reference product prior to a clinical trial. However, in practice this may not be easy, because the variability of a reference product may be unknown. This point is an advantage of the proposed design, because relative distance rather than absolute difference is employed to assess biosimilarity.

As mentioned earlier, there are many possible choices for specific forms of distance. For the assessment of bioequivalence for small-molecule drug products, average bioequivalence uses $d_2(T,R)=|\mu_T/\mu_R|$ and the population and the individual bioequivalences employ $d_4(T,R)=E(Y_T-Y_R)^2$. Since different distances may produce different conclusions for biosimilarity, it is of interest to develop statistical tests for several difference distances which have often been used in the statistical literature. It seems that the absolute mean difference used as the distance in this chapter does not incorporate the variance. Another natural choice of the distance is the standardized absolute mean difference $d_1^s(T,R)=|\mu_T-\mu_R|/\sigma$. However, since the common variance is assumed, the common standard deviation σ is cancelled out in the relative distance. Therefore, actually this chapter uses the standardized absolute mean difference as the distance. It is of interest to develop statistical tests when the common variance assumption does not hold.

In this chapter, the distance between a biosimilar product and an innovator biological product is defined as $d_1(t,R)=|\mu_T-(\mu_{R_1}+\mu_{R_2})/2|$. But, there are also other ways of defining the distance such as

$$d_1(T,R)' = \max\left(|\mu_T-\mu_{R_1}|,|\mu_T-\mu_{R_2}|\right)$$

and

$$d_1(T,R)'' = \min\left(|\mu_T-\mu_{R_1}|,|\mu_T-\mu_{R_2}|\right).$$

It is interesting to develop appropriate statistical tests for these new distances.

Note that the randomization ratio $2:1$ between n_1 and n_2 is employed in this chapter. However, a general randomization ratio $k:1$ can be used. Finding an optimal value of k might also be an interesting future study.

6

General Approach for Assessing Biosimilarity

6.1 Background

As discussed in the previous chapters, the assessment of bioequivalence and/or biosimilarity is very sensitive to bioequivalence/biosimilarity criteria. The one-size-fits-all criterion for the assessment of bioequivalence for small-molecule drug products has been criticized and considered not to be appropriate for the assessment of biosimilarity. However, little or no information regarding what criteria are most appropriate for the assessment of biosimilarity is available in regulatory guidances. Without a well-defined and widely accepted biosimilarity criterion, it is difficult to demonstrate that the test product is highly similar to the reference product. To overcome this problem, Kang and Chow (2013) suggested considering the evaluation of relative distance between $T-R$ and $R-R$ and proposed useful statistical methods for the assessment of biosimilarity based on the defined relative distance as described in the previous section. The methods proposed by Kang and Chow, however, still depend upon the selection of biosimilarity criteria.

Chow et al. (2011) proposed a general approach for assessing biosimilarity based on the concept of comparing the reproducibility probability in a $T-R$ study as compared to that of an $R-R$ study. Chow et al. (2011) referred to their proposed general approach as the local biosimilarity index for a given domain. Chow et al. (2011) claimed that the proposed biosimilarity index can take variability into consideration and it is insensitive to the selection of biosimilarity criteria. Based on the local biosimilarity index, a totality biosimilarity index for providing the totality-of-the-evidence can be obtained across functional structures or domains for the development of biosimilar products. As indicated by Chow et al. (2013), a similar idea can be applied to obtain a switching index and/or alternating index for the assessment of drug interchangeability under certain study designs for switching and/or alternating.

Alternatively, Tsou et al. (2012) proposed a consistency approach for the statistical evaluation of similarity between a biosimilar product and the innovator biologic using the idea from Tsou et al. (2011) for the assessment of similarity between a bridging study conducted in a new region and studies conducted in the original region. Tsou et al.'s (2012) consistency approach was developed based on either a response for therapeutic efficacy or a response for adverse effects. The consistency approach is useful for the evaluation of drug interchangeability under certain assumptions.

In the next section, the assessment of reproducibility probability under different study designs is briefly described. The development of the biosimilarity index, based on the concept of reproducibility probability proposed by Chow (2010) and Chow et al. (2011), is given in Section 6.3. Section 6.4 studies the relationship between the biosimilarity criterion and variability. The biosimilarity index based on the Bayesian approach is outlined in Section 6.5. A general consistency approach for assessing biosimilarity is outlined in Section 6.6. Brief concluding remarks are given in the last section of this chapter.

6.2 Reproducibility Probability

For marketing approval of a new drug product, the U.S. Food and Drug Administration (FDA) requires that at least two adequate and well-controlled clinical trials be conducted to provide substantial evidence regarding the effectiveness of the drug product under investigation. The purpose of conducting the second trial is to study whether the observed clinical result from the first trial is reproducible on the same target patient population. Let H_0 be the null hypothesis that the mean response of the drug product is the same as the mean response of a control (e.g., a placebo) and H_a be the alternative hypothesis. An observed result from a clinical trial is said to be significant if it leads to the rejection of H_0. It is often of interest to determine whether clinical trials that produced significant clinical results provide substantial evidence to assure that the results will be reproducible in a future clinical trial with the same study protocol. Under certain circumstance, the FDA Modernization Act (FDAMA) of 1997 includes a provision (Section 115 of FDAMA) to allow data from one adequate and well-controlled clinical trial investigation and confirmatory evidence to establish the effectiveness of the drug and biological candidates for approval by a risk/benefit assessment. Suppose that the null hypothesis H_0 is rejected if and only if $|T| > c$, where c is a positive known constant and T is a test statistic. This is usually related to a two-sided alternative hypothesis. The discussion for a one-sided alternative hypothesis is similar. In statistical theory, the probability of observing a significant clinical result when H_a is indeed true is referred to as the power of the test procedure. If the statistical model under H_a is a parametric model, then the power is

$$P(|T| > c \mid H_a) = P(|T| > c \mid \theta),$$ (6.1)

where θ is an unknown parameter or vector of parameters. Suppose now that one clinical trial has been conducted and the result is significant. What is the probability that the second trial will produce a significant result, that is, if the significant result from the first trial is reproducible? Mathematically, if the two trials are independent, the probability of observing a significant result from the second trial when H_a is true is still given by Equation 6.1, regardless of whether the result from the first trial is significant or not. However, information from the first clinical trial should be useful in the evaluation of the probability of observing a significant result in the second trial. This leads to the concept of the reproducibility probability, which is different from the power defined by Equation 6.1.

In general, the reproducibility probability is a person's subjective probability of observing a significant clinical result from a future trial, when he/she observes significant results from one or several previous trials. For example, Goodman (1992) considered the reproducibility probability as the probability in Equation 6.1 with θ replaced by its estimate based on the data from the previous trial(s). In other words, the reproducibility probability can be defined as an estimated power of the future trial using the data from the previous trial(s). In Section 6.2, we study how to evaluate the reproducibility probability using this approach, under several study designs. When the reproducibility probability is used to provide an evidence of the effectiveness of a drug product, the estimated power approach may produce a rather optimistic result. A more conservative approach is to define the reproducibility probability as a lower confidence bound of the power of the second trial. This will be studied in Section 6.3. Perhaps a more sensible definition of the reproducibility probability can be obtained by using the Bayesian approach. Under the Bayesian approach, the unknown parameter θ is a random vector with a prior distribution $\pi(\theta)$ assumed to be known. Thus, the reproducibility probability can be defined as the conditional probability of $|T| > c$ in the future trial, given the data set x observed from the previous trial(s), that is,

$$P\left(|T| > c \mid x\right) = \int P\left(|T| > c \mid \theta\right) \pi(\theta \mid x) d\theta, \qquad (6.2)$$

where $T = T(Y)$ is based on the data set y from the future trial and $\pi(\theta|X)$ is the posterior density of θ, given X. In practice, the reproducibility probability is useful when the clinical trials are conducted sequentially. It provides important information for regulatory agencies in deciding whether it is necessary to require the second clinical trial when the result from the first clinical trial is strongly significant. On the other hand, if the second trial is necessary, the reproducibility probability can be used for sample size adjustment of the second trial. To study the reproducibility probability, we need to specify the test procedure, that is, the form of the test statistic T. We consider several different study designs.

6.2.1 Two Samples with Equal Variances

Suppose that a total of $n=n_1+n_2$ patients are randomly assigned to two groups, a treatment group and a control group. In the treatment group, n_1 patients receive the treatment (or a test drug) and produce responses $x_{11},...,x_{1n_1}$. In the control group, n_2 patients receive the placebo (or a reference drug) and produce responses $x_{21},...,x_{2n_2}$. This design is a typical two-group parallel design in clinical trials. We assume that x_{ij}'s are independent and normally distributed with means μ_i, $i = 1, 2$, and a common variance σ^2. Suppose that the hypotheses of interest are

$$H_0 : \mu_1 - \mu_2 = 0 \quad \text{vs.} \quad H_a : \mu_1 - \mu_2 \neq 0. \tag{6.3}$$

The discussion for a one-sided H_a is similar.

Consider the commonly used two-sample t-test which rejects H_0 if and only if $|T| > t_{0.975,n-2}$, where $t_{0.975,n-2}$ is the 97.5th percentile of the t-distribution with $n-2$ degrees of freedom

$$T = \frac{\bar{x}_1 - \bar{x}_2}{\sqrt{\left((n_1-1)s_1^2 + (n_2-1)s_2^2\right)/(n-2)}\sqrt{(1/n_1)+(1/n_2)}} \tag{6.4}$$

and $\bar{x}_i$ and s_i^2 are, respectively, the sample mean and variance based on the data from the ith treatment group. The power of T for the second trial is

$$p(\theta) = P\left(|T(y)| > t_{0.975,n-2}\right)$$

$$= 1 - \Im_{n-2}(t_{0.975,n-2} \mid \theta) + \Im_{n-2}(-t_{0.975,n-2} \mid \theta), \tag{6.5}$$

where

$$\theta = \frac{\mu_1 - \mu_2}{\sigma\sqrt{((1/n_1)+(1/n_2))}} \tag{6.6}$$

and $\Im_{n-2}(\cdot \mid \theta)$ denotes the distribution function of the non-central t-distribution with $n - 2$ degrees of freedom and the non-centrality parameter θ. Note that $p(\theta) = p(|\theta|)$.

Values of $P(\theta)$ as a function of $|\theta|$ are provided in Table 6.1. Using the idea of replacing θ by its estimate $T(x)$, where T is defined by Equation 6.4, we obtain the following reproducibility probability:

$$\hat{P} = 1 - \Im_{n-2}(t_{0.975,n-2} \mid T(x)) + \Im_{n-2}(-t_{0.975,n-2} \mid T(x)), \tag{6.7}$$

TABLE 6.1

Values of the Power Function $p(\theta)$ in Equation 6.5

$|\theta|$	Total Sample Size							
	10	20	30	40	50	60	100	∞
1.96	0.407	0.458	0.473	0.480	0.484	0.487	0.492	0.500
2.02	0.429	0.481	0.496	0.504	0.508	0.511	0.516	0.524
2.08	0.448	0.503	0.519	0.527	0.531	0.534	0.540	0.548
2.14	0.469	0.526	0.542	0.550	0.555	0.557	0.563	0.571
2.20	0.490	0.549	0.565	0.573	0.578	0.581	0.586	0.594
2.26	0.511	0.571	0.588	0.596	0.601	0.604	0.609	0.618
2.32	0.532	0.593	0.610	0.618	0.623	0.626	0.632	0.640
2.38	0.552	0.615	0.632	0.640	0.645	0.648	0.654	0.662
2.44	0.573	0.636	0.654	0.662	0.667	0.670	0.676	0.684
2.50	0.593	0.657	0.675	0.683	0.688	0.691	0.697	0.705
2.56	0.613	0.678	0.695	0.704	0.708	0.711	0.717	0.725
2.62	0.632	0.698	0.715	0.724	0.728	0.731	0.737	0.745
2.68	0.652	0.717	0.735	0.743	0.747	0.750	0.756	0.764
2.74	0.671	0.736	0.753	0.761	0.766	0.769	0.774	0.782
2.80	0.690	0.754	0.771	0.779	0.783	0.786	0.792	0.799
2.86	0.708	0.772	0.788	0.796	0.800	0.803	0.808	0.815
2.92	0.725	0.789	0.805	0.812	0.816	0.819	0.824	0.830
2.98	0.742	0.805	0.820	0.827	0.831	0.834	0.839	0.845
3.04	0.759	0.820	0.835	0.842	0.846	0.848	0.853	0.860
3.10	0.775	0.834	0.849	0.856	0.859	0.862	0.866	0.872
3.16	0.790	0.848	0.862	0.868	0.872	0.874	0.879	0.884
3.22	0.805	0.861	0.874	0.881	0.884	0.886	0.890	0.895
3.28	0.819	0.873	0.886	0.892	0.895	0.897	0.901	0.906
3.34	0.832	0.884	0.897	0.902	0.905	0.907	0.911	0.916
3.40	0.844	0.895	0.907	0.912	0.915	0.917	0.920	0.925
3.46	0.856	0.905	0.916	0.921	0.924	0.925	0.929	0.932
3.52	0.868	0.914	0.925	0.929	0.932	0.933	0.936	0.940
3.58	0.879	0.923	0.933	0.937	0.939	0.941	0.943	0.947
3.64	0.889	0.931	0.940	0.944	0.946	0.947	0.950	0.953
3.70	0.898	0.938	0.946	0.950	0.952	0.953	0.956	0.959
3.76	0.907	0.944	0.952	0.956	0.958	0.959	0.961	0.965
3.82	0.915	0.950	0.958	0.961	0.963	0.964	0.966	0.969
3.88	0.923	0.956	0.963	0.966	0.967	0.968	0.970	0.973
3.94	0.930	0.961	0.967	0.970	0.971	0.972	0.974	0.977

Source: Shao, J. and Chow, S.C., *Stat. Med.*, 21, 1727, 2002.

which is a function of $|T(x)|$. When $|T(x)| > t_{0.975,n-2}$,

$$\hat{P} \approx \begin{cases} 1 - \Im_{n-2}(t_{0.975,n-2} \,|\, T(x)) & \text{if } T(x) > 0 \\ \Im_{n-2}(-t_{0.975,n-2} \,|\, T(x)) & \text{if } T(x) < 0. \end{cases} \tag{6.8}$$

If $\Im_{n-2}$ is replaced by the normal distribution and $t_{0.975,n-2}$ is replaced by the normal percentile, then Formula 6.8 is the same as that in Goodman (1992) who studied the case where the variance σ^2 is known. Table 6.1 can be used to find the reproducibility probability $\hat{P}$ in Equation 6.7 with a fixed sample size n. For example, if $|T(x)| = 2.9$ was observed in a clinical trial with $n = n_1 + n_2 = 40$, then the reproducibility probability is 0.807. If $T(x) = 2.9$ was observed in a clinical trial with $n = 36$, then an extrapolation of the results in Table 6.1 (for $n = 30$ and 40) leads to a reproducibility probability of 0.803.

6.2.2 Two Samples with Unequal Variances

Consider the problem of testing Hypotheses 6.3 under the two-group parallel design without the assumption of equal variances. That is, x_{ij}'s are independently distributed as $N(\mu_i, \sigma_i^2)$, $i = 1, 2$. When $\sigma_1^2 \neq \sigma_2^2$, there exists no exact testing procedure for the hypotheses in Equation 5.3. When both n_1 and n_2 are large, an approximate 5% level test rejects H_0 when $|T| > z_{0.975}$, where

$$T = \frac{\bar{x}_1 - \bar{x}_2}{\sqrt{(s_1^2/n_1) + (s_2^2/n_2)}}. \tag{6.9}$$

Since T is approximately distributed as $N(\theta, 1)$ with

$$\theta = \frac{\mu_1 - \mu_2}{\sqrt{(\sigma_1^2/n_1) + (\sigma_2^2/n_2)}}, \tag{6.10}$$

the reproducibility probability, obtained by using the estimated power approach, is given by

$$\hat{P} = \Phi(T(x) - z_{0.975}) + \Phi(-T(x) - z_{0.975}). \tag{6.11}$$

When the variances under different treatments are different and the sample sizes are not large, a different study design, such as a matched-pair parallel design or a 2 × 2 crossover design is recommended. A matched-pair parallel design involves m pairs of matched patients. One patient in each pair is assigned to the treatment group and the other is assigned to the control group. Let x_{ij} be the observation from the jth pair and the ith group. It is assumed that the differences $x_{1j} - x_{2j}$, $j = 1, ..., m$, are independent and identically distributed as $N(\mu_1 - \mu_2, \sigma_D^2)$. Then, the null hypothesis H_0 is rejected at the 5% level of significance if $|T| > t_{0.975, m-1}$, where

$$T = \frac{\sqrt{m}(\bar{x}_1 - \bar{x}_2)}{\hat{\sigma}_D^2} \tag{6.12}$$

and $\hat{\sigma}_D^2$ is the sample variance based on the differences $x_{1j} - x_{2j}$, $j = 1, ..., m$. Note that T has the non-central t-distribution with $m-1$ degrees of freedom and the non-centrality parameter

$$\theta = \frac{\sqrt{m}(\mu_1 - \mu_2)}{\sigma_D^2}. \tag{6.13}$$

Consequently, the reproducibility probability obtained by using the estimated power approach is given by Equation 6.7 with T defined by Equation 6.12 and $n - 2$ replaced by $m - 1$.

Suppose that the study design is a 2×2 cross-over design in which n_1 patients receive the treatment at the first period and the placebo at the second period and n_2 patients receive the placebo at the first period and the treatment at the second period. Let x_{lij} be the normally distributed observation from the jth patient at the ith period and lth sequence. Then the treatment effect μ_D can be unbiasedly estimated by

$$\hat{\mu}_D = \frac{\bar{x}_{11} - \bar{x}_{12} - \bar{x}_{21} + \bar{x}_{22}}{2} \sim N\left(\mu_D, \frac{\sigma_D^2}{4}\left(\frac{1}{n_1} + \frac{1}{n_2}\right)\right),$$

where
$\bar{x}_{li}$ is the sample mean based on x_{lij}, $j = 1, ..., n_l$
$\sigma_D^2 = \text{var}(x_{l1j} - x_{l2j})$

An unbiased estimator of σ_D^2 is

$$\hat{\sigma}_D^2 = \frac{1}{n_1 + n_2 - 2} \sum_{l=1}^{2} \sum_{j=1}^{m} (x_{l1j} - x_{l2j} - \bar{x}_{l1} + \bar{x}_{l2})^2,$$

which is independent of $\hat{\mu}_D$ and distributed as $\sigma_D^2/(n_1 + n_2 - 2)$ times the chi-square distribution with $n_1 + n_2 - 2$ degrees of freedom. Thus, the null hypothesis $H_0 : \mu_D = 0$ is rejected at the 5% level of significance if $|T| > t_{0.975,n-2}$, where $n = n_1 + n_2$ and

$$T = \frac{\hat{\mu}_D}{\hat{\sigma}_D/2\sqrt{(1/n_1)+(1/n_2)}}. \tag{6.14}$$

Note that T has the non-central t-distribution with $n-2$ degrees of freedom and the non-centrality parameter

$$\theta = \frac{\mu_D}{\sigma_D/2\sqrt{(1/n_1)+(1/n_2)}}. \tag{6.15}$$

Consequently, the reproducibility probability obtained by using the estimated power approach is given by Equation 6.7 with T defined by Equation 6.14.

6.2.3 Parallel-Group Designs

Parallel-group designs are often adopted in clinical trials to compare more than one treatment with a placebo control or to compare one treatment, one placebo control and one active control. Let $a \geq 3$ be the number of groups and x_{ij} be an observation from the jth patient in the ith group, $j = 1, \ldots, n_i, i = 1, \ldots, a$. Assume that x_{ij}'s are independently distributed as $N(\mu_i, \sigma^2)$. The null hypothesis H_0 is then $H_0 : \mu_1 = \mu_2 = \cdots = \mu_a$, which is rejected at the 5% level of significance if $T > F_{0.95;a-1,n-a}$, where $F_{0.95;a-1,n-a}$ is the 95th percentile of the F-distribution with $a-1$ and $n-a$ degrees of freedom, $n = n_1 + n_2 + \cdots + n_a$,

$$T = \frac{SST/(a-1)}{SSE/(n-a)}, \tag{6.16}$$

and

$$SST = \sum_{i=1}^{a} n_i(\bar{x}_i - \bar{x})^2, \quad SSE = \sum_{i=1}^{a}\sum_{j=1}^{n_i} (x_{ij}-\bar{x}_i)^2,$$

where
    $\bar{x}_i$ is the sample mean based on the data in the ith group
    $\bar{x}$ is the overall sample mean

Note that T has the non-central F-distribution with $a-1$ and $n-a$ degrees of freedom and the non-centrality parameter

$$\theta = \sum_{i=1}^{a} \frac{n_i(\mu_i - \bar{\mu})^2}{\sigma^2},$$

where $\bar{\mu} = \sum_{i=1}^{a} n_i\mu_i/n$. Let $\Im_{\alpha-1,v-\alpha}(\cdot|\theta)$ be the distribution function of T. Then, the power of the second clinical trial is

$$P(T(y) > F_{0.95;a-1,n-a}) = 1 - \Im_{a-1,n-a}(F_{0.95;a-1,n-a}\,|\,\theta).$$

Thus, the reproducibility probability obtained by using the estimated power approach is

$$\hat{P} = 1 - \Im_{a-1,n-a}(F_{0.95;a-1,n-a}\,|\,T(x)),$$

where $T(x)$ is the observed T based on the data x from the first clinical trial.

6.3 Development of the Biosimilarity Index

Chow (2010) proposed the development of a composite index for assessing the biosimilarity of follow-on biologics based on the facts that (1) the concept of biosimilarity for biological products (made of living cells) is very different from that of bioequivalence for drug products, and (2) biological products are very sensitive to small changes in the variation during the manufacturing process (i.e., it might have a drastic change in clinical outcome). Although some research on the comparison of moment-based criteria and probability-based criteria for the assessment of (1) average biosimilarity and (2) the variability of biosimilarity for some given study endpoints by applying the criteria for bioequivalence are available in the literature (see, e.g., Chow et al., 2010; Hsieh et al. 2010), universally acceptable criteria for biosimilarity are not available in the regulatory guidelines/guidances. Thus, Chow (2010) and Chow et al. (2011) proposed a biosimilarity index based on the concept of the probability of reproducibility as follows:

Step 1: Assess the average biosimilarity between the test product and the reference product based on a given biosimilarity criterion. For the purpose of an illustration, consider a bioequivalence criterion as a biosimilarity criterion. That is, biosimilarity is claimed if the 90% confidence interval of the ratio of means of a given study endpoint falls within the biosimilarity limits of (80%, 125%) or (−0.2231, 0.2231) based on log-transformed data or based on raw (original) data.

Step 2: Once the product passes the test for biosimilarity in Step 1, calculate the reproducibility probability based on the observed ratio (or observed mean difference) and variability. Thus, the calculated reproducibility probability will take the variability and the sensitivity of heterogeneity in variances into consideration for the assessment of biosimilarity.

Step 3: We then claim biosimilarity if the calculated 95% confidence lower bound of the reproducibility probability is larger than a pre-specified number p_0, which can be obtained based on an estimate of reproducibility probability for a study comparing a "reference product" to itself (the "reference product"). We will refer to such a study as an R–R study. Alternatively, we can then claim (local) biosimilarity if the 95% confidence lower bound of the biosimilarity index is larger than p_0.

In an R–R study, define

$$P_{TR} = P\left(\begin{array}{c}\text{Concluding average biosimilarity between the test and the}\\ \text{reference products in a future trial given that the average}\\ \text{biosimiliarity based on the ABE criterion has been}\\ \text{established in the first trial}\end{array}\right) \quad (6.17)$$

Alternatively, a reproducibility probability for evaluating the biosimilarity of the same two reference products based on the ABE criterion is defined as

$$P_{RR} = P\left(\begin{array}{c}\text{Concluding average biosimiliarity of the two same reference}\\ \text{products in a future trial given that the average biosimilarity}\\ \text{based on the ABE criterion has been established in}\\ \text{the first trial}\end{array}\right) \quad (6.18)$$

Since the idea of the biosimilarity index is to show that the reproducibility probability is higher in a study for comparing "a reference product" with "the reference product" than the study for comparing a follow-on biologic with the innovative (reference) product, the criterion of an acceptable reproducibility probability (i.e., p_0) for the assessment of biosimilarity can be obtained based on the R–R study. For example, if the R–R study suggests the reproducibility probability of 90%, that is, $P_{RR}=90\%$, the criterion of the reproducibility probability for the biosimilarity study could be chosen as 80% of the 90%, which is $p_0=80\% \times P_{RR}=72\%$.

The biosimilarity index described earlier has the advantages that (1) it is robust with respect to the selected study endpoint, biosimilarity criteria, and study design; and (2) the probability of reproducibility will reflect the sensitivity of heterogeneity in variance.

Note that the proposed biosimilarity index can be applied to different functional areas (domains) of biological products such as pharmacokinetics (PK), biological activities, biomarkers (e.g., pharmacodynamics), immunogenicity, manufacturing process, efficacy, etc. An overall biosimilarity index or totality biosimilarity index across domains can be similarly obtained as follows:

Step 1: Obtain $\hat{P}_i$, the probability of reproducibility for the ith domain, $i = 1, ..., K$.

Step 2: Define the biosimilarity index $\hat{p} = \sum_{i=1}^{K} w_i \hat{p}_i$, where w_i is the weight for the ith domain.

Step 3: Claim global biosimilarity if we reject the null hypothesis that $p \leq p_0$, where p_0 is a pre-specified acceptable reproducibility probability. Alternatively, we can claim (global)biosimilarity if the 95% confidence lower bound of p is larger than p_0.

Let T and R be the parameters of interest (e.g., a PK response) with means μ_T and μ_R, for a test product and a reference product, respectively. Thus, the interval hypotheses for testing the ABE of two products can be expressed as

$$H_0 : \theta'_L \geq \frac{\mu'_T}{\mu'_R} \quad \text{or} \quad \theta'_u \leq \frac{\mu'_T}{\mu'_R} \quad \text{vs.} \quad H_a : \theta'_L < \frac{\mu'_T}{\mu'_R} < \theta'_u,$$

where (θ'_L, θ'_u) is the ABE limit. For in vivo bioequivalence testing, (θ'_L, θ'_u) is chosen to be (80%, 125%). The aforementioned hypotheses can be re-expressed as

$$H_0 : \theta_L \geq \mu_T - \mu_R \quad \text{or} \quad \theta_u \leq \mu_T - \mu_R \quad \text{vs.} \quad H_a : \theta_L < \mu_T - \mu_R < \theta_u,$$

where
μ_T and μ_R are the means of log-transformed data which are equal to the log-transformed values of μ'_T and μ'_R
(θ_L, θ_u) is $(-0.2231, 0.2231)$, which is equal to the log-transformed values of (80%, 125%)

To calculate the reproducibility probability under the interval hypotheses mentioned earlier, the probability of P_{TR} can be expressed when considering a parallel design (since it is a common design for biological products) as follows:

$$P(\delta_L, \delta_u)$$

$$= P(T_L(\overline{Y}_T, \overline{Y}_R, s_T, s_R) > t_{\alpha,dfp} \quad \text{and} \quad T_U(\overline{Y}_T, \overline{Y}_R, s_T, s_R) < -t_{\alpha,dfp} \mid \delta_L, \delta_u), \quad (6.19)$$

where s_T, s_R, n_T, and n_R are the sample standard deviations and sample sizes for the test and reference formulations, respectively. The value of *dfp* can be calculated by

$$dfp = \frac{((s_T^2/n_1)+(s_R^2/n_2))^2}{((s_T^2/n_T)^2/(n_T-1))+((s_R^2/n_T)^2/(n_R-1))}$$

$$T_L(\bar{Y}_T,\bar{Y}_R,\hat{\sigma}_T,\hat{\sigma}_R)=\frac{(\bar{Y}_T-\bar{Y}_R)-\theta_L}{\sqrt{(s_T^2/n_T)+(s_R^2/n_R)}} \qquad T_U(\bar{Y}_T,\bar{Y}_R,\hat{\sigma}_T,\hat{\sigma}_R)=\frac{(\bar{Y}_T-\bar{Y}_R)-\theta_U}{\sqrt{(s_T^2/n_T)+(s_R^2/n_R)}}$$

$$\delta_L = \frac{\mu_T-\mu_R-\theta_L}{\sqrt{(\sigma_T^2/n_T)+(\sigma_R^2/n_R)}} \quad \text{and} \quad \delta_U = \frac{\mu_T-\mu_R-\theta_U}{\sigma_d\sqrt{(\sigma_T^2/n_T)+(\sigma_R^2/n_R)}}. \tag{6.20}$$

σ_T^2 and σ_R^2 are the variances for test and reference formulations, respectively.

The vectors (T_L, T_U) can be shown to follow a bivariate non-central *t*-distribution with n_1+n_2-2 and *dfp* degrees of freedom, correlation of 1, and non-centrality parameters δ_L and δ_U (Phillips, 1990; Owen, 1965). Owen (1965) showed that the integral of the earlier bivariate non-central *t*-distribution can be expressed as the difference of the integrals between two univariate non-central *t*-distributions. Therefore, the power function in Equation 6.19 can be obtained by

$$P(\delta_L,\delta_U)=Q_f(t_U,\delta_U;0,R)-Q_f(t_L,\delta_L;0,R), \tag{6.21}$$

where

$$Q_f(t,\delta;0,R)=\frac{\sqrt{2\pi}}{\Gamma(f/2)2^{(f-2)/2}}\int_0^R G(tx/\sqrt{f}-\delta)x^{f-1}G'(x)dx$$

$$R=(\delta_L-\delta_U)\sqrt{f}/(t_L-t_U), \quad G'(x)=\frac{1}{\sqrt{2\pi}}e^{-x^2/2}, \quad G(x)=\int_{-\infty}^x G'(t)dt,$$

and

$$t_L=t_{\alpha,dfp}, \quad t_U=-t_{\alpha,dfp}, \quad \text{and} \quad f=dfp \text{ for parallel design.}$$

Note that when $0<\theta_U=-\theta_L$, $P(\delta_L,\delta_U)=P(-\delta_U,-\delta_L)$.

Figure 6.1 presents the relationship of the reproducibility and variability under various sample sizes and ratios of means. The reproducibility

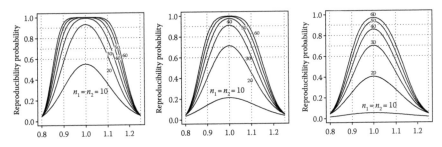

FIGURE 6.1
Reproducibility probability curves based on the estimation approach for sample sizes $n_T = n_R = 10, 20, 30, 40, 50,$ and 60 at the 0.05 level of significance and $(\theta'_L, \theta'_U) = (80\%, 125\%)$ when $\sigma_T = 0.2, 0.3, 0.4$ and $\sigma_R = 0.2$.

probabilities increase when the sample size increases and the means ratio is close to 1, while it decreases when the variability increases for the same setting of sample size and means ratio which shows the impact of variability on reproducibility probabilities.

Since the true values of δ_L and δ_U are unknown, using the idea of replacing δ_L and δ_U in Equation 6.20 by their estimates based on the sample from the first study, the estimated reproducibility probability can be obtained as

$$\hat{P}(\hat{\delta}_L, \hat{\delta}_U) = Q_f(t_L, \hat{\delta}_U; 0, \hat{R}) - Q_f(t_U, \hat{\delta}_L; 0, \hat{R}), \qquad (6.22)$$

where

$$\hat{\delta}_L = \frac{\overline{Y}_T - \overline{Y}_L - \theta'_L}{\sqrt{(s_T^2/n_T) + (s_R^2/n_R)}}, \quad \hat{\delta}_U = \frac{\overline{Y}_T - \overline{Y}_L - \theta'_U}{\sqrt{(s_T^2/n_T) + (s_R^2/n_R)}}, \quad \hat{R} = (\hat{\delta}_L - \hat{\delta}_U)\sqrt{\frac{f}{t_L - t_U}}.$$

6.4 Relationship of the Biosimilarity Criterion versus Variability

As described in the previous section, the pre-specified criterion for claiming biosimilarity between a test product and a reference product, that is, p_0, is chosen based on the reproducibility probability P_{RR}, which is obtained from an R–R study. The values of p_0 may differ for different reference products since each of reference products has its own specific reproducibility probability. Thus, P_{RR} is related to the variability associated with the reference product. A simulation study was conducted to investigate the impact of variability on the selected p_0. The parameter settings of the simulation study were $n_R = 24, 36, 72; \sigma_R = 0.1, 0.15; (\theta_L, \theta_U) = (-0.2231, 0.2231)$.

TABLE 6.2

P_{BE} and $P_{RR,RR}$ and Average versus Variability-Based Estimation Approach

σ_R	$\sqrt{\sigma_R^2 + \sigma_R^2}$	avg.					avg.					avg.				
		P_{BE}	$P_{RR,RR}$	$\hat{P}_{RR,RR}$	$p_{0,0.7}$	$p_{0,0.8}$	P_{BE}	$P_{RR,RR}$	$\hat{P}_{RR,RR}$	$p_{0,0.7}$	$p_{0,0.8}$	P_{BE}	$P_{RR,RR}$	$\hat{P}_{RR,RR}$	$p_{0,0.7}$	$p_{0,0.8}$
0.1	0.14	1.0000	1.0000	1.0000	0.7000	0.8000	1.0000	1.0000	1.0000	0.7000	0.8000	1.0000	1.0000	1.0000	0.7000	0.8000
0.1	0.21	1.0000	0.9994	0.9886	0.7000	0.8000	1.0000	1.0000	0.9991	0.7000	0.8000	1.0000	1.0000	1.0000	0.7000	0.8000
0.1	0.28	1.0000	0.9694	0.9198	0.7000	0.8000	1.0000	0.9976	0.9556	0.7000	0.8000	1.0000	1.0000	0.9999	0.7000	0.8000

Key: P_{BE}, probability of claiming biosimilarity based on the BE criterion; P_{RR}, reproducibility probability of R–R comparison study; avg. $\hat{P}_{RR,RR}$, average of the estimated reproducibility probability of R–R comparison study.

Note that since there are the same two products, the means and variabilities of the two reference products are assumed the same in the simulations. In addition, the correlation coefficient of the intra-subject variabilities of the two products was set to be 1, which resulted in t zero subject-by-formulation interaction. A total of 1000 random samples were generated for each parameter combination. The simulation results given in Table 6.2 show that P_{BE}, which is the probability of claiming biosimilarity based on the BE criterion, is higher than the reproducibility probability of P_{RR}. The average of estimated reproducibility probabilities denoted by avg. $\hat{P}_{RR}$ is close to the true reproducibility probability of P_{RR} for the R–R comparison. The difference setting of intra-subject variabilities results only in a small change in avg. $\hat{P}_{RR}$ since the subject-by-formulation interaction is assumed to be 0. As expected, the P_{RR} and agv. $\hat{P}_{RR}$ decrease as the total variability of σ_d and $\sqrt{\sigma_R^2 + \sigma_R^2}$ increase. The P_{RR} and agv. $\hat{P}_{RR}$ increase when the sample size increases. The two values of p_0 (i.e., corresponding to 70% and 80% of P_{RR}) are presented in the table for researchers' reference to choose an appropriate value of p_0 for their own products. If we define $d = p_0/p_{RR}$, then d can be used to address the degree of similarity and consequently the question "*How similar is similar?*"

6.5 Biosimilarity Index Based on the Bayesian Approach

The calculation of the reproducibility probability given earlier is based on the estimation approach by replacing the unknown parameters using their estimates. An alternative definition of the reproducibility probability is proposed by Goodman (1992) and Shao and Chow (2002). Let $p(\theta)$ be the power function, where θ is an unknown parameter or a vector of parameters. Under this Bayesian approach, θ is random with a prior distribution assumed to be known. The reproducibility probability can be viewed as the posterior mean of the power function for a future trial

$$\int p(\theta)\pi(\theta \,|\, x)d\theta, \tag{6.23}$$

where $\pi(\theta|x)$ is the posterior density of θ, given the data set x observed for the previous trial(s).

Two Bayesian versions of reproducibility probability will be derived by (1) assuming that (μ_T, μ_R) is random and the variance is fixed, and (2) (μ_T, μ_R) is fixed and the variance is random in Sections 6.5.1 and 6.5.2, respectively.

6.5.1 μ_T, μ_R Is Random and the Variance Is Fixed

In statistical theory, the probability of observing a significant result when H_1 is indeed true is referred to as the power of the test procedure. The power is given by

$$P(T_L(\bar{X}_T, \bar{X}_R) > z_\alpha, T_U(\bar{X}_T, \bar{X}_R) < -z_\alpha \mid \mu_T, \mu_R)$$

$$= \Phi\left[-\frac{(\mu_T - \mu_R) - \theta_U}{\sigma\sqrt{1/n_T + 1/n_R}} - z_\alpha \right] + \Phi\left[\frac{(\mu_T - \mu_R) - \theta_L}{\sigma\sqrt{1/n_T + 1/n_R}} - z_\alpha \right] - 1,$$

where

$$T_L(\bar{X}_T, \bar{X}_R) = \frac{(\bar{X}_T - \bar{X}_R) - \theta_L}{\sigma\sqrt{1/n_T + 1/n_R}}, \quad T_U(\bar{X}_T, \bar{X}_R) = \frac{(\bar{X}_T - \bar{X}_R) - \theta_U}{\sigma\sqrt{1/n_T + 1/n_R}},$$

σ is a common variance for the test and reference products. As indicated by Goodman (1992) and Shao and Chow (2002), the reproducibility probability can be viewed as the posterior mean of the power function for the future trial. Under the Bayesian approach, the unknown parameter (μ_T, μ_R) is random with a prior distribution $\pi(\mu_T, \mu_R)$ assumed to be known. Thus, the reproducibility probability can be defined as the conditional probability $P(T_L > z_\alpha, T_U < -z_\alpha \mid x)$ in the future trial, given the observation x from the previous trial. Here $T_L = T_L(y)$ and $T_U = T_U(y)$ are based on the data $\mathbf{y}$ from the future trial. We can use the posterior mean of the power function to estimate reproducibility probability based on Equation 6.22, that is,

$$\hat{P}_{TR} = P(T_L > z_\alpha, T_U < -z_\alpha \mid x)$$

$$= \iint P(T_L(\bar{X}_T, \bar{X}_R) > z_\alpha, T_U(\bar{X}_T, \bar{X}_R) < -z_\alpha \mid \mu_T, \mu_R)$$

$$\cdot \pi(\mu_T, \mu_R \mid x) d\mu_T d\mu_R. \tag{6.24}$$

Under the Bayesian approach, it is essential to construct the posterior density $\pi(\mu_T, \mu_R \mid x)$ in Formula 6.24, given the data x from the previous trial. Consider first that σ^2 is known, a commonly used prior for $\pi(\mu_T, \mu_R)$ is the non-informative prior $\pi(\mu_T, \mu_R)$. Consequently, $\hat{P}_{TR,TR}$ can be derived by

$$\hat{P}_{TR,TR} = \Phi\left(-\frac{T_U(\bar{X}_T, \bar{X}_R) - z_\alpha}{\sqrt{2}} \right) + \Phi\left(\frac{T_L(\bar{X}_T, \bar{X}_R) - z_\alpha}{\sqrt{2}} \right) - 1.$$

6.5.2 Both (μ_T, μ_R) and the Variance Are Random

For the more realistic situation where σ^2 is unknown, we need a prior for σ^2. A commonly used non-informative prior for σ^2 is the Lebegue density $\pi(\sigma^2) = \sigma^{-2}$. If σ^2 is unknown, the pooled sample variance is

$$S^2 = \frac{\sum_{i=1}^{n_T} (X_{Ti} - \bar{X}_T)^2 + \sum_{i=1}^{n_R} (X_{Ri} - \bar{X}_R)^2}{n_1 + n_2 - 2},$$

where X_{Ti} and X_{Ri} are the log-transformed values for the test and reference products, respectively, and the power is given by

$$P(\delta_L, \delta_U) = P(T_L(\bar{X}_T, \bar{X}_R, S) > t_{\alpha, n_1 + n_2 - 2}, T_U(\bar{X}_T, \bar{X}_R, S) < -t_{\alpha, n_1 + n_2 - 2} \mid \delta_L, \delta_U), \quad (6.25)$$

where

$$T_L(\bar{X}_T, \bar{X}_R, S) = \frac{(\bar{X}_T - \bar{X}_R) - \theta_L}{S\sqrt{1/n_T + 1/n_R}}, \quad T_U(\bar{X}_T, \bar{X}_R, S) = \frac{(\bar{X}_T - \bar{X}_R) - \theta_U}{S\sqrt{1/n_T + 1/n_R}},$$

and

$$\delta_L = \frac{(\mu_T - \mu_R) - \theta_L}{S\sqrt{1/n_T + 1/n_R}}, \quad \delta_U = \frac{(\mu_T - \mu_R) - \theta_U}{S\sqrt{1/n_T + 1/n_R}}.$$

Assume that the priors for μ_T, μ_R and σ^2 are independent. Under the assumption, we can obtain that the posterior density for $(\mu_T - \mu_R \mid \sigma^2, x)$ is normally distributed given by

$$\pi(\mu_T - \mu_R \mid \sigma^2, x) \sim N(\bar{X}_T - \bar{X}_R, \sigma^2(1/n_1 + 1/n_2)),$$

and the posterior density for $(\sigma^2 \mid x)$ is the inverted gamma function IG (α, β), given by

$$\pi(\sigma^2 \mid x) = \frac{1}{\Gamma(\alpha)\beta^\alpha} \frac{1}{(\sigma^2)^{\alpha+1}} e^{-1/(\beta\sigma^2)}, \quad 0 < \sigma^2 < \infty,$$

where $\alpha = (n_1 + n_2 - 2)$ and $\beta = (n_1 + n_2 - 2)S^2/2$. Therefore, the posterior mean of $p(\delta_L, \delta_U)$ is

$$\hat{P}_{TR} = \int_0^\infty \left[\int_{-\infty}^\infty p(\delta_L, \delta_U)\pi(\mu_T - \mu_R \mid \sigma^2, x)d(\mu_T - \mu_R) \right] \pi(\sigma^2 \mid x)d\sigma^2, \quad (6.26)$$

which is the reproducibility probability under the Bayesian approach. The probability of $\hat{P}_{TR}$ in Equation 6.26 can be evaluated numerically. The Monte Carlo method can be applied to approximate $\hat{P}_{TR}$.

Estimates of the proposed biosimilarity index associated with a given σ and model configurations are then computed through Monte Carlo simulation based on 1000 replicate data sets. One thousand estimates are computed, the average and SE of the estimate can be calculated. The results of the simulation studies are presented in Table 6.3 and Figure 6.2.

TABLE 6.3

P_{BE} and $\hat{P}_{RR,RR}$ versus Variability Based on the Bayesian Approach When (μ_T, μ_R) Is Random and the Variance Is Fixed

| | $n_T = n_R = 12$ | | | $n_T = n_R = 24$ | | | $n_T = n_R = 36$ | | | $n_T = n_R = 48$ | | |
| | | $\hat{P}_{RR,RR}$ | | | $\hat{P}_{RR,RR}$ | | | $\hat{P}_{RR,RR}$ | | | $\hat{P}_{RR,RR}$ | |
σ	P_{BE}	Mean	SE	P_{BE}	Mean	SE	P_{BE}	Mean	SE	P_{BE}	Mean	SE
0.05	0.30	0.97	0.08	0.36	0.99	0.06	0.35	0.99	0.05	0.39	0.99	0.06
0.10	0.28	0.93	0.13	0.31	0.96	0.10	0.33	0.97	0.10	0.35	0.97	0.09
0.15	0.22	0.85	0.15	0.27	0.92	0.13	0.31	0.94	0.12	0.29	0.94	0.12
0.20	0.17	0.75	0.14	0.25	0.88	0.14	0.25	0.90	0.14	0.28	0.92	0.13
0.25	0.10	0.64	0.08	0.20	0.82	0.13	0.23	0.88	0.14	0.27	0.91	0.13
0.30	0.03	0.54	0.03	0.16	0.72	0.12	0.21	0.81	0.15	0.23	0.85	0.16
0.35	0.00	NA	NA	0.11	0.66	0.08	0.16	0.76	0.12	0.20	0.82	0.14
0.40	0.00	NA	NA	0.04	0.57	0.04	0.12	0.67	0.10	0.17	0.76	0.13
0.45	0.00	NA	NA	0.02	0.51	0.01	0.10	0.62	0.07	0.12	0.71	0.10
0.50	0.00	NA	NA	0.00	NA	NA	0.07	0.57	0.04	0.08	0.65	0.07

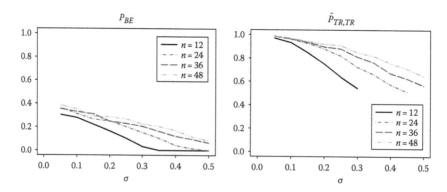

FIGURE 6.2
Reproducibility probability curves based on the Bayesain approach when (μ_T, μ_R) is random and the variance is fixed.

6.6 Consistency Approach

Tsou et al. (2011) proposed a consistency approach to the evaluation of bridging studies. Following a similar idea, Tsou et al. (2012) developed a consistency criterion for the assessment of biosimilar products. For the purpose of illustration, for simplicity, we focus only on the trials comparing a test product and a placebo control.

6.6.1 Response for Therapeutic Efficacy

Suppose that there were K historical reference studies for the approval of an innovator product. Based on the K historical reference studies, the innovator product has been already approved in a traditional trial due to its proven efficacy against placebo control. For evaluating the similarity of a biosimilar product to the innovator product, a clinical trial was conducted to compare the difference in efficacy between the biosimilar and the innovator product.

Let x_{ij} be some efficacy responses for the jth patient receiving the innovator product in the ith historical reference trial, $i = 1, ..., K$, and $j = 1, ..., m_i$, and y_{ij} the efficacy responses for the jth patient receiving the placebo control in the ith historical reference trial, $i = 1, ..., K$, and $j = 1, ..., n_i$. Assume that a higher score indicates better therapeutic efficacy and that both x_{ij}'s and y_{ij}'s are normally distributed for simplicity. Then the treatment group difference in means for the ith study is

$$w_i = \bar{x}_i - \bar{y}_i, \tag{6.27}$$

where $\bar{x}_i = 1/m_i \sum_{j=1}^{m_i} x_{ij}$ and $\bar{y}_i = 1/n_i \sum_{j=1}^{n_i} y_{ij}$ are the sample means of the m_i and n_i observations in the innovator product and the placebo group, respectively. With sufficient sample sizes, $w_i \sim N(\Delta, \sigma_i^2)$ is assumed approximately, that is, a normal distribution with mean Δ and variance σ_i^2, where the estimate of σ_i^2, $\hat{\sigma}_i^2 = s_i^2 ((1/m_i) + (1/n_i))$, and s_i is the estimate of standard deviation of the ith original trial, $i = 1, ..., K$. Here, Δ represents the true parameter of the treatment difference. Let $\mathbf{w} = (w_1, ..., w_K)$ be the results of the K reference studies.

Let x_{Br} and y_{Bs} be the efficacy responses for patients r and s receiving the biosimilar product and the placebo control, respectively, in the new trial conducted for evaluating biosimilarity, $r = 1, ..., m_B$, and $s = 1, ..., n_B$. Similar to Equation 6.27, let v be the treatment group difference between the means for the new trial. That is,

$$v = \bar{x}_B - \bar{y}_B,$$

where $\overline{x_B} = 1/m_B \sum_{r=1}^{m_B} x_{Br}$ and $\overline{y_B} = 1/n_B \sum_{s=1}^{n_B} y_{Bs}$. We are here to assess whether v can reasonably be thought of as in consistency with the K previous results. Similar to Tsou et al. (2011), we construct the predictive probability function, $p(v|w)$, which provides a measure of plausibility of v given the previous results w. In addition, we also construct $p(w_i|w)$, for $i = 1, ..., K$. We say that the result v is consistent with the reference result w if and only if

$$p(v|w) \geq \rho \min\{p(w_i|w), \quad i = 1, ..., k\}, \tag{6.28}$$

for some pre-specified $\rho > 0$. Here ρ represents the magnitude of the consistency trend. We assume $0.9 \leq \rho \leq 1$ or specify $\rho = 1$ because a biosimilar product is required to be "highly similar" to the reference product.

With a vague prior of $c\Delta$, the posterior probability density function (pdf) for Δ, given the reference set w, $p(\Delta|w)$, is given by

$$p(\Delta|w) \propto p(\Delta)l(\Delta|w)$$

$$\propto \exp\left\{-\frac{1}{2}\sum_{i=1}^{K}\frac{1}{\sigma_i^2}(\Delta - w_i)^2\right\}$$

$$\propto \exp\left\{-\frac{1}{2}\left(\sum_{i=1}^{K}\frac{1}{\sigma_i^2}\right)\left(\Delta - \frac{\sum_{i=1}^{K} w_i/\sigma_i^2}{\sum_{i=1}^{K} 1/\sigma_i^2}\right)^2\right\},$$

where $l(\Delta|w) = \prod_{i=1}^{K}(1/\sqrt{2\pi}\sigma_i)\exp\{-(1/2)(w_i - \Delta)^2/\sigma_i^2\}$ denotes the likelihood function. Consequently, $\Delta|w$ is normally distributed with mean $\overline{w}$ and variance Σ^2 where

$$\overline{w} = \frac{\sum_{i=1}^{K} w_i/\sigma_i^2}{\sum_{i=1}^{K} 1/\sigma_i^2}$$

and $\sum^2 = \left(\sum_{i=1}^{K} 1/\sigma_i^2\right)^{-1}$. That is, $\Delta|w \sim N(\overline{w}, \Sigma^2)$.

Assume the result v in the new trial is also asymptotically distributed as a normal distribution with mean C and variance σ_B^2. The estimate of σ_B^2 is $\hat{\sigma}_B^2 = s_B^2((1/m_B)+(1/n_B))$, where s_B is the estimate of standard deviation of the efficacy response in the new trial. The joint pdf for v and the mean parameter Δ, given w, is given by

$$p(v, \Delta \mid w) = p(v \mid \Delta, w)p(\Delta \mid w),\tag{6.29}$$

where

$p(v \mid w) = 1/\sqrt{2\pi\sigma_B} \exp\{-(1/2)(v - \Delta)^2/\sigma_B^2\}$ is the conditional pdf for v, given Δ and w

$p(\Delta \mid w)$ is the posterior pdf for Δ

By integrating Equation 6.29 with respect to Δ, the predictive probability density function (Aitchison and Dunsmore, 1975) can be represented by

$$p(v \mid w) = \int p(v, \Delta \mid w)d\Delta$$

$$= \int p(v, \Delta \mid w)p(\Delta \mid w)d\Delta$$

$$\propto \int \exp\left\{-\frac{1}{2}\left[\frac{1}{\sigma_B^2}(v - \Delta)^2 + \frac{1}{\sum^2}(\Delta - \bar{w})^2\right]\right\}d\Delta$$

$$\propto \int \exp\left\{-\frac{1}{2}\left[\left(\frac{1}{\sigma_B^2} + \frac{1}{\sum^2}\right)\left(\Delta - \frac{(v/\sigma_B^2) + \left(\bar{w}/\sum^2\right)}{(v/\sigma_B^2) + \left(1/\sum^2\right)}\right)^2\right.\right.$$

$$\left.\left. + \frac{1}{\sigma_B^2 + \sum^2}(v - \bar{w})^2\right]\right\}d\Delta$$

$$\propto \int \exp\left\{-\frac{1}{2\left(\sigma_B^2 + \sum^2\right)}(v - \bar{w})^2\right\}.$$

Consequently, we can derive that $v \mid w \sim N(\bar{w}, \tau_B^2)$ and $w_i \mid w \sim N(\bar{w}, \tau_i^2)$, where

$$\tau_B^2 = \sum\nolimits^2 + \sigma_B^2$$

and

$$\tau_B^2 = \sum\nolimits^2 + \sigma_i^2,$$

for $i = 1, \ldots, K$. The estimator of τ_B^2 is

$$\hat{\tau}_B^2 = \hat{\Sigma}^2 + \hat{\sigma}_B^2 = \left(\sum_{i=1}^{K} 1/\hat{\sigma}_B^2\right)^{-1} + s_B^2\left((1/m_B)+(1/n_B)\right)$$

and the estimator of τ_B^2 is

$$\hat{\tau}_B^2 = \hat{\Sigma}^2 + \hat{\sigma}_i^2 = \left(\sum_{i=1}^{K} 1/\hat{\sigma}_i^2\right)^{-1} + s_i^2\left((1/m_i)+(1/n_i)\right),$$

where the estimator of Σ^2 is

$$\hat{\Sigma}^2 = \left(\sum_{i=1}^{K} 1/\hat{\sigma}_i^2\right)^{-1}. \text{ Let } p_i = (1/\tau_i)\exp\left\{-(1/2\tau_i^2)(w_i - \bar{w})^2\right\}$$

and $p_0 = \min\{p_i, i = 1, \ldots, K\}$. Then the consistency criterion

$$p(v \,|\, w) \geq \rho \min\left\{p(w_i \,|\, w), \quad \text{for } i = 1, \ldots, K\right\}$$

holds if and only if

$$(v - \bar{w})^2 \leq -2\tau_B^2 \ln(\rho\tau_B p_0).$$

The proposed approach described in this chapter is to assess whether the comparative response of the biosimilar product to the placebo is consistent with the comparative response of the innovator product to the placebo. A simplified version of the proposed approach could be considered. It could be sufficient to compare directly the average response of the biosimilar product with the average response of the originator product from the study of the latter which deviates (after standardization) most from its average. Consequently, placebos may not be needed.

6.6.2 Response for Adverse Effects

The proposed approach could be applied to responses not only for therapeutic efficacy but also for adverse effects. Let x_{ij} be some responses for adverse effects for the jth patient receiving the innovator product in the ith historical reference trial, $i = 1, \ldots, K$ and $j = 1, \ldots, m_i$. Assume that the higher score indicates a more severe adverse effect of the tested drug. Here we want to compare directly the average response of the biosimilar product with the average response of the originator product without placebos in the trials. Using similar notation and assuming that x_{ij}'s are normally distributed, the sample mean of the m_i observations in the innovator product for the ith study is $w_i = 1/m \sum_{j=1}^{m_i} x_{ij}$. With sufficient sample sizes, $w_i \sim N(\Delta, \sigma_i^2)$ approximately, where the estimate of σ_i^2, $\hat{\sigma}_i^2 = s_i^2/m_i$, and s_i is the estimate of the standard deviation of the ith original trial, $i = 1, \ldots, K$. Let $w = (w_1, \ldots, w_K)$ be the results of the K reference studies. Similarly, let x_{Br} be the responses for adverse effects for patients r receiving the biosimilar product in the new trial conducted for evaluating the similarity of the biosimilar product, $r = 1, \ldots, m_B$. Let v be the sample means of the m_B observations for the new trial. That is, $v = 1/m_B \sum_{r=1}^{m_B} x_{Br}$. Our goal is to assess whether v can reasonably be thought of as being consistent with the K previous results. Similar to Section 2.1, we construct the predictive probability functions, $p(v|w)$ and $p(w_i|w)$, for $i = 1, \ldots, K$. Since the higher score indicates more a severe adverse effect of the tested drug in this case, we say that the result v is consistent with the reference result w if and only if

$$p(v \mid w) \leq \frac{1}{\rho} \max\left\{p(w_i \mid w), \quad i = 1, \ldots, K\right\},$$

for some pre-specified $0.9 \leq \rho \leq 1$ or specified $\rho = 1$. Similarly, it can be shown that the consistency criterion

$$p(v \mid w) \leq \frac{1}{\rho} \max\left\{p_1, p_2, \ldots, p_K\right\}$$

holds if and only if

$$(v - \bar{w})^2 \geq -2\tau_B^2 \ln\left(\tau_B \frac{p_{\max}}{\rho}\right),$$

where

$$\bar{w} = \frac{\sum_{i=1}^{K}(w_i/\sigma_i^2)}{\sum_{i=1}^{K}(1/\sigma_i^2)}$$

$$\Sigma^2 = \left(\sum_{i=1}^{K}\frac{1}{\sigma_i^2}\right)^{-1}$$

$$p_i = \frac{1}{\tau_i}\exp\left\{-\frac{1}{2\tau_i^2}(w_i - \bar{w})^2\right\}$$

$$p_{\max} = \max\left\{p_i, i = 1, \ldots, K\right\}$$

$$\tau_B^2 = \Sigma^2 + \sigma_B^2$$

$$\tau_i^2 = \Sigma^2 + \sigma_i^2, \quad \text{for } i = 1, \ldots, K$$

6.6.3 Sample Size Determination

In this section, we focus only on the response for therapeutic efficacy. For the determination of sample size for the new clinical trial, let n represent the numbers of patients studied per treatment group in the new trial. We assume that both efficacy responses for the test product and the placebo control for the new clinical trial are normally distributed with variance σ^2. At the design stage, we assume that σ^2 is known. Consequently, the treatment group difference in means v in the new clinical trial is also normally distributed with mean Δ and variance $\sigma_B^2 = 2\sigma^2/n$. Proceeding similarly, τ_B^2 in Section 6.2 will become

$$\tau_B^2 = \Sigma^2 + \sigma_B^2 = \left(\sum_{i=1}^{K} \frac{1}{\sigma_i^2}\right)^{-1} + \frac{2\sigma^2}{n}.$$

Again the consistency criterion

$$p(v\,|\,w) \geq \rho\min\{p(w_i\,|\,w), \quad \text{for } i = 1,\dots,K\}$$

holds if and only if

$$(v-\bar{w})^2 \leq -2\tau_B^2 \ln(\rho\tau_B p_0).$$

Let $R = \{v : (v-\bar{w})^2 \leq -2\tau_B^2 \ln(\rho\tau_B p_0)\}$ be the expanse of all consistent trials. Therefore, the cover of this consistency expanse can be expressed by the predictive probability

$$p(R) = \int_R p(v\,|\,w)\,dv$$

$$= p\{(v-\bar{w})^2 \leq -2\tau_B^2 \ln(\rho\tau_B p_0)\}$$

$$= p\left(\frac{-\sqrt{-2\tau_B^2 \ln(\rho\tau_B p_0)}}{\tau_B} \leq \frac{v-\bar{w}}{\tau_B} \leq \frac{\sqrt{-2\tau_B^2 \ln(\rho\tau_B p_0)}}{\tau_B}\right)$$

$$= 1 - 2\Phi\left(-\sqrt{-2\ln(\rho\tau_B p_0)}\right),$$

where $\Phi(\cdot)$ is the cumulative distribution function of standard normal distribution. The sample size per treatment group, n, is determined to ensure that the cover probability of consistency expanse be at least γ, say, for example, 80%. That is,

$$p(R) = 1 - 2\Phi\left(-\sqrt{-2\ln(\rho\tau_B p_0)}\right) \geq \gamma. \qquad (6.30)$$

As a result, Equation 6.30 holds if

$$\Phi\left(-\sqrt{-2\ln(\rho\tau_B p_0)}\right) \leq \frac{1-\gamma}{2}.$$

Therefore,

$$\tau_B \leq \frac{1}{\rho p_0} \exp\left\{-\frac{1}{2} Z^2_{1-\gamma/2}\right\}.$$

Then the sample size n can be determined by finding the smallest n such that

$$n \geq \frac{2\sigma^2}{(1/\rho p_0)^2 \exp\left\{-Z^2_{1-y/2}\right\} - \Sigma^2}. \qquad (6.31)$$

Note that the denominator may be negative. Our experience shows that the possibility of getting negative denominator can be reduced when $K \geq 2$.

6.7 Concluding Remarks

Biological products or medicines are therapeutic agents made of a living system or organism. As a number of biological products will be due to expire in the next few years, the potential opportunity for developing the follow-on products of these originator products may result in the reduction of these products and provide more choices to medical doctors and patients for getting similar treatment care with lower cost. However, the price reductions versus the originator biological products remain to be determined, as the advantage of a slightly cheaper price may be outweighed by the hypothetical increased risk of side effects from biosimilar molecules that are not exact copies of their originators. Unlike traditional, small-molecule drug products, the characteristics and development of biological products are more complicated and sensitive to many factors. Any small change in the manufacturing process may result in a change in the therapeutic effect of the biological products.

The traditional bioequivalence criterion for average bioequivalence of small-molecule drug products may not be suitable for the evaluation of biosimilarity of biological products. Therefore, in this chapter, we evaluate the biosimilar index proposed by Chow et al. (2011) for the assessment of the (average) biosimilarity between innovator and reference products. Both results based on the estimation and Bayesian approaches demonstrate that the proposed method based on the biosimilar index can reflect the characteristics and impact of variability on the therapeutic effect of biological products. However, the estimated reproducibility probability based on the Bayesian approach depends on the choice of the prior distributions. If a different prior such as an informative prior is used, a sensitivity analysis may be performed to evaluate the effects of different prior distributions.

The other advantage of the proposed method is that it can be applied to different functional areas (domains) of biological products such as PK, biological activities, biomarkers (e.g., pharmacodynamics), immunogenicity, manufacturing process, efficacy, etc., since it is developed based on the probability of reproducibility. Further research will be employed for the development of the statistical testing approach for the evaluation of biosimilarity across domains.

Current methods for the assessment of bioequivalence for drug products with identical active ingredients are not applicable to follow-on biologics due to fundamental differences. The assessment of biosimilarity between follow-on biologics and innovator products in terms of surrogate endpoints (e.g., PK parameters and/or pharmacodynamic responses) or biomarkers (e.g., genomic markers) requires the establishment of the Fundamental Biosimilarity Assumption in order to bridge the surrogate endpoints and/or biomarker data to clinical safety and efficacy.

Unlike conventional drug products, follow-on biologics are very sensitive to small changes in variation during the manufacturing process, which have been shown to have an impact on the clinical outcome. Thus, it is a concern whether current criteria and regulatory requirements for the assessment of bioequivalence for drugs with small-molecules can also be applied to the assessment of biosimilarity of follow-on biologics. It is suggested that current, existing criteria for the evaluation of bioequivalence, similarity, and biosimilarity be scientifically/statistically evaluated in order to choose the most appropriate approach for assessing biosimilarity of follow-on biologics. It is recommended that the selected biosimilarity criteria should be able to address (1) the sensitivity due to small variations in both location (bias) and scale (variability) parameters and (2) the degree of similarity, which can reflect the assurance for drug interchangeability.

Under the established Fundamental Biosimilarity Assumption and the selected biosimilarity criteria, it is also recommended that appropriate statistical methods (e.g., comparing distributions and the development of biosimilarity index) be developed under valid study designs (e.g., Design A and Design B described earlier) for achieving the study objectives (e.g., the establishment of biosimilarity at specific domains or drug interchangeability) with a desired statistical inference (e.g., power or confidence interval). To ensure the success of studies conducted for the assessment of biosimilarity of follow-on biologics, regulatory guidelines/guidances need to be developed. Product-specific guidelines/guidances published by the European Medicines Agency (EMA) have been criticized for not having standards. Although product-specific guidelines/guidances do not help to establish standards for the assessment of biosimilarity, they do provide the opportunity for accumulating valuable experience/information for establishing standards in the future. Thus, several numerical studies are recommended including simulations, meta-analysis, and/or sensitivity analysis, in order to (1) provide a better understanding of these product-specific guidelines/guidances and (2) check the validity of the Fundamental Biosimilarity Assumption, which is the legal basis for assessing μ'_T/μ'_R (original scale) biosimilarity of follow-on biologics.

7

Non-Inferiority versus Equivalence/Similarity

7.1 Background

In clinical research and development, the method of hypothesis testing is usually employed to test for the treatment effect of a test treatment under investigation. The purpose is not only to detect whether there is a treatment effect that is of clinical importance but also to assure that the detected treatment effect (or observed difference) is of statistical meaning (i.e., it has achieved statistical significance) in the sense that it is not by chance alone and is reproducible under the same experimental conditions. Commonly employed hypothesis testing includes testing for equality, testing for non-inferiority, testing for superiority, and testing for equivalence/similarity. Under a given, valid study design, sample sizes required for achieving the study objectives are different depending upon the hypotheses (i.e., equality, non-inferiority, superiority, and equivalence/similarity hypotheses) to be tested. In the following, whenever equivalence will be discussed, the similarity of two products will be equally considered.

For hypothesis testing in clinical investigation, the following questions are probably the most commonly asked by clinical scientists:

1. Is testing for non-inferiority equivalent to testing for equivalence?
2. What is the difference between the non-inferiority margin and equivalence limit?
3. What is the impact on sample size when switching hypotheses is tested?
4. What is the relationship among the hypotheses for testing non-inferiority, superiority, and/or equivalence?

In this chapter, we will make an attempt to address these questions. In the subsequent sections (Sections 7.2–7.5), hypotheses for testing equality, non-inferiority, superiority, and equivalence are described. The relationship among testing for non-inferiority, superiority, and equivalence is studied in Section 7.6. Section 7.7 examines the impact on sample size requirement when there is a switch of the hypotheses to be tested. Also included in this section is an example concerning a switch from testing equivalence to testing non-inferiority. Some concluding remarks are given in the last section.

7.2 Testing for Equality

In clinical investigations of a test treatment for treating patients with certain diseases, a commonly employed approach for the demonstration of the efficacy and safety of the test treatment is first to show that there is a difference between the test treatment and a control (e.g., placebo control) by testing the null hypothesis of no treatment difference. After the rejection of the null hypothesis of no treatment difference, the investigator is then to show that there is at least 80% power for correctly detecting a clinically meaningful difference if such a difference truly exists.

For testing the null hypothesis that there is no treatment difference (or testing for equality), statistical hypotheses can be formulated as follows:

$$H_0 : \mu_T = \mu_S \quad \text{vs.} \quad H_a : \mu_T \neq \mu_S, \tag{7.1}$$

where μ_T and μ_S are the means for the test treatment and the control (e.g., placebo control or standard of care), respectively. In practice, we would reject the null hypothesis in favor of the alternative hypothesis, and conclude that there is a treatment difference. Once we have rejected the null hypothesis of no treatment difference, we can then evaluate the power under the alternative hypothesis. The power is the probability of correctly detecting a difference when such a difference truly exists.

If we let $\delta = \mu_T - \mu_S$, then the aforementioned hypotheses can be rewritten as follows:

$$H_0 : \delta = 0 \quad \text{vs.} \quad H_a : \delta \neq 0. \tag{7.2}$$

In practice, δ may be referred to as a *statistical* difference if it has achieved statistical significance at a pre-specified level of significance (say 5%). In other words, a statistical difference is a difference which is not observed by chance alone. On the other hand, δ may be referred to as a *clinical* difference if it is of clinical importance.

In clinical trials, one of the controversial issues regarding hypothesis testing for equality is that both a statistical difference and a clinical difference

TABLE 7.1

Relationship between Statistical Difference
and Clinical Difference

		Clinical Difference	
		Yes	No
Statistical difference	Yes	No confusion	[a]
	No	[a]	No confusion

[a] Inconsistencies between clinical difference and statistical difference may be due to small sample size or large variability associated with the observations.

do not translate to each other. In practice, it is not uncommon to have the following situations: (1) the observed difference is of no clinical importance but has reached statistical significance and (2) the observed difference is of clinical importance and yet it does not reach statistical significance. To overcome this dilemma, a typical approach is to power the study by selecting an appropriate sample size for achieving a desired power to detect a clinically meaningful difference at a pre-specified level of significance (see, e.g., Chow et al., 2008). In other words, we power the study to detect a clinical difference (of clinical meaning) with statistical meaning (i.e., achieving statistical significance). The relationship between a statistical difference and a clinical difference is exhibited in Table 7.1.

The other controversial issue is the use of a one-sided test *versus* a two-sided test for detecting a clinical difference with statistical meaning. The alternative hypothesis under Equation 7.1 is two-sided in the sense that the mean of the test treatment could be either larger than or smaller than that of the control or standard of care. For a one-sided test, the significance level would be the same as the nominal level of significance, while the significance level would be half of the nominal level of significance for a two-sided test.

7.3 Testing for Non-Inferiority

Unlike testing for equality (i.e., no treatment difference), the purpose of testing for non-inferiority is to show that the test treatment is not inferior to or at least as effective as a standard therapy or an active agent. Situations where it is applicable are (1) the test treatment is less toxic, (2) the test treatment is easier to administer, (3) the test treatment is less expensive, and (4) the test treatment has other clinical benefits.

The null hypothesis is that the test treatment is inferior to the standard therapy, while the alternative hypothesis is that the test treatment is at least

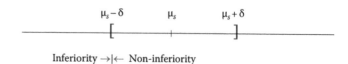

FIGURE 7.1
Testing for non-inferiority.

as effective as the standard care or therapy. Let $\mu_T > \mu_S$ indicate improvement. Thus, hypothesis testing for non-inferiority can be expressed as follows:

$$H_0 : \mu_T - \mu_S \leq -\delta \quad \text{vs.} \quad H_a : \mu_T - \mu_S > -\delta, \tag{7.3}$$

where $\delta > 0$ is the non-inferiority margin. To provide a better understanding, the concept of testing for non-inferiority is illustrated in Figure 7.1.

Statistically, we would like to reject the null hypothesis and conclude that the difference between the test drug and the standard therapy is less than a clinically meaningful difference (i.e., non-inferiority margin), and hence the test drug is as effective as the standard therapy.

One of the most controversial issues in non-inferiority trials is probably the selection of non-inferiority margin. A different choice of non-inferiority margin may affect the method of analyzing clinical data and consequently may alter the conclusion of the clinical study. As pointed out in the guideline by the International Conference on Harmonization (ICH), the determination of non-inferiority margins should be based on both statistical reasoning and clinical judgment (ICH, 2000). Despite the existence of some studies (e.g., Tsong et al., 1999; Hung et al., 2003; Laster and Johnson, 2003; Phillips, 2003; Chow and Shao, 2006), there is no established rule or gold standard for the determination of non-inferiority margins in active control trials until a recent draft guidance distributed by the U.S. Food and Drug Administration (FDA) for comments (FDA, 2010). The determination of non-inferiority margin will be discussed in Section 7.7.

7.4 Testing for Superiority

For testing superiority, the purpose is to show that the test drug is superior to a standard therapy or an active control agent, which has been approved by the regulatory agencies. The null hypothesis is that the test treatment is not superior to the standard therapy, while the alternative hypothesis is that the test treatment is superior to the standard therapy. Let $\mu_T > \mu_S$ indicate improvement of the test treatment as compared to the standard therapy. Thus, hypothesis testing for non-inferiority can be expressed as follows:

$$H_0 : \mu_T - \mu_S \leq \delta \quad \text{vs.} \quad H_a : \mu_T - \mu_S > \delta, \tag{7.4}$$

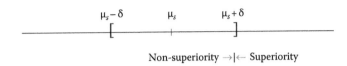

FIGURE 7.2
Testing for superiority.

where $\delta \geq 0$ is the superiority margin. When $\delta = 0$, the aforementioned hypotheses are to test for *statistical* superiority. On the other hand, when $\delta > 0$, it is referred to as hypotheses for testing *clinical* superiority. It should be noted that in some cases, non-inferiority margin need not be the same as the superiority margin (i.e., symmetric with respect to the treatment effect of the standard therapy). To provide a better understanding, the concept of testing for superiority is illustrated in Figure 7.2.

Similarly, the concept is to reject the null hypothesis and conclude that the test treatment is superior to the standard therapy; that is, the difference between the test treatment and the standard therapy is larger than a clinically meaningful difference (i.e., superiority margin), and hence the test treatment is superior to the standard therapy.

For investigation of a newly developed test treatment, hypothesis testing for clinical superiority of the test treatment over a placebo control is often employed. However, for active control trials comparing a test treatment and an active control agent (which has been approved by the regulatory agencies) or a standard therapy, hypothesis testing for both statistical ($\delta = 0$) or clinical ($\delta > 0$) superiority are usually not preferred by the regulatory agencies unless there is some strong evidence in clinical benefits (in terms of safety, efficacy, and risk benefits) of the test treatment under investigation. The endorsement of superiority of the test treatment by the regulatory agencies will force the approved active control agent to be withdrawn from the marketplace.

In practice, it is suggested that non-inferiority hypotheses be tested first. The superiority hypotheses can then be tested once non-inferiority has been established. In this case, we do not pay statistical penalty due to the closed testing procedure.

7.5 Testing for Equivalence

In clinical investigation, the purpose of testing for equivalence is to show that the test treatment can reach the same therapeutic effect as that of a standard therapy (or an active agent) or that they are therapeutically equivalent. In practice, situations in which equivalence is tested could involve (i) testing for therapeutic equivalence between a test treatment and a standard therapy

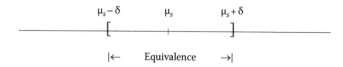

FIGURE 7.3
Testing for equivalence.

or an active control agent and (ii) testing for bioequivalence between an innovator drug product and its generic copies.

The null hypothesis is that the test treatment is not equivalent to the standard therapy, while the alternative hypothesis is that the test treatment is equivalent to the standard therapy. Let $\mu_T > \mu_S$ indicate improvement of the test treatment as compared to the standard therapy. Thus, hypothesis testing for equivalence can be expressed as follows:

$$H_0 : |\mu_T - \mu_S| \geq \delta \quad \text{vs.} \quad H_a : |\mu_T - \mu_S| < \delta, \tag{7.5}$$

where $\delta > 0$ is the equivalence limit. To provide a better understanding, the concept of testing for equivalence is illustrated in Figure 7.3.

The rejection of the null hypothesis suggests that there is no clinically meaningful difference between the test drug and the standard therapy and hence we conclude that the test drug is superior to the standard therapy.

Note that there is a slight difference between testing for therapeutic equivalence and testing for bioequivalence. Testing for therapeutic equivalence is often conducted based on a two-sided test at the 5% level of significance, while testing for bioequivalence is always conducted based on a two one-sided tests procedure at the 5% level of significance (FDA, 1988, 2003). In other words, the significance level used for testing therapeutic equivalence (based on a two-sided test) is 5%, while the significance level used for testing bioequivalence (based on two one-sided tests) is 10%. For further study regarding the relationship between testing for therapeutic equivalence and testing for bioequivalence, the note by Chow and Shao (2002) is helpful.

7.6 Relationship among Testing for Non-Inferiority, Superiority, and Equivalence

Figure 7.4 summarizes the relationship among different types of hypothesis testing including testing for non-inferiority, testing for superiority, and testing for equivalence. As can be seen from Figure 7.4, testing for non-inferiority

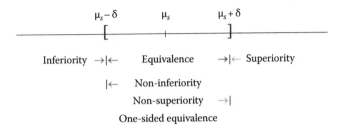

FIGURE 7.4
Relationship among testing for non-inferiority, superiority, and equivalence.

and testing for superiority (or non-superiority) are sometimes referred to as testing for one-sided equivalence.

Testing for non-inferiority includes testing for equivalence and testing for superiority. In other words, we may test for equivalence or test for superiority once the non-inferiority has been established. Thus, non-inferiority does not imply equivalence. It should be noted that testing for non-inferiority/superiority is often employed based on a one-sided test procedure at the 5% level of significance, which is equivalent to one of a two-sided test procedure at the 10% level of significance. Thus, it is suggested that a one-sided test procedure at the 2.5% level of significance, which is equivalent to a two-sided test procedure at the 5% level of significance, should be used for testing non-inferiority.

Similarly, testing for superiority includes testing for equivalence and testing for non-inferiority. In other words, we may test for equivalence or test for non-inferiority if we fail to reject the null hypothesis of non-superiority. It should also be noted that superiority does not imply equivalence. In practice, it is also suggested that a one-sided test procedure at the 2.5% level of significance should be used for testing superiority, which is equivalent to a two-sided test procedure at the 5% level of significance. To provide a better understanding of the relationship between testing for non-inferiority/superiority and equivalence, Figure 7.5 also provides the corresponding hypotheses underneath the figures. It should be noted that the hypotheses are derived assuming that $\mu_T - \mu_S > 0$ is considered an *improvement*. If $\mu_T - \mu_S > 0$ is considered *worsening*, the hypotheses need to be modified.

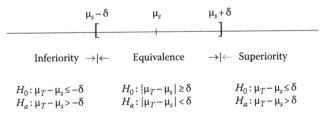

FIGURE 7.5
Hypotheses for testing non-inferiority, superiority, and equivalence.

7.7 Determination of the Non-Inferiority Margin

Let θ_T, θ_A, and θ_P be the unknown population efficacy parameters associated with the test therapy, the active control agent, and the placebo, respectively. Also, let $\Delta \geq 0$ be a non-inferiority margin. Without loss of generality, we assume that a large value of population efficacy parameter is desired. The hypotheses for non-inferiority can be formulated as

$$H_0 : \theta_T - \theta_A \leq -\Delta \quad \text{vs.} \quad H_a : \theta_T - \theta_A > -\Delta. \tag{7.6}$$

If Δ is a fixed pre-specified value, then standard statistical methods can be applied to testing Hypotheses 7.6. In practice, however, Δ is often unknown. There exists an approach that constructs the value of Δ based on a placebo-controlled historical trial. For example, $\Delta = a$ fraction of the lower limit of the 95% confidence interval for $\theta_A - \theta_P$ could be based on some historical trial data (see, e.g., CBER/FDA, 1999). Although this approach is intuitively conservative, it is not statistically valid because (1) if the lower confidence limit is treated as a fixed value, then the variability in historical data is ignored, and (2) if the lower confidence limit is treated as a statistic, then this approach violates the basic frequentist statistical principle, that is, the hypotheses being tested should not involve any estimates from current or past trials (Hung et al., 2003).

From the statistical point of view, the ICH E10 Guideline suggests that the non-inferiority margin Δ should be chosen to satisfy at least the following two criteria:

Criterion 1: We want the ability to claim that the test therapy is non-inferior to the active control agent and is superior to the placebo (even though the placebo is not considered in the active control trial).

Criterion 2: The non-inferiority margin should be suitably conservative, that is, variability should be taken into account.

A fixed Δ (i.e., if it does not depend on any parameter) is rarely suitable under criterion 1. Let $\delta > 0$ be a superiority margin if a placebo-controlled trial is conducted to establish the superiority of the test therapy over a placebo control. Since the active control is an established therapy, we may assume that $\theta_A - \theta_P > \delta$. However, when $\theta_T - \theta_A > -\Delta$ (i.e., the test therapy is non-inferior to the active control) for a fixed Δ, we cannot ensure that $\theta_T - \theta_P > \delta$ (i.e., the test therapy is superior to the placebo) unless $\Delta = 0$. Thus, it is reasonable to consider non-inferiority margins depending on unknown parameters. Hung et al. (2003) summarized the approach of using the non-inferiority margin of the form

$$\Delta = \gamma(\theta_A - \theta_P), \tag{7.7}$$

where γ is a fixed constant between 0 and 1. This is based on the idea of preserving a certain fraction of the active control effect $\theta_A - \theta_P$. The smaller $\theta_A - \theta_P$ is, the smaller Δ is. How to select the proportion of γ, however, was not discussed.

Chow and Shao (2006) derived a non-inferiority margin satisfying criterion 1. Let $\delta > 0$ be a superiority margin if a placebo control is added to the trial. Suppose that the non-inferiority margin Δ is proportional to δ, that is, $\Delta = r\delta$, where r is a known value chosen in the beginning of the trial. To be conservative, r should be ≤ 1. If the test therapy is not inferior to the active control agent and is superior over the placebo, then both

$$\theta_T - \theta_A > -\Delta \quad \text{and} \quad \theta_T - \theta_P > \delta \tag{7.8}$$

should hold. Under the worst scenario, that is, $\theta_T - \theta_A$ achieves its lower bound $-\Delta$, the largest possible Δ satisfying Equation 7.8 is given by

$$\Delta = \theta_A - \theta_P - \delta,$$

which leads to

$$\Delta = \frac{r}{1+r}(\theta_A - \theta_P). \tag{7.9}$$

From Equations 7.7 and 7.9, $\gamma = r/(r + 1)$. If $0 < r \leq 1$, then $0 < \gamma \leq 1/2$.

The previously described argument in determining Δ takes Criterion 1 into account, but is not conservative enough, since it does not consider the variability. Let $\hat{\theta}_T$ and $\hat{\theta}_P$ be sample estimators of θ_T and θ_P, respectively, based on data from a placebo-controlled trial. Assume that $\hat{\theta}_T - \hat{\theta}_P$ is normally distributed with mean $\theta_T - \theta_P$ and standard error SE_{T-P} (which is true under certain conditions or approximately true under the central limit theorem for large sample sizes). When $\theta_T = \theta_A - \Delta$,

$$P(\hat{\theta}_T - \hat{\theta}_P < \delta) = \Phi\left(\frac{\delta + \Delta - (\theta_A - \theta_P)}{SE_{T-P}}\right), \tag{7.10}$$

where Φ denotes the standard normal distribution function. If Δ is chosen according to Equation 7.9 and $\theta_T = \theta_A - \Delta$, then the probability that $\hat{\theta}_T - \hat{\theta}_P$ is less than δ is equal to 1/2. In view of Criterion 2, a value much smaller than 1/2 for this probability is desired, because it is the probability that the estimated test therapy effect is not superior over that of the placebo. Since the probability in Equation 7.10 is an increasing function of Δ, the smaller Δ (the more conservative choice of the non-inferiority margin) is, the smaller the chance that $\hat{\theta}_T - \hat{\theta}_P$ is less than δ. Setting the probability on the left-hand side of Equation 7.10 to ε with $0 < \varepsilon \leq 1/2$, we obtain that

$$\Delta = \theta_A - \theta_P - \delta - z_{1-\varepsilon}SE_{T-P},$$

where $z_a = \Phi^{-1}(a)$. Since $\delta = \Delta/r$, we obtain that

$$\Delta = \frac{r}{1+r}(\theta_A - \theta_P - z_{1-\varepsilon}SE_{T-P}). \tag{7.11}$$

Figure 7.6 provides an illustration for the selection of the non-inferiority margin according to this idea. Comparing Equations 7.7 and 7.11, we obtain that

$$\gamma = \frac{r}{1+r}\left(1 - \frac{z_{1-\varepsilon}SE_{T-P}}{\theta_A - \theta_P}\right),$$

that is, the proportion γ in Equation 7.7 is a decreasing function of a type of noise-to-signal ratio (or coefficient of variation).

The non-inferiority margin Equation 7.11 can also be derived from a slightly different point of view. Suppose that we actually conduct a placebo-controlled trial with superiority margin δ to establish the superiority of the

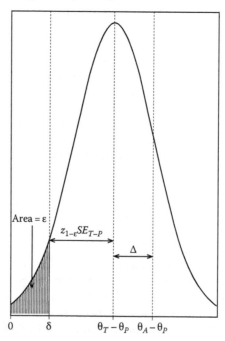

FIGURE 7.6

Selection of non-inferiority margin Δ (the solid curve is the probability density of $\hat{\theta}_T - \hat{\theta}_P$).

test therapy over the placebo. Then, the power of the large-sample *t*-test for hypotheses $\theta_T - \theta_P \leq \delta$ vs. $\theta_T - \theta_P > \delta$ is approximately equal to

$$\Phi\left(\frac{\theta_T - \theta_P - \delta}{SE_{T-P}} - z_{1-\alpha}\right),$$

where α is the level of significance. Assume the worst scenario $\hat{\theta}_T = \hat{\theta}_A - \Delta$ and that β is a given desired level of power. Then, setting the power to β leads to

$$\frac{\theta_A - \theta_P - \delta - \Delta}{SE_{T-P}} - z_{1-\alpha} = z_\beta,$$

$$\Delta = \frac{r}{1+r}\left[\theta_A - \theta_P - (z_{1-\alpha} + z_\beta)SE_{T-P}\right]. \tag{7.12}$$

Comparing Equations 7.11 with 7.12, we have $z_{1-\beta} = z_{1-\alpha} + z_\beta$. For $\alpha = 0.05$, the following table gives some examples with different values of β, ε, and $z_{1-\varepsilon}$ (Table 7.2). We now summarize the aforementioned discussions as follows:

1. The non-inferiority margin proposed by Chow and Shao (2006) given in Equation 7.12 takes variability into consideration; that is, Δ is a decreasing function of the standard error of $\hat{\theta}_T - \hat{\theta}_P$. It is an increasing function of the sample sizes, since SE_{T-P} decreases as sample sizes increase. Choosing a non-inferiority margin depending on the sample sizes does not violate the basic frequentist statistical principle. In fact, it cannot be avoided when variability of sample estimators is considered. Statistical analysis, including sample size calculation in the trial planning stage, can still be performed. In the limiting case ($SE_{T-P} \rightarrow 0$), the non-inferiority margin in Equation 7.12 is the same as that in Equation 7.10.

2. The ε value in Equation 7.12 represents a degree of conservativeness. An arbitrarily chosen ε may lead to highly conservative tests. When sample sizes are large (SE_{T-P} is small), one can afford a small ε. A reasonable value of ε and sample sizes can be determined in the planning stage of the trial.

TABLE 7.2

Various β, ε, and $z_{1-\varepsilon}$ for $\alpha = 0.05$

β	ε	$z_{1-\varepsilon}$
0.36	0.1000	1.282
0.50	0.0500	1.645
0.60	0.0290	1.897
0.70	0.0150	2.170
0.75	0.0101	2.320
0.80	0.0064	2.486

3. The non-inferiority margin in Equation 7.12 is non-negative if and only if $\theta_A - \theta_P \geq z_{1-\varepsilon} SE_{T-P}$; that is, the active control effect is substantial or the sample sizes are large. We might take our non-inferiority margin to be the larger of the quantity in Equation 7.12 and 0 to force the non-inferiority margin to be non-negative. However, it may be wise not to do so. Note that if θ_A is not substantially larger than θ_P, then non-inferiority testing is not justifiable since, even if $\Delta = 0$, concluding H_a does not imply the test therapy is superior to the placebo. Using Δ in Equation 7.12, testing hypotheses converts to testing the superiority of the test therapy over the active control agent when Δ is actually negative. In other words, when $\theta_A - \theta_P$ is smaller than a certain margin, our test automatically becomes a superiority test and the property $P(\hat{\theta}_T - \hat{\theta}_P < \delta) = \varepsilon$ (with $\delta = |\Delta|/r$) still holds.

4. In many applications, there are no historical data. In such cases parameters related to placebo are not estimable, and, hence, a non-inferiority margin not depending on these parameters is desired. Since the active control agent is a well-established therapy, let us assume that the power of the level α test showing that the active control agent is superior to placebo by the margin δ is at the level η. This means that approximately

$$\theta_A - \theta_P \geq \delta + (z_{1-\alpha} + z_\eta)SE_{A-P}.$$

Replacing $\theta_A - \theta_P - \delta$ in Equation 7.12 by its lower bound given in the previous expression, we obtain the non-inferiority margin

$$\Delta = (z_{1-\alpha} + z_\eta)SE_{A-P} - z_{1-\varepsilon}SE_{T-P}.$$

To use this non-inferiority margin, we need some information about the population variance of the placebo group. As an example, consider the parallel design with two treatments, the test therapy and the active control agent. Assume that the same two-group parallel design would have been used if a placebo-controlled trial had been conducted. Then $SE_{A-P} = \sqrt{\sigma_A^2/n_A + \sigma_P^2/n_P}$ and $SE_{T-P} = \sqrt{\sigma_T^2/n_T + \sigma_P^2/n_P}$, where σ_k^2 is the asymptotic variance for $\sqrt{n_k}(\hat{\theta}_k - \theta_k)$ and n_k is the sample size under treatment k. If we assume $\sigma_P/\sqrt{n_P} = c$, then

$$\Delta = (z_{1-\alpha} + z_\eta)\sqrt{\frac{\sigma_A^2}{n_A} + c^2} - z_{1-\varepsilon}\sqrt{\frac{\sigma_T^2}{n_T} + c^2}. \tag{7.13}$$

Formula 7.13 can be used in two ways. One way is to replace c in Formula 7.13 by an estimate. When no information from the placebo control is available, a suggested estimate of c is the smaller of the estimates of $\sigma_T/\sqrt{n_T}$ and $\sigma_A/\sqrt{n_A}$. The other way is to carry out a sensitivity analysis by using Δ in Formula 7.13 for a number of c values.

The 2010 FDA draft guidance defines two non-inferiority margins, namely, M_1 and M_2, where M_1 is defined as the entire effect of the active control assumed to be present in the non-inferiority study and M_2 is referred to as the largest clinically acceptable difference (degree of inferiority) of the test drug compared to the active control. As indicated in the 2010 FDA draft guidance, M_1 is based on (1) the treatment effect estimated from the historical experience with the active control drug, (2) the assessment of the likelihood that the current effect of the active control is similar to the past effect (the constancy assumption), and (3) the assessment of the quality of the non-inferiority trial, particularly looking for defects that could reduce a difference between the active control and the new drug. On the other hand, M_2 is a clinical judgment which can never be larger than M_1, even if for active control drugs with small effects, a clinical judgment might argue that a larger difference is not clinically important. Ruling out a difference between the active control and the test drug that is larger than M_1 is a critical finding that supports the conclusion of effectiveness.

7.8 Sample Size Requirement When There Is a Switch in Hypothesis Testing

In practice, it is not uncommon to switch from a superiority hypothesis to a non-inferiority hypothesis in order to increase the probability of success of the intended clinical trial. A typical approach is to test for non-inferiority and then test for superiority after the non-inferiority has been established. In this case, we do not have to pay for statistical penalty due to *closed* testing procedure. In some case, the investigator may switch from testing for equivalence to testing for non-inferiority (one-sided equivalence). The switch in hypotheses will have an impact on the sample size required for achieving study objectives at a desired power and at a pre-specified level of significance. In this section, a couple of examples are presented to illustrate the impact on sample size requirement when such a switch occurs.

7.8.1 Switch from Equivalence Hypotheses to Non-Inferiority/Superiority Hypotheses

As indicated in Chow et al. (2008), the problem of testing superiority and non-inferiority can be unified by the following hypotheses:

$$H_0 : \mu_T - \mu_S \leq \lambda \quad \text{vs.} \quad H_a : \mu_T - \mu_S > \lambda, \tag{7.14}$$

where λ is the superiority or non-inferiority margin. When $\lambda > 0$, the rejection of the null hypothesis indicates the superiority of test treatment over the standard therapy. When $\lambda < 0$, the rejection of the null hypothesis indicates the non-inferiority of the test treatment against the standard therapy. Thus, the sample size needed to achieve power $1 - \beta$ at the α level of significance can be obtained as follows:

$$n_1 = kn_2,$$

$$n_2 = \frac{(z_\alpha + z_\beta)^2 \sigma^2 (1 + (1/k))}{(\epsilon - \lambda)^2}, \tag{7.15}$$

where $k = n_1/n_2$, $\epsilon = \mu_T - \mu_S$, and σ is the standard deviation of the standard therapy. On the other hand, for testing equivalence, the sample size required to achieve the power $1 - \beta$ at the α level of significance is given by

$$n_1 = kn_2,$$

but

$$n_2 = \frac{(z_\alpha + z_\beta)^2 \sigma^2 (1 + (1/k))}{(\lambda - |\epsilon|)^2}. \tag{7.16}$$

Let $k = 1$ and assume that sample sizes in each treatment group are the same. Thus, the sample size requirement when switching from an equivalence hypothesis to a superiority hypothesis or a non-inferiority hypothesis can be evaluated by the following factor:

$$R = \left(\frac{z_\alpha + z_{\beta/2}}{z_\alpha + z_\beta} \right)^2 \left(\frac{\epsilon - \lambda}{\lambda - |\epsilon|} \right)^2, \tag{7.17}$$

where R is the ratio of Equations 7.15 and 7.16.

7.8.2 Example

Note that when $\epsilon = \mu_T - \mu_S = 0$, Equation 7.9 reduces to

$$R = \left(\frac{z_\alpha + z_{\beta/2}}{z_\alpha + z_\beta} \right)^2. \tag{7.18}$$

Based on Equation 7.18, the impact of a sample size requirement when switching from testing equivalence to testing non-inferiority can be evaluated. Table 7.3 summarizes the sample size reduction from testing equivalence to

TABLE 7.3

Sample Size Requirement when
Switching Equivalence Hypothesis
to Non-Inferiority Hypothesis

A	β	Power (%)	Sample Size Reduction (%)
0.10	0.1	90	23.3
	0.2	80	31.4
0.05	0.1	90	20.9
	0.2	80	27.8
0.01	0.1	90	17.5
	0.2	80	22.9

Note: α is the level of significance;
power $= (1 - \beta) \times 100\%$.

testing non-inferiority with various powers at several levels of significance. For example, there is a 27.8% sample size reduction if we switch from testing equivalence to testing non-inferiority for maintaining an 80% power at 5% level of significance.

7.8.3 Remarks

The impact on sample size requirement for a given switch in hypotheses under a valid study design for various data types (such as continuous, discrete or binary, or time-to-event data) can be similarly evaluated at different powers and levels of significance with respect to different variabilities associated with the observations.

7.9 Concluding Remarks

As indicated in Figures 7.1 through 7.4, testing for non-inferiority includes both testing for equivalence and testing for superiority. Testing for superiority does not imply testing for equivalence. Testing for non-inferiority has the opportunity to test for superiority after the non-inferiority has been established.

For testing non-inferiority/equivalence, the selection of non-inferiority margin/equivalence limit is the key to the success of clinical investigation. In comparative active control clinical trials, non-inferiority margin is the same as the equivalence limit. According to the ICH guideline, the non-inferiority margin should be both clinically and statistically justifiable. More specifically, the non-inferiority margin should be chosen in such a way that it is superior to the placebo control but non-inferior to the standard therapy or active control agent. For this purpose, the draft guidance by the FDA is useful. For testing bioequivalence/biosimilarity, however, the current bioequivalence limit in terms of the ratio of geometric means of the primary pharmacokinetic responses such as the area under the blood or plasma concentration–time curve (AUC) or the maximum concentration (C_{max}) is 80% to 125%, which is a one-size-fits-all criterion for all drug products.

Sample size requirements for testing non-inferiority and equivalence (similarity) are different. The impact on the sample size requirement when there is a switch in hypotheses to be tested depends upon the selected non-inferiority margin and the true difference between the test treatment and the standard therapy.

8

Statistical Test for Biosimilarity in Variability

8.1 Introduction

As indicated in Chapter 2, current regulatory requirements for assessment of bioequivalence focus on average bioavailability, which ignore the associated variability of bioavailability (FDA, 2003; Chen et al., 1996; Chow and Liu, 2008). It is a concern that standard methods for evaluation of small-molecule drug products may not be suitable for biological products due to some fundamental differences between small-molecule drug products and biological products (see, e.g., Fox, 2010). These fundamental differences include that (1) the biological products are made of living cells; (2) the biological products have heterogeneous structures, which are difficult to characterize; (3) the biological products are variable and sensitive to certain conditions such as pH, light, and temperature; and (4) the biological products are usually injected and prescribed by specialists. In practice, large variability is often more likely to occur during the manufacturing process of biological products than that of the traditional small-molecules due to variability in the biologic mechanisms, inputs, and relatively large number of complex steps in the process. Variability in the products could lead to lower efficacy or potential safety risks for some patients, and have a significant impact on clinical outcomes of follow-on biologics (FOBs). Therefore, incorporating variance equivalence assessments should be an important part of determining biosimilarity between biological products.

The manufacturing process of a biological products usually involves five steps of cell expansion, cell production, recovery (through filtration or centrifugation), purification, and formulation, which is a very complicated process. A small variation which occurs at each step may lead to structure difference in the final product, and consequently result in differences in efficacy and safety of the biological products. As a result, in addition to the assessment of average biosimilarity, Chow et al. (2010a) indicated that the statistical methodology for comparing the variabilities should be developed for assessing biosimilarity between biological products as the variability has a significant impact on clinical performance of FOBs. Under a crossover design, the classical Pitman–Morgan's adjusted F-test is usually considered. Yang et al. (2013) proposed an F-type test for testing homogeneity of variances of FOBs. The F-type test, however, is known to be sensitive to the normality of the underlying assumption of population distribution. When the distributions are non-normal, the actual size of the test can be much higher than the assumed level of significance. Thus, Zhang et al. (2013) considered two types of non-parametric methods for comparing variabilities between biosimilar products, which include the Conover's squared ranks test (Conover, 1973, 1999) and Levene's type of tests (Levene, 1960; Brown and Forsythe, 1974). Alternatively, Hsieh et al. (2010) considered an approach for comparing variabilities between biosimilar products based on the probability-based criterion, following the idea of Tse et al. (2006) for evaluating average biosimilarity between FOBs. The comparison was also made for comparing the relative performance of moment-based method and probability-based method in average bioequivalence. The results indicated that the probability-based criterion is not only a much more stringent criterion but also sensitive to any small change in variability. This justified the use of a statistical method for evaluating biosimilarity in variability of biological products.

In the next two sections, the classical Pitman–Morgan's test for assessment of bioequivalence of small-molecule drugs under a crossover design and an F-type test for testing homogeneity of variances of FOBs under a parallel-group design are briefly introduced. Two types of non-parametric tests are described in Section 8.3. Also included in this section are some simulation studies for evaluation of the relative performances of the methods. Section 8.4 discusses probability-based criterion and its corresponding statistical hypotheses. Also included in this section are the corresponding statistical testing procedures proposed by Hsieh et al. (2010). The numerical study is also employed to investigate the relationship between the probability-based criterion in variability and various combinations of the essential parameters. Some concluding remarks and recommendation are given in the last section.

8.2 Pitman–Morgan's Adjusted Test for Comparing Variabilities

In bioavailability and bioequivalence studies, the most commonly used test for equality of variabilities under a crossover design is probably the so-called Pitman–Morgan's adjusted F-test. Let Y_T and Y_R be the parameters of interest (e.g., pharmacokinetic responses) for the test (T) product and the reference (R) product with means μ_T and μ_R, and variances V_T and V_R, respectively. The hypothesis for testing equality of variabilities of the two products can be expressed as

$$H_0 : V_T = V_R \quad \text{vs.} \quad H_a : V_T \neq V_R.$$

To test the hypothesis, let's denote independent samples observed on subject i from sequence k as (Y_{iTk}, Y_{iRk}) from a crossover study with $i = 1, \ldots, n_k$ and $k = 1, 2$. Pitman (1939) and Morgan (1939) proposed a test statistic based on the correlation between the crossover differences and the subject totals, which can be expressed as

$$F_{PM} = \frac{(n_1 + n_2 - 2)(F_{TR} - 1)^2}{4 F_{TR}(1 - r_{TR}^2)},$$

where $F_{TR} = S_{TT}^2 / S_{RR}^2$, $r_{TR} = S_{TR}/S_{TT}S_{RR}$ and S_{TT}^2, S_{RR}^2, and S_{TR} are the sample variances and covariance of Y_{iTk} and Y_{iRk}. On the other hand, if one is interested in testing equivalence between variabilities between drug products, the hypotheses for testing equivalence between variabilities can be expressed as

$$H_0 : \theta_L \geq \frac{V_T}{V_R} \quad \text{or} \quad \theta_U \leq \frac{V_T}{V_R} \quad \text{vs.} \quad H_a : \theta_L < \frac{V_T}{V_R} < \theta_U, \tag{8.1}$$

where (θ_L, θ_U) is the biosimilarity margin for the ratio of variances. It can be decomposed into two one-sided hypotheses as

$$H_{01} : \theta_L \geq \frac{V_T}{V_R} \quad \text{vs.} \quad H_{a1} : \theta_L < \frac{V_T}{V_R}$$

$$H_{02} : \theta_U \leq \frac{V_T}{V_R} \quad \text{vs.} \quad H_{a2} : \theta_U > \frac{V_T}{V_R} \tag{8.2}$$

or

$$H_{01} : \theta_L V_R \geq V_T \quad \text{vs.} \quad H_{a1} : \theta_L V_R < V_T$$

$$H_{02} : \theta_U V_R \leq V_T \quad \text{vs.} \quad H_{a2} : \theta_U V_R > V_T,$$

given that V_T and V_R are always positive. To test the two one-sided hypotheses, Liu and Chow (1992) extended the idea of Pitman–Morgan's adjusted

F-test by defining the pairs of $(Y_{iTk}, \theta_L Y_{iRk})$ and $(Y_{iTk}, \theta_U Y_{iRk})$. The test statistics are then calculated similarly using the pairs as

$$F_{PML} = \frac{(n_1 + n_2 - 3)[S_{TT}^2 - \theta_L S_{RR}^2 + (\theta_L - 1)S_{TR}]^2}{(\theta_L + 1)^2 (S_{TT}^2 S_{RR}^2 - S_{TR}^2)}$$

and

$$F_{PMU} = \frac{(n_1 + n_2 - 3)[S_{TT}^2 - \theta_U S_{RR}^2 + (\theta_U - 1)S_{TR}]^2}{(\theta_U + 1)^2 (S_{TT}^2 S_{RR}^2 - S_{TR}^2)}.$$

8.3 *F*-Type Test under Parallel Design

The Pitman–Morgan's test for comparing variabilities described in the previous section was derived under a crossover design. For assessment of biosimilar products, a parallel design is often recommended due to the fact that most biological products have relatively long half-lives. Therefore, statistical test for evaluation of the similarity in variability between biosimilar products under a parallel design is needed. For this purpose, Yang et al. (2013) applied similar idea to the two-sample F-test of equal variance to measure equivalence in variability under a parallel design. The test is described in the following text.

Consider a parallel design for evaluating the biosimilarity in variability of the test product with the reference product. Let's denote independent samples of T_i and R_j as the observations of T and R with $i = 1, \ldots, n_T$ and $j = 1, \ldots, n_R$. To test the two one-sided hypotheses

$$H_{01} : \theta_L \geq \frac{V_T}{V_R} \quad \text{vs.} \quad H_{\alpha 1} : \theta_L < \frac{V_T}{V_R}$$

$$H_{02} : \theta_U \leq \frac{V_T}{V_R} \quad \text{vs.} \quad H_{\alpha 2} : \theta_U > \frac{V_T}{V_R}$$

in the extended F-test procedure, we define

$$\begin{cases} L_j = \sqrt{\theta_L}\, R_j, & j = 1, \ldots, n_R \\ U_j = \sqrt{\theta_U}\, R_j, & j = 1, \ldots, n_R \end{cases} \tag{8.3}$$

so that $\text{Var}(L_j) \equiv V_L = \theta_L V_R$ and $\text{Var}(U_j) \equiv V_U = \theta_U V_R$. Then, the hypotheses are equivalent to

$$H_{01} : V_L \geq V_T \quad \text{vs.} \quad H_{\alpha 1} : V_L < V_T$$

$$H_{02} : V_U \leq V_T \quad \text{vs.} \quad H_{\alpha 2} : V_U > V_T.$$

Apply the one-sided F-test for equal variances. H_{01} is rejected at the α level of significance if

$$F_L = \frac{\sum_{i=1}^{n_T} (T_i - \bar{T})^2/(n_T - 1)}{\sum_{j=1}^{n_R} (L_j - \bar{L})^2/(n_R - 1)} = \frac{s_T^2}{s_L^2} > F(\alpha; n_T - 1, n_R - 1),$$

and H_{02} is rejected if

$$F_U = \frac{\sum_{i=1}^{n_T} (T_i - \bar{T})^2/(n_T - 1)}{\sum_{j=1}^{n_R} (U_j - \bar{U})^2/(n_R - 1)} = \frac{s_T^2}{s_U^2} < F(1 - \alpha; n_T - 1, n_R - 1).$$

We then conclude that V_T and V_R are equivalent with significance level of α if both H_{01} and H_{02} are rejected.

8.4 Non-Parametrics Methods

Under normality assumption, the extended F-test described earlier is expected to be the most powerful test. However, when the distributions are non-normal, the actual size of the F-test can be much higher than the assumed level of significance. Therefore, Zhang et al. (2013) consider two non-parametric tests for evaluation of biosimilarity in variability between FOBs. One is the squared rank type of test (Conover, 1999) and the other one is based on Levene's type of test (Levene, 1960). These are distribution-free tests and hopefully will overcome the difficulty of extended F-test when the underlying population distribution is non-normal.

8.4.1 Conover's Squared Rank Test

When the normality assumption of T and R is not true, the first non-parametric test we considered is the squared rank test proposed by Conover (1980). It is a powerful non-parametric test for equality of variances based on joint ranks of $(T_i - \bar{T})^2$, $i = 1, \ldots, n_T$, and $(R_j - \bar{R})^2$, $j = 1, \ldots, n_R$. In practice, we do not need to square the deviations to obtain the required rankings because the same order is achieved by ranking the absolute deviations. Therefore, let's denote $u_i(T) = $ rank of $|T_i - \bar{T}|$ and $u_j(R) = $ rank of $|R_j - \bar{R}|$. Then the test statistic is as follows

$$Z_{calc} = \frac{\sum_{i=1}^{n_T} [u_i(T)]^2 - n_T \bar{u}}{s}, \tag{8.4}$$

where

$$\bar{u} = \frac{1}{n_T + n_R} \left(\sum_{i=1}^{n_T} [u_i(T)]^2 + \sum_{j=1}^{n_R} [u_j(R)]^2 \right)$$

$$s = \sqrt{\frac{n_T n_R \left(\sum_{i=1}^{n_T} [u_i(T)]^4 + \sum_{j=1}^{n_R} [u_j(R)]^4 - (n_T + n_R)\bar{u}^2 \right)}{(n_T + n_R)(n_T + n_R - 1)}}.$$

Quantiles of the exact distribution of $\sum_{i=1}^{n_T} [u_i(T)]^2 \equiv$ sum of squared ranks in one sample and a large sample approximation are given in Table A9 of Conover's book (1999). But for reasonably large sample sizes, Z is approximately a standard normal distribution. Therefore, for a one-sided level α test of

$$H_0 : V_R = V_T \quad \text{vs.} \quad H_\alpha : V_R < V_T,$$

we reject the null hypothesis if $Z_{calc} > Z(\alpha)$, where $Z(\alpha)$ is the α upper quantile of the standard normal distribution. For a one-sided level α test,

$$H_0 : V_R = V_T \quad \text{vs.} \quad H_\alpha : V_R > V_T,$$

we reject null hypothesis if $Z_{calc} < Z(1 - \alpha)$. To test the biosimilarity of variability as expressed in Equation 8.2, we again define L_j and U_j as in Equation 8.3 so that $V_L = \theta_L V_R$ and $V_U = \theta_U V_R$. Then the Hypothesis 8.2 is equivalent to

$$H_{01} : V_L \geq V_T \quad \text{vs.} \quad H_{\alpha 1} : V_L < V_T$$

$$H_{02} : V_U \leq V_T \quad \text{vs.} \quad H_{\alpha 2} : V_U > V_T.$$

H_{01} is then rejected at the α level of significance if $Z_{calc,L} > Z(\alpha)$; and H_{02} is rejected if $Z_{calc,U} < Z(1 - \alpha)$, where $Z_{calc,L}$ and $Z_{calc,U}$ are calculated as in Equation 8.4 with (T_i, L_j) and (T_i, U_j), respectively. We conclude that V_T and V_R are equivalent with significance level of α if both H_{01} and H_{02} are rejected.

8.4.2 Levene's Type of Test

Another non-parametric test is the Levene's type of test initiated by Levene (1960). The original Levene's test considers the hypothesis of

$$H_0 : V_T = V_R \quad \text{vs.} \quad H_\alpha : V_T \neq V_R.$$

The test statistic is defined as

$$W = \frac{(n_T + n_R - 2)[n_T(\bar{Z}_T - \bar{Z})^2 + n_R(\bar{Z}_R - \bar{Z})^2]}{\sum_{i=1}^{n_T}(Z_{Ti} - \bar{Z}_T)^2 + \sum_{j=1}^{n_R}(Z_{Rj} - \bar{Z}_R)^2}, \tag{8.5}$$

where Z_{Ti} and Z_{Rj} can have one of the following three definitions based on different centrality parameters used:

1. $Z_{Ti} = |T_i - \bar{T}|$ and $Z_{Rj} = |R_j - \bar{R}|$ where $\bar{T}$ and $\bar{R}$ are the means of each treatment group.
2. $Z_{Ti} = |T_i - \tilde{T}|$ and $Z_{Rj} = |R_j - \tilde{R}|$ where $\tilde{T}$ and $\tilde{R}$ are the medians of each treatment group. When median is used, it is actually the Brown–Forsythe Levene's type of test.
3. $Z_{Ti} = |T_i - \bar{T}'|$ and $Z_{Rj} = |R_j - \bar{R}'|$ where $\bar{T}'$ and $\bar{R}'$ are the trimmed means of each treatment group.

$\bar{Z}_T$ and $\bar{Z}_R$ are the group means of Z_{Ti} and Z_{Rj}, respectively; and $\bar{Z}$ is the overall mean of all Z_{Ti} and Z_{Rj}.

The Levene test rejects the hypothesis that variances are equal if $W > F(\alpha; 1, n_T + n_R - 2)$, where $F(\alpha; 1, n_T + n_R - 2)$ is the upper critical value of the F distribution with the specified degrees of freedom at a significance level of α.

Levene's test constructed the test statistic as F distribution, which generally doesn't distinguish direction of the alternative. However, in the case of two samples, such a test is equivalent to the t-test. Therefore, we are able to extend the Levene's test to the two one-sided hypotheses testing when comparing the FOB with reference drug where only two groups are involved. That is, we construct

$$t_L = \sqrt{W_L},$$

where W_L is the Levene's test statistic obtained from comparing T_i and L_j and

$$t_U = \sqrt{W_U},$$

where W_U is the Levene's test statistic obtained from comparing T_i and U_j

H_{01} is then rejected at the α level of significance if $t_L > t(\alpha; n_T + n_R - 2)$; and H_{02} is rejected if $t_U < t(1 - \alpha; n_T + n_R - 2)$. We conclude that V_T and V_R are equivalent with significance level of α if both H_{01} and H_{02} are rejected.

8.4.3 Simulation Studies

In order to compare the performance of the two types of non-parametric tests with the extended F-test under a parallel design, Zhang et al. (2013) conducted several simulation studies in terms of (1) type I error rate, which is the maximum of the probability of concluding biosimilarity when variance ratio is less than or equal to θ_L or is greater than or equal to θ_U, and (2) power, which is the probability of correctly concluding biosimilarity when variance ratio is close to 1.

Simulation studies were conducted under various settings. Each setting contains 10,000 repetitions, and each repetition consists of random samplings from a particular distribution of reference group and from treatment group which has the same distribution family as the reference group but different variances. Then the test statistics from extended F-test, Conover's test, and Levene's test with mean are calculated from each repetition and the number of times rejecting null hypothesis (i.e., concluding biosimilarity) using different biosimilarity margins of (θ_L, θ_U) from the 10,000 repetitions are recorded for comparison in terms of power or type I error.

The distributions explored here are the Normal distributions, t distributions, Laplace distributions, Chi-square distributions, Weibull distributions, and zero-inflated Poisson distribution. The sample sizes used are 50 (not shown here) and 100 for each group, and the biosimilarity margins tested are $(\theta_L, \theta_U) = (0.5, 2); (0.5, 1.5); (0.67, 1.5)$ (not shown here). The simulation results are summarized in Tables 8.1 through 8.7.

In the first set of simulations, Normal distribution is used. The extended F-test performed the best as expected. The proposed non-parametric tests are less powerful but the relative efficiency is reasonably good. For example, when biosimilarity margin (0.5, 2) is used, the relative power between Conover's and extended F-test is $0.8172/0.9251 = 88\%$; and is $0.88/0.9251 = 95\%$ between Levene's and extended F-test. The type I error is well controlled by all three tests (0.0527, 0.0511, and 0.0533 from extended F-test, Conover's, and Levene's tests, respectively). When narrowing the biosimilarity margin from (0.5, 2) to (0.5, 1.5), the probability of concluding biosimilar drops quickly, where Levene's test is still relatively comparable to the extended F-test. When the biosimilarity margin of (0.67, 1.5) is used, the probability of concluding biosimilar drops dramatically and close to 0 in most cases even when the two groups are the same.

From Table 8.2 where central t distribution is used, surprisingly none of the tests is sensitive to changes in variance ratio. Further investigation is needed to understand why and to find tests that are suitable for such cases. However, at least one message is even with such small deviation from Normal distribution, the tests could fail to show the robustness.

TABLE 8.1

Normal Distribution with Sample Size = 100

Reference Group	Test Group	Variance Ratio	Biosimilarity Margin = (0.5, 2)			Biosimilarity Margin = (0.5, 1.5)		
			Conover's Test	F-Test	Levene's Test	Conover's Test	F-Test	Levene's Test
N(100, 100)	N(100, 25)	0.25	0	0	0	0	0	0
N(100, 100)	N(100, 50)	0.50	0.0511	0.0473	0.0511	0.0547	0.0516	0.0552
N(100, 100)	N(100, 67)	0.67	0.352	0.4259	0.3893	0.3203	0.4138	0.3684
N(100, 100)	N(100, 75)	0.75	0.5407	0.6397	0.591	0.4479	0.6044	0.5318
N(100, 100)	N(100, 80)	0.80	0.6438	0.7619	0.7002	0.5121	0.6893	0.6038
N(100, 100)	N(100, 100)	1.00	0.8172	0.9251	0.88	0.4519	0.6082	0.535
N(100, 100)	N(100, 125)	1.25	0.6366	0.7538	0.6947	0.1823	0.2244	0.2028
N(100, 100)	N(100, 133)	1.33	0.5333	0.6398	0.5917	0.1247	0.147	0.1333
N(100, 100)	N(100, 150)	1.50	0.3355	0.4053	0.3698	0.0498	0.0498	0.0491
N(100, 100)	N(100, 200)	2.00	0.0501	0.0527	0.0533	0.0019	0.0013	0.0015
N(100, 100)	N(100, 400)	4.00	0	0	0	0	0	0

TABLE 8.2

Central t Distribution with Sample Size = 100

Reference Group d.f.	Test Group d.f.	Variance Ratio	Biosimilarity Margin = (0.5, 2)			Biosimilarity Margin = (0.5, 1.5)		
			Conover's Test	F-Test	Levene's Test	Conover's Test	F-Test	Levene's Test
4	7.882353	0.67	0.6018	0.5116	0.5297	0.3474	0.4365	0.3583
4	6	0.75	0.6262	0.5943	0.5863	0.3344	0.4728	0.3376
4	5.333333	0.8	0.6400	0.6409	0.6059	0.3180	0.4676	0.3260
4	4.5	0.9	0.6409	0.6687	0.6138	0.2860	0.4424	0.2769
4	4	1	0.6266	0.6585	0.5957	0.2577	0.4084	0.2415
4	3.666667	1.1	0.6185	0.6315	0.5690	0.2313	0.3640	0.2000
4	3.333333	1.25	0.5965	0.5889	0.5274	0.2042	0.3115	0.1606
4	3.204819	1.33	0.5784	0.5525	0.4943	0.1953	0.2884	0.1449
4	3	1.5	0.5425	0.5000	0.4399	0.1731	0.2432	0.1229
4	2.666667	2	0.5049	0.3941	0.3407	0.1352	0.1735	0.0753
4	2.285714	4	0.3888	0.2329	0.1903	0.0796	0.0835	0.0319

Note: d.f., degrees of freedom.

TABLE 8.3

Simulation: Laplace Distribution (Lap(μ,b)) with Sample Size = 100 where μ Is the Location Parameter and b Is the Dispersion Parameter

Reference Group	Test Group	Variance Ratio	Biosimilarity Margin = (0.5, 2)			Biosimilarity Margin = (0.5, 1.5)		
			Conover's Test	F-Test	Levene's Test	Conover's Test	F-Test	Levene's Test
Lap(10, 2)	Lap(10, 1)	0.25	0	5.00E−04	0	0	7.00E−04	0
Lap(10, 2)	Lap(10, 1.4142)	0.5	0.053	0.1425	0.0524	0.0271	0.1372	0.0362
Lap(10, 2)	Lap(10, 1.6371)	0.67	0.2274	0.4375	0.2577	0.0951	0.3756	0.1541
Lap(10, 2)	Lap(10, 1.7321)	0.75	0.3236	0.5731	0.3796	0.1180	0.4698	0.2008
Lap(10, 2)	Lap(10, 1.7889)	0.8	0.3708	0.6434	0.4487	0.1358	0.5013	0.2262
Lap(10, 2)	Lap(10, 2)	1	0.4722	0.7509	0.5743	0.1285	0.4653	0.2091
Lap(10, 2)	Lap(10, 2.2361)	1.25	0.3873	0.6358	0.4526	0.0704	0.2828	0.1097
Lap(10, 2)	Lap(10, 2.3065)	1.33	0.3247	0.5787	0.3817	0.0572	0.2328	0.0812
Lap(10, 2)	Lap(10, 2.4495)	1.5	0.2160	0.4329	0.2501	0.0269	0.1361	0.0394
Lap(10, 2)	Lap(10, 2.8284)	2	0.0491	0.1436	0.0512	0.0041	0.0238	0.0042
Lap(10, 2)	Lap(10, 4)	4	0	7.00E−04	0	0	0	0

TABLE 8.4

Chi-Square Distribution with Sample Size = 100

Reference Group d.f.	Test Group d.f.	Variance Ratio	Biosimilarity Margin = (0.5, 2)				Biosimilarity Margin = (0.5, 1.5)			
			Conover's Test	F-Test	Levene's Test		Conover's Test	F-Test	Levene's Test
4	1	0.25	1.00E–04	0.0067	1.00E–04		0	0.0064	1.00E–04
4	2	0.50	0.0529	0.1709	0.0570		0.0452	0.1507	0.0470
4	3	0.75	0.5126	0.5535	0.4509		0.4393	0.4587	0.3359
4	4	1.00	0.7840	0.7517	0.7095		0.4744	0.4664	0.3690
4	5	1.25	0.6154	0.6466	0.5749		0.2270	0.2885	0.1892
4	6	1.50	0.3337	0.4291	0.3176		0.0583	0.1224	0.0575
4	8	2.00	0.0524	0.1226	0.0564		0.0046	0.0163	0.0054
4	16	4.00	0	0	0		0	0	0

Note: degrees of freedom

TABLE 8.5

Weibull Distribution ($W(\lambda, \kappa)$) with Sample Size = 100 where λ Is the Scale Parameter and κ Is the Shape Parameter

Reference Group	Test Group	Variance Ratio	Biosimilarity Margin = (0.5, 2)			Biosimilarity Margin = (0.5, 1.5)		
			Conover's Test	F-Test	Levene's Test	Conover's Test	F-Test	Levene's Test
W(10, 30)	W(5, 30)	0.25	0	1.00E-04	0	1.00E-04	0	0
W(10, 30)	W(6, 30)	0.36	0.0038	0.0072	0.0033	0.0036	0.0069	0.003
W(10, 30)	W(7, 30)	0.49	0.0599	0.0918	0.0564	0.0582	0.0882	0.0525
W(10, 30)	W(8, 30)	0.64	0.3006	0.3724	0.2943	0.2714	0.3550	0.2680
W(10, 30)	W(9, 30)	0.81	0.6296	0.6924	0.6364	0.4677	0.5671	0.4769
W(10, 30)	W(10, 30)	1	0.7639	0.8222	0.7757	0.4236	0.5266	0.4327
W(10, 30)	W(11, 30)	1.21	0.6509	0.7173	0.6550	0.2357	0.3146	0.2355
W(10, 30)	W(12, 30)	1.44	0.4197	0.4931	0.4149	0.0926	0.1377	0.0864
W(10, 30)	W(13, 30)	1.69	0.2065	0.2612	0.1950	0.0288	0.0463	0.0259
W(10, 30)	W(14, 30)	1.96	0.0827	0.1183	0.0767	0.0061	0.0109	0.0045
W(10, 30)	W(15, 30)	2.25	0.0293	0.0456	0.0239	0.0011	0.0028	0.001

TABLE 8.6

Weibull Distribution ($W(\lambda,\kappa)$) with Sample Size = 100 where λ Is the Scale Parameter and κ Is the Shape Parameter

Reference Group	Test Group	Variance Ratio	Biosimilarity Margin = (0.5, 2)			Biosimilarity Margin = (0.5, 1.5)		
			Conover's Test	F-Test	Levene's Test	Conover's Test	F-Test	Levene's Test
W(10, 30)	W(9.9109, 60.7)	0.25	0	0	0	0	1.00E-04	0
W(10, 30)	W(9.9448, 42.7)	0.50	0.0692	0.1066	0.0642	0.0658	0.1110	0.0628
W(10, 30)	W(9.9667, 36.8)	0.67	0.3626	0.4444	0.3613	0.3148	0.4015	0.3136
W(10, 30)	W(9.9630, 34.7)	0.75	0.5275	0.6065	0.5278	0.4208	0.5210	0.4251
W(10, 30)	W(9.9749, 33.6)	0.80	0.6145	0.6800	0.6171	0.4567	0.5579	0.4657
W(10, 30)	W(10, 30)	1.00	0.7619	0.8248	0.7771	0.4246	0.5185	0.4275
W(10, 30)	W(10.0170, 26.75)	1.25	0.6085	0.6829	0.6183	0.2048	0.2778	0.2067
W(10, 30)	W(10.0187, 25.9)	1.33	0.5257	0.6018	0.5307	0.1438	0.2001	0.1389
W(10, 30)	W(10.0318, 24.35)	1.50	0.3454	0.4321	0.3495	0.0645	0.1034	0.0622
W(10, 30)	W(10.0658, 21)	2.00	0.0663	0.1038	0.0630	0.0042	0.0086	0.0033
W(10, 30)	W(10.1736, 14.67)	4.00	0	2.00E-04	0	0	0	0

TABLE 8.7

Zero-Inflated Poisson Distribution (ZIP(λ, p_0)) with Sample Size = 100 where λ Is the Poisson Parameter and p_0 Is the Probability of Zero

Reference Group	Test Group	Variance Ratio	Biosimilarity Margin = (0.5, 2)			Biosimilarity Margin = (0.5, 1.5)		
			Conover's Test	F-Test	Levene's Test	Conover's Test	F-Test	Levene's Test
ZIP(5, 0.3)	ZIP(3.75, 0.06667)	0.5	0.0192	0.0306	0.0113	0.0195	0.0304	0.0116
ZIP(5, 0.3)	ZIP(4.175, 0.1617)	0.67	0.3968	0.4039	0.2847	0.3998	0.4053	0.2917
ZIP(5, 0.3)	ZIP(4.375, 0.2)	0.75	0.6923	0.6642	0.5725	0.6730	0.6528	0.5610
ZIP(5, 0.3)	ZIP(4.5, 0.2222)	0.8	0.8245	0.7951	0.7304	0.8075	0.7589	0.7093
ZIP(5, 0.3)	ZIP(4.75, 0.26316)	0.9	0.9601	0.9408	0.9276	0.9136	0.8051	0.8290
ZIP(5, 0.3)	ZIP(5, 0.3)	1	0.9855	0.9757	0.9753	0.8919	0.6685	0.7342
ZIP(5, 0.3)	ZIP(5.25, 0.3333)	1.1	0.9826	0.9511	0.9516	0.8135	0.4426	0.5083
ZIP(5, 0.3)	ZIP(5.625, 0.3778)	1.25	0.9417	0.8047	0.7865	0.6295	0.1649	0.1952
ZIP(5, 0.3)	ZIP(5.825, 0.3991)	1.33	0.9017	0.6886	0.6577	0.5226	0.0846	0.0907
ZIP(5, 0.3)	ZIP(6.25, 0.44)	1.5	0.7854	0.3938	0.3486	0.3175	0.0158	0.0165
ZIP(5, 0.3)	ZIP(7.5, 0.5333)	2	0.3412	0.0204	0.0168	0.0496	1.00E–04	3.00E–04

In the third set of simulations (Table 8.3), Laplace distribution (also known as double exponential distribution) is used. As we can see from Table 8.3, for symmetric distribution as Laplace, when the normal assumption is violated, F-test failed to show robustness. However, both Conover and Levene's tests successfully maintain the type I error, while Levene test is a little bit more powerful than Conover's under this case.

In the fourth set of simulations (Table 8.4), central chi-square distribution with degrees of freedom of 4 is used in the reference group, and central chi-square distribution with different degrees of freedom is used in the test arm to reflect the different variance ratios. The power of the Conover's test is comparable to the F-test (0.784 vs. 0.7517 at biosimilarity margin of (0.5, 2); and 0.4744 vs. 0.4664 for biosimilarity margin (0.5, 1.5)), although Levene's test is not that powerful under this situation. However, F-test failed to control the type I error (0.1709) when biosimilarity margin = (0.5, 2), as noticed in the previous papers. While at the same time, the non-parametric tests still maintained the proposed type I error (0.0529 from Conover's test and 0.057 from Levene's test). Therefore, under this situation where the underlying distribution is asymmetric with long tailed, non-parametric Conover's test performs the best.

In the fifth set of simulations (Tables 8.5 and 8.6) where Weibull distribution is used, we explore two scenarios. In the first scenario, the scale parameter changes in the test group to create different variances while the shape parameter stays same as the reference. Therefore, different variances from the two groups imply different means as well. In the second scenario, both scale and shape parameters change in the test group, so variances are changed but mean is still about same as the reference group. The simulation results are summarized later.

When a biosimilarity margin of (0.5, 2) is used, the power of the non-parametric tests is comparable to that of the F-test (0.76–0.79 vs. 0.82–0.83) in both scenarios. But again F-test failed to control the type I error (around 0.1 in both scenarios) as noticed in the previous papers, while the non-parametric tests are a little bit better (0.6–0.8 in the first scenario and around 0.6 in the second scenario). When a biosimilarity margin of (0.5, 1.5) is used, similar pattern was observed.

Finally, a non-continuous distribution, zero-inflated Poisson, was explored in the simulation (Table 8.7).

8.4.4 Remarks

Simulation results indicate that under the given distribution assumption of normality, the two types of non-parametric tests have relatively good efficiency as compared to the parametric method. However, when the underlying distribution is deviated from normal, the parametric F-test incorrectly concludes biosimilarity far too often, thus failing to control the type I error (not robust). Under such situations, the two types of non-parametric methods provide considerable improvement over the robustness while maintaining comparable power.

The reported sample sizes used in simulations are 50 and 100 in each group. We tried smaller sample size (e.g., $N = 36$) in which none of the methods can achieve ideal power. It suggests that to assess biosimilarity in variabilities, adequate sample size is generally required. From the simulation, we also noticed that the biosimilarity margin of (0.67, 1.5) is too stringent for all these tests of variability. The margin (0.5, 2) is symmetric around the variance ratio of 1, therefore resulting in roughly symmetric power/type I error rate around 1. However, considering small variance (ratio < 1) of FOB should not be penalized same as ratio > 1, some people may prefer the asymmetric biosimilarity margin of (0.5, 1.5). Further discussion will be needed in choosing the proper biosimilarity margin for evaluating variabilities. Finally, the proposed non-parametric methods and extended F-test presented in this manuscript are all based on parallel design of a clinical study. They do not distinguish inter- and intra-subject variability and variability due to possible subject-by-treatment interaction, which are known to have an impact on drug interchangeability. Further research is desired to address these motivating questions in assessing FOBs.

8.5 Alternative Methods

8.5.1 Probability-Based Criterion and Statistical Hypothesis

As a parallel design is often considered for assessment of biosimilarity between biological products, in this section, biosimilarity in variability will be evaluated under a parallel-group design. Let X and Y be the parameters of interest (e.g., pharmacokinetic response) which follow a normal distribution with variances V_X and V_Y, respectively. Let X_i and Y_i be the observations of X and Y with $i = 1, ..., n_X$ and $i = 1, ..., n_Y$. Thus, the maximum likelihood estimators (MLE) of V_X and V_Y are given by $\hat{V}_X = \sum_{i=1}^{n_X} (X_i - \bar{X})^2/n_X$ and $\hat{V}_Y = \sum_{i=1}^{n_Y} (Y_i - \bar{Y})^2/n_Y$, respectively. Following the similar idea of a probability-based index for the statistical quality control/assurance process for traditional Chinese medicine proposed by Tse et al. (2006), a probability-based criterion for assessment of the biosimilarity in variability can be proposed as

$$p_{PB} = P\left(1-\delta < \frac{\hat{V}_X}{\hat{V}_Y} < 1+\delta\right) \tag{8.6}$$

$$= P\left(\frac{\hat{V}_X}{\hat{V}_Y} < 1+\delta\right) - P\left(\frac{\hat{V}_X}{\hat{V}_Y} < 1-\delta\right) \tag{8.7}$$

$$= P\left(\hat{V}_X - (1+\delta)\hat{V}_Y < 0\right) - P\left(\hat{V}_X - (1-\delta)\hat{V}_Y < 0\right), \tag{8.8}$$

where $0 < \delta < 1$ is the biosimilarity limit in variability for the probability-based method. Equation 8.8 is the expression which converts the ratio of variabilities in Equation 8.7 into their linear combination. We will refer to p_{PB} as the biosimilarity index in variability.

The probability-based method for testing biosimilarity in variability can be obtained based on the index of p_{PB} by considering the following hypotheses:

$$H_0 : p_{PB} \le p_0 \quad \text{vs.} \quad H_a : p_{PB} > p_0, \tag{8.9}$$

where p_0 is the biosimilarity limit. The biosimilarity in variability of two biological products is claimed if the $100(1 - \alpha)\%$ upper confidence limit of p_{PB} is greater than p_0.

8.5.2 Statistical Testing Procedure

With respect to constructing the $(1 - \alpha) \times 100\%$ upper limit of p_{PB} for testing the hypothesis (4), since it is known that the linear combination of the MLE of the variances for two independent normal distributions has an asymptotic normal distribution, we can construct the $(1 - \alpha) \times 100\%$ upper limit of p_{PB} stated by considering the expression of p_{PB} in terms of the form of the linear combination in Equation 8.3. The expected values and variances of the random variables of $\hat{V}_X - (1 + \delta)\hat{V}_Y$ and $\hat{V}_X - (1 - \delta)\hat{V}_Y$ can be obtained as follows:

$$E\left[\hat{V}_X - (1+\delta)\hat{V}_Y\right] = \frac{n_X - 1}{n_X} V_X - \frac{n_Y - 1}{n_Y}(1+\delta)V_Y$$

$$\text{Var}\left[\hat{V}_X - (1+\delta)\hat{V}_Y\right] = \frac{2(n_X - 1)}{n_X^2} V_X^2 + \frac{2(n_Y - 1)}{n_Y^2}(1+\delta)^2 V_Y^2$$

$$E\left[\hat{V}_X - (1-\delta)\hat{V}_Y\right] = \frac{n_X - 1}{n_X} V_X - \frac{n_Y - 1}{n_Y}(1-\delta)V_Y \tag{8.10}$$

$$\text{Var}\left[\hat{V}_X - (1-\delta)\hat{V}_Y\right] = \frac{2(n_X - 1)}{n_X^2} V_X^2 + \frac{2(n_Y - 1)}{n_Y^2}(1-\delta)^2 V_Y^2.$$

For the large n_X and n_Y, the central limit theorem leads to Equation 8.3 as

$$p_{PB} = \Phi\left(\frac{-E\left[\hat{V}_X - (1+\delta)\hat{V}_Y\right]}{\sqrt{\text{Var}\left[\hat{V}_X - (1+\delta)\hat{V}_Y\right]}}\right) - \Phi\left(\frac{-E\left[\hat{V}_X - (1-\delta)\hat{V}_Y\right]}{\sqrt{\text{Var}\left[\hat{V}_X - (1-\delta)\hat{V}_Y\right]}}\right), \tag{8.11}$$

By the invariance principle, the MLE of p_{PB} can be obtained as

$$\hat{p}_{PB} = \Phi\left(\frac{-\hat{E}\left[\hat{V}_X - (1+\delta)\hat{V}_Y\right]}{\sqrt{\widehat{Var}\left[\hat{V}_X - (1+\delta)\hat{V}_Y\right]}}\right) - \Phi\left(\frac{-\hat{E}\left[\hat{V}_X - (1-\delta)\hat{V}_Y\right]}{\sqrt{\widehat{Var}\left[\hat{V}_X - (1-\delta)\hat{V}_Y\right]}}\right) \quad (8.12)$$

by substituting V_X and V_Y using $\hat{V}_X$ and $\hat{V}_Y$ into Equation 8.6, respectively.

Moreover, expanding $\hat{p}_{PB}$ by its Taylor expansion function at p, that is, $\hat{V}_X = V_X$ and $\hat{V}_Y = V_Y$, $E(\hat{p}_{PB})$ and $Var(\hat{p}_{PB})$ can be expressed as $p_{PB} + B(p_{PB}) + o(n^{-1})$ and $C(p_{PB}) + o(n^{-1})$, respectively. The asymptomatic normal distribution of $\hat{p}_{PB}$ can be obtained as

$$\frac{\hat{p}_{PB} - p_{PB} - B(\hat{p}_{PB})}{\sqrt{C(\hat{p}_{PB})}} \to N(0,1), \quad (8.13)$$

where $B(\hat{p}_{PB})$ and $C(\hat{p}_{PB})$ are the MLEs of $B(p_{PB})$ and $C(p_{PB})$ by substituting $\hat{V}_X$ and $\hat{V}_Y$ for V_X and V_Y, respectively. $B(p_{PB})$, $C(p_{PB})$, and the derivation of Equation 8.14 are given later.

Considering the definition of $\hat{p}_{PB}$, its Taylor expansion at p_{PB} can be obtained as

$$\hat{p}_{PB} = p_{PB} + \frac{\partial \hat{p}_{PB}}{\partial V_X}(\hat{V}_X - V_X) + \frac{\partial \hat{p}_{PB}}{\partial V_Y}(\hat{V}_Y - V_Y)$$

$$+ \frac{1}{2}\frac{\partial^2 \hat{p}_{PB}}{\partial V_X^2}(\hat{V}_X - V_X)^2 + \frac{1}{2}\frac{\partial^2 \hat{p}_{PB}}{\partial V_Y^2}(\hat{V}_Y - V_Y)^2 + O(n^{-2}).$$

Taking its expectation and variance,

$$E(\hat{p}_{PB}) = p_{PB} - \frac{\partial \hat{p}_{PB}}{\partial V_X}\frac{V_X}{n_X} - \frac{\partial \hat{p}_{PB}}{\partial V_Y}\frac{V_Y}{n_Y} + \frac{\partial^2 \hat{p}_{PB}}{\partial V_X^2}\frac{V_X^2}{n_X} + \frac{\partial^2 \hat{p}_{PB}}{\partial V_Y^2}\frac{V_Y^2}{n_Y} + O(n^{-2})$$

$$Var(\hat{p}_{PB}) = \left(\frac{\partial \hat{p}_{PB}}{\partial V_X}\right)^2\left(\frac{2V_X^2}{n_X}\right) + \left(\frac{\partial \hat{p}_{PB}}{\partial V_Y}\right)^2\left(\frac{2V_Y^2}{n_Y}\right) + \left(\frac{\partial^2 \hat{p}_{PB}}{\partial V_X^2}\right)^2\left(\frac{2}{n_X^2}\right)\left(1 + \frac{1}{n_X} - \frac{2}{n_X^2}\right)V_X^4$$

$$+ \left(\frac{\partial^2 \hat{p}_{PB}}{\partial V_Y^2}\right)^2\left(\frac{2}{n_Y^2}\right)\left(1 + \frac{1}{n_Y} - \frac{2}{n_Y^2}\right)V_Y^4 + \left(\frac{\partial \hat{p}_{PB}}{\partial V_X}\right)\left(\frac{\partial^2 \hat{p}_{PB}}{\partial V_X^2}\right)\left(\frac{4}{n_X^2}\right)\left(1 - \frac{1}{n_X}\right)V_X^3$$

$$+ \left(\frac{\partial \hat{p}_{PB}}{\partial V_Y}\right)\left(\frac{\partial^2 \hat{p}_{PB}}{\partial V_Y^2}\right)\left(\frac{4}{n_Y^2}\right)\left(1 - \frac{1}{n_Y}\right)V_Y^3$$

$$B(p_{PB}) = -\frac{\partial p_{PB}}{\partial V_X}\frac{V_X}{n_X} - \frac{\partial p_{PB}}{\partial V_Y}\frac{V_Y}{n_Y} + \frac{\partial^2 p_{PB}}{\partial V_X^2}\frac{V_X^2}{n_X} + \frac{\partial^2 p_{PB}}{\partial V_Y^2}\frac{V_Y^2}{n_Y}$$

$$C(p_{PB}) = \left(\frac{\partial \hat{p}_{PB}}{\partial V_X}\right)^2\left(\frac{2V_X^2}{n_X}\right) + \left(\frac{\partial \hat{p}_{PB}}{\partial V_Y}\right)^2\left(\frac{2V_Y^2}{n_Y}\right) + \left(\frac{\partial^2 \hat{p}_{PB}}{\partial V_X^2}\right)^2\left(\frac{2}{n_X^2}\right)\left(1 + \frac{1}{n_X} - \frac{2}{n_X^2}\right)V_X^4$$

$$+ \left(\frac{\partial^2 \hat{p}_{PB}}{\partial V_Y^2}\right)^2\left(\frac{2}{n_Y^2}\right)\left(1 + \frac{1}{n_Y} - \frac{2}{n_Y^2}\right)V_Y^4 + \left(\frac{\partial \hat{p}_{PB}}{\partial V_X}\right)\left(\frac{\partial^2 \hat{p}_{PB}}{\partial V_X^2}\right)\left(\frac{4}{n_X^2}\right)\left(1 - \frac{1}{n_X}\right)V_X^3$$

$$+ \left(\frac{\partial \hat{p}_{PB}}{\partial V_Y}\right)\left(\frac{\partial^2 \hat{p}_{PB}}{\partial V_Y^2}\right)\left(\frac{4}{n_Y^2}\right)\left(1 - \frac{1}{n_Y}\right)V_Y^3 + O(n^{-2}),$$

where

$$\frac{\partial \hat{p}_{PB}}{\partial V_X} = -\phi(z_1)\left[V_Y\left(l_1 V_X^2 + m_1 V_Y^2\right)^{-\frac{3}{2}}\left(k_1 l_1 V_X - j_1 m_1 V_Y\right)\right]$$

$$+ \phi(z_2)\left[V_Y\left(l_2 V_X^2 + m_2 V_Y^2\right)^{-\frac{3}{2}}\left(k_2 l_2 V_X - j_2 m_2 V_Y\right)\right],$$

$$\frac{\partial \hat{p}_{PB}}{\partial V_Y} = \phi(z_1)\left[V_X\left(l_1 V_X^2 + m_1 V_Y^2\right)^{-\frac{3}{2}}\left(k_1 l_1 V_X - j_1 m_1 V_Y\right)\right]$$

$$- \phi(z_2)\left[V_X\left(l_2 V_X^2 + m_2 V_Y^2\right)^{-\frac{3}{2}}\left(k_2 l_2 V_X - j_2 m_2 V_Y\right)\right],$$

$$\frac{\partial^2 \hat{p}_{PB}}{\partial V_X^2} = z_1\phi(z_1)\left[V_Y^2\left(l_1 V_X^2 + m_1 V_Y^2\right)^{-3}\left(k_1 l_1 V_X - j_1 m_1 V_Y\right)^2\right.$$

$$\left. - l_1 V_Y\left(l_1 V_X^2 + m_1 V_Y^2\right)^{-\frac{5}{2}}\left(2k_1 l_1 V_X^2 - 3j_1 m_1 V_X V_Y - k_1 m_1 V_Y^2\right)\right]$$

$$- z_2\phi(z_2)\left[V_Y^2\left(l_2 V_X^2 + m_2 V_Y^2\right)^{-3}\left(k_2 l_2 V_X - j_2 m_2 V_Y\right)^2\right.$$

$$\left. - l_2 V_Y\left(l_2 V_X^2 + m_2 V_Y^2\right)^{-\frac{5}{2}}\left(2k_2 l_2 V_X^2 + 3j_2 m_2 V_X V_Y - k_2 m_2 V_Y^2\right)\right],$$

$$\frac{\partial^2 \hat{p}_{PB}}{\partial V_Y^2} = z_1 \phi(z_1) \left[V_X^2 \left(l_1 V_X^2 + m_1 V_Y^2 \right)^{-3} \left(k_1 l_1 V_X - j_1 m_1 V_Y \right)^2 \right.$$

$$\left. + m_1 V_X \left(l_1 V_X^2 + m_1 V_Y^2 \right)^{-\frac{5}{2}} \left(j_1 l_1 V_X^2 + 3 k_1 l_1 V_X V_Y - 2 j_1 m_1 V_Y^2 \right) \right]$$

$$- z_2 \phi(z_2) \left[V_X^2 \left(l_2 V_X^2 + m_2 V_Y^2 \right)^{-3} \left(k_2 l_2 V_X - j_2 m_2 V_Y \right)^2 \right.$$

$$\left. + m_2 V_X \left(l_2 V_X^2 + m_2 V_Y^2 \right)^{-\frac{5}{2}} \left(j_2 l_2 V_X^2 + 3 k_2 l_2 V_X V_Y - 2 j_2 m_2 V_Y^2 \right) \right]$$

$$j_1 = j_2 = -\frac{n_X - 1}{n_X}$$

$$k_1 = \frac{n_Y - 1}{n_Y}(1 + \delta), \quad k_2 = \frac{n_Y - 1}{n_Y}(1 - \delta)$$

$$l_1 = l_2 = \frac{2(n_X - 1)}{n_X^2}$$

$$m_1 = \frac{2(n_Y - 1)}{n_Y^2}(1 + \delta)^2, \quad m_2 = \frac{2(n_Y - 1)}{n_Y^2}(1 - \delta)^2$$

$$z_1 = \frac{j_1 V_X + k_1 V_Y}{\sqrt{l_1 V_X^2 + m_1 V_Y^2}}, \quad z_2 = \frac{j_2 V_X + k_2 V_Y}{\sqrt{l_2 V_X^2 + m_2 V_Y^2}}.$$

The null hypothesis in Equation 8.9 will be rejected and the biosimilarity concluded if

$$\hat{p}_{PB} > p_0 + B(\hat{p}_{PB}) + Z_\alpha \sqrt{C(\hat{p}_{PB})}. \tag{8.14}$$

8.5.3 Probability-Based Criteria versus n_X, n_Y, and δ

As p_{PB} is the function of n_X, n_Y, δ and the ratio of V_X and V_Y, a numerical study is employed to investigate the relationship of p_{PB} with these parameters. Since the second expression of p_{PB} in Equation 8.11 can be reformulated as follows:

$$p_{PB} = P\left(\frac{\hat{V}_X}{\hat{V}_Y} < 1+\delta\right) - P\left(\frac{\hat{V}_X}{\hat{V}_Y} < 1-\delta\right)$$

$$= P\left(\frac{\dfrac{n_X\hat{V}_X}{(n_X-1)V_X}}{\dfrac{n_Y\hat{V}_Y}{(n_Y-1)V_Y}} < (1+\delta)\frac{n_X(n_Y-1)\ V_Y}{n_Y(n_X-1)\ V_X}\right) - P\left(\frac{\dfrac{n_X\hat{V}_X}{(n_X-1)V_X}}{\dfrac{n_Y\hat{V}_Y}{(n_Y-1)V_Y}} < (1-\delta)\frac{n_X(n_Y-1)\ V_Y}{n_Y(n_X-1)\ V_X}\right)$$

$$= P\left(F_{n_X-1,n_Y-1} < (1+\delta)\frac{n_X(n_Y-1)\ V_Y}{n_Y(n_X-1)\ V_X}\right) - P\left(F_{n_X-1,n_Y-1} < (1-\delta)\frac{n_X(n_Y-1)\ V_Y}{n_Y(n_X-1)\ V_X}\right),$$

$$(8.15)$$

where F_{n_X-1,n_Y-1} is the random variable of F-distribution with $n_X - 1$ and $n_Y - 1$ degrees of freedom, the true value of p_{PB} can be obtained via Equation 8.15. Table 8.8 presents the values of p_{PB} which achieve 0.65 under various combinations of n_X, n_Y, and δ when the true ratio of V_X and V_Y is equal to 0.75, 1.00, and 1.75, respectively. n_X and n_Y are chosen to be the same value denoted by n in the table for the convenience of the discussion. As shown in the table, p_{PB} cannot reach 0.65 for all V_X/V_Y and n when δ is the smallest value of 0.1. In addition, p_{PB} increases when the sample size and δ increase. With respect to impact of V_X/V_Y on p_{PB}, the p_{PB} at $V_X/V_Y = 1.25$ are smaller than those at $V_X/V_Y = 0.75$ and 1.00 for all combinations of δ and n. It may mean that the probability index p_0 needs to be set as a higher value for assessing the biosimilarity if the variability of the follow-on product is greater than that of the originator product. On the other hand, the p_{PB} at $V_X/V_Y = 0.75$ is greater than that at $V_X/V_Y = 1.00$ when δ is greater than 0.5, while the results are opposite if δ is less than 0.5. If δ is set as 0.2, only the combinations of $V_X/V_Y = 1.00$ with the sample size ≥ 100 can achieve a p_{PB} of 0.65.

Table 8.8 provides the idea for selecting the appropriate combination of n_X, n_Y, δ for performing the proposed statistical testing procedure according to the need of the researcher. For instance, if the researcher is considering that V_X and V_Y are comparable (i.e., the true ratio of V_X and V_Y is around 1.00), the sample size of $n_X = n_Y = 150$ is suggested for a biosimilarity limit δ of 0.2 and the biosimilarity index at least $p_0 = 75\%$.

TABLE 8.8

Values of p_{PB} under Various Combinations of n_X, n_Y, and δ

V_X/V_Y	n	0.1	0.2	0.3	0.4	0.5	0.6	0.7	0.8	0.9
0.75	24	—	—	—	0.6306	0.7794	0.8926	0.9560	0.9784	0.9849
	36	—	—	—	0.7092	0.8604	0.9526	0.9871	0.9942	0.9963
	50	—	—	—	0.7657	0.9119	0.9804	0.9967	0.9987	0.9993
	100	—	—	0.6306	0.8646	0.9772	0.9989	0.9999	0.9999	0.9999
	150	—	—	0.6624	0.9127	0.9931	0.9999	0.9999	0.9999	0.9999
	200	—	—	0.6864	0.9418	0.9978	0.9999	1.0000	1.0000	1.0000
	250	—	—	0.7067	0.9605	0.9993	0.9999	1.0000	1.0000	1.0000
1.00	24	—	—	—	0.6730	0.7794	0.8501	0.8919	0.9168	0.9345
	36	—	—	0.6311	0.7701	0.8605	0.9112	0.9391	0.9568	0.9692
	50	—	—	0.7115	0.8404	0.9119	0.9475	0.9669	0.9789	0.9867
	100	—	0.6827	0.8645	0.9463	0.9772	0.9899	0.9956	0.9981	0.9992
	150	—	0.7793	0.9297	0.9786	0.9931	0.9978	0.9993	0.9998	0.9999
	200	—	0.8422	0.9614	0.9908	0.9978	0.9995	0.9999	0.9999	0.9999
	250	—	0.8850	0.9780	0.9959	0.9993	0.9999	0.9999	0.9999	0.9999
1.25	24	—	—	—	—	0.6509	0.7165	0.7661	0.8058	0.8388
	36	—	—	—	0.6139	0.6996	0.7650	0.8163	0.8572	0.8898
	50	—	—	—	0.6476	0.7363	0.8046	0.8574	0.8973	0.9269
	100	—	—	—	0.7129	0.8170	0.8894	0.9361	0.9644	0.9808
	150	—	—	—	0.7550	0.8665	0.9335	0.9692	0.9866	0.9945
	200	—	—	0.6088	0.7876	0.9003	0.9588	0.9847	0.9948	0.9984
	250	—	—	0.6214	0.8141	0.9245	0.9740	0.9922	0.9979	0.9995

8.5.4 Simulation Study

The simulation study is conducted to evaluate the performance of the proposed probability-based asymptotic testing procedure in terms of empirical sizes and powers. The empirical sizes are evaluated under the following parameter settings: $n_X = n_Y = 24, 36, 50, 100, 150, 200, 250$; $\delta = 0.1, 0.2, 0.3, 0.4,$ $0.5, 0.6, 0.7, 0.8, 0.9$; $\mu_X = \mu_Y = 0$, where μ_X and μ_Y are the population means for X and Y, respectively. In addition, (V_X, V_Y) are set as $(0.75, 1.00)$, $(1.00, 1.00)$, and $(1.25, 1.00)$ for getting the true ratio of V_X and V_Y as $0.75, 1.00,$ and 1.25. For each combination, 10,000 random samples are generated. For the 5% nominal significance level, a simulation study with 10,000 random samples implies that 95% of the empirical sized evaluated at the allowable margins will be within 0.0457 and 0.0543 if the proposed methods can adequately control the size at the nominal level of 0.05. Tables 8.9 through 8.12 present the empirical sizes at $V_X/V_Y = 0.75, 1.00,$ and 1.25, respectively. The p_0 in the tables are calculated by Equation 8.15. The results show the empirical size increases when δ increases if the sample size is fixed. On the other hand, the empirical size is greater than 0 only at $V_X/V_Y = 1.25$ when δ ranges from 0.1 to 0.4. In addition, all empirical sizes at $V_X/V_Y = 1.25$ are greater than 0 when δ ranges from 0.5 to 0.9 except for which at $\delta = 0.5$ and sample size = 24, while only 17.1% (6/35) and 77.1% of empirical sizes are greater than 0 at $V_X/V_Y = 0.75$ and 1.00, respectively. Moreover, the empirical sizes at $V_X/V_Y = 0.75$ are greater than 0 at $\delta = 0.3$ and 0.4, while the empirical sizes at $V_X/V_Y = 1.00$ are all equal to zero for the same value of δ. Comparing the corresponding p_0 among three ratios of V_X and V_Y when δ and n are fixed, the order of value of p_0 is $V_X/V_Y = 1.25 < V_X/V_Y = 1.00 < V_X/V_Y = 0.75$ when δ ranges from 0.5 to 0.9. With respect to the δ less than 0.5, the value of p_0 at $V_X/V_Y = 0.75$ is less than $V_X/V_Y = 1.00$. Through the earlier discussion, it can be found that the higher p_0 result in the lower empirical sizes. This may be the reason why the null hypothesis in Equation 8.9 is harder to reject when p_0 is higher, in particular for p_0 close to 1. However, all empirical sizes cannot be adequately controlled at the 5% nominal level since all of them are out of (0.0457, 0.0543) for all combination of parameters.

As it can be found that the empirical size is the function of δ, p_0, and n from the results of Tables 8.9 through 8.11, an alternative simulation study is employed to investigate the desirable δ and p_0 for which the empirical size can be adequately controlled at the 5% nominal level for each of the selected sample sizes. Table 8.12 presents the results of the simulation for the cases of $p_0 \geq 0.6$. As shown in the table, for achieving the 5% nominal level, δ decreases while the corresponding p_{PB} increases when the sample size increases. In addition, the minimum δ for which the empirical size can be adequately controlled are 0.533 at $n = 200$, 0.425 at $n = 250$, and 0.513 at $n = 24$ when $V_X/V_Y = 0.75, 1.00,$ and 1.25, respectively. The larger sample size and small V_X/V_Y do not guarantee the smaller value of δ. This shows that δ, n, and V_X/V_Y not only have impact on the empirical size simultaneously but may also have different ways of impact under different combinations.

TABLE 8.9

Empirical Sizes when $V_X/V_Y = 0.75$

n	0.1	0.2	0.3	0.4	0.5	0.6	0.7	0.8	0.9
24	—	—	—	0.6306 0.0000	0.7794 0.0000	0.8926 0.0000	0.9560 0.0000	0.9784 0.0000	0.9849 0.0000
36	—	—	—	0.7092 0.0000	0.8604 0.0000	0.9526 0.0000	0.9871 0.0000	0.9942 0.0000	0.9963 0.0549
50	—	—	—	0.7657 0.0000	0.9119 0.0000	0.9804 0.0000	0.9967 0.0000	0.9987 0.0000	0.9993 0.0685
100	—	—	0.6306 0.1608	0.8646 0.1465	0.9772 0.0000	0.9989 0.0000	0.9999 0.0000	0.9999 0.0000	0.9999 0.0475
150	—	—	0.6624 0.1928	0.9127 0.2068	0.9931 0.0988	0.9999 0.0000	0.9999 0.0000	0.9999 0.0000	0.9999 0.0000
200	—	—	0.6864 0.2018	0.9418 0.2340	0.9978 0.1618	0.9999 0.0000	1.0000 0.0000	1.0000 0.0000	1.0000 0.0000
250	—	—	0.7067 0.2052	0.9605 0.2601	0.9993 0.1980	0.9999 0.0000	1.0000 0.0000	1.0000 0.0000	1.0000 0.0000

TABLE 8.10

Empirical Sizes when $V_X/V_Y = 1.00$

n	0.1		0.2		0.3		0.4		0.5		0.6		0.7		0.8		0.9	
24	—	—	—	—	—	—	0.6730	0.0000	0.7794	0.0000	0.8501	0.0000	0.8919	0.0000	0.9168	0.1600	0.9345	0.2030
36	—	—	—	—	0.6311	0.0000	0.7701	0.0000	0.8605	0.0000	0.9112	0.0000	0.9391	0.0997	0.9568	0.1989	0.9692	0.1998
50	—	—	—	—	0.7115	0.0000	0.8404	0.0000	0.9119	0.0000	0.9475	0.0000	0.9669	0.1641	0.9789	0.2139	0.9867	0.1989
100	—	—	0.6827	0.0000	0.8645	0.0000	0.9463	0.0000	0.9772	0.0000	0.9899	0.1724	0.9956	0.2233	0.9981	0.2084	0.9992	0.1878
150	—	—	0.7793	0.0000	0.9297	0.0000	0.9786	0.0000	0.9931	0.0986	0.9978	0.2089	0.9993	0.2219	0.9998	0.2129	0.9999	0.1784
200	—	—	0.8422	0.0000	0.9614	0.0000	0.9908	0.0000	0.9978	0.1655	0.9995	0.2321	0.9999	0.2237	0.9999	0.2002	0.9999	0.1727
250	—	—	0.8850	0.0000	0.9780	0.0000	0.9959	0.0000	0.9993	0.1974	0.9999	0.2430	0.9999	0.2127	0.9999	0.1984	0.9999	0.1733

TABLE 8.11

Empirical Sizes when $V_X/V_Y = 1.25$

n	0.1	0.2	0.3	0.4	0.5	0.6	0.7	0.8	0.9
24	—	—	—	—	0.6509 / 0.0000	0.7165 / 0.1427	0.7661 / 0.2027	0.8058 / 0.2190	0.8388 / 0.2232
36	—	—	—	0.6139 / 0.0727	0.6996 / 0.1519	0.7650 / 0.1956	0.8163 / 0.2263	0.8572 / 0.2271	0.8898 / 0.2331
50	—	—	—	0.6476 / 0.1447	0.7363 / 0.1953	0.8046 / 0.2082	0.8574 / 0.2337	0.8973 / 0.2337	0.9269 / 0.2255
100	—	—	—	0.7129 / 0.1983	0.8170 / 0.2286	0.8894 / 0.2337	0.9361 / 0.2429	0.9644 / 0.2433	0.9808 / 0.2434
150	—	—	—	0.7550 / 0.2139	0.8665 / 0.2371	0.9335 / 0.2440	0.9692 / 0.2532	0.9866 / 0.2449	0.9945 / 0.2529
200	—	—	0.6088 / 0.1907	0.7876 / 0.2174	0.9003 / 0.2410	0.9588 / 0.2536	0.9847 / 0.2489	0.9948 / 0.2579	0.9984 / 0.2530
250	—	—	0.6214 / 0.1935	0.8141 / 0.2319	0.9245 / 0.2507	0.9740 / 0.2543	0.9922 / 0.2616	0.9979 / 0.2602	0.9995 / 0.2499

TABLE 8.12

(δ, p_0) for Controlling the Empirical Sizes
Adequately at 5% Nominal Level

V_X/V_Y	n	δ	p_0	Empirical Size
0.75	24	0.923	0.9859	0.0472
	24	0.924	0.9859	0.0512
	36	0.900	0.9964	0.0509
	50	0.880	0.9992	0.0460
	50	0.885	0.9992	0.0532
	100	0.465	0.9523	0.0504
	100	0.855	0.9999	0.0470
	100	0.860	0.9999	0.0507
	100	0.865	0.9999	0.0523
	100	0.872	0.9999	0.0539
	100	0.875	0.9999	0.0534
	100	0.890	0.9999	0.0502
	100	0.900	0.9999	0.0487
	100	0.921	0.9999	0.0477
	100	0.930	0.9999	0.0464
	150	0.511	0.9953	0.0541
	200	0.533	0.9996	0.0482
1.00	24	0.756	0.9047	0.0521
	36	0.680	0.9346	0.0479
	50	0.631	0.9546	0.0481
	100	0.536	0.9830	0.0496
	150	0.485	0.9918	0.0504
	200	0.450	0.9955	0.0472
	250	0.425	0.9973	0.0473
1.25	24	0.513	0.6606	0.0480
	24	0.514	0.6613	0.0468
	24	0.515	0.6620	0.0493
	24	0.516	0.6627	0.0503
	24	0.517	0.6635	0.0519
	24	0.518	0.6642	0.0536

Figure 8.1 presents the empirical power curves versus δ for true $V_X/V_Y = 0.75$, 1.00, and 1.25, respectively, with $n = 150$. The p_0 in statistical Hypothesis 8.9 is set as 0.75. The figure shows that all three power curves increase when δ increases. It can be also found that the empirical power at $V_X/V_Y = 0.75$ reaches 0.05 (i.e., the 5% nominal level) at the earliest, while that at $V_X/V_Y = 1.00$ reaches 0.05 at the latest. In addition, the power curve at $V_X/V_Y = 1.25$ is lower than both power curves at $V_X/V_Y = 0.75$

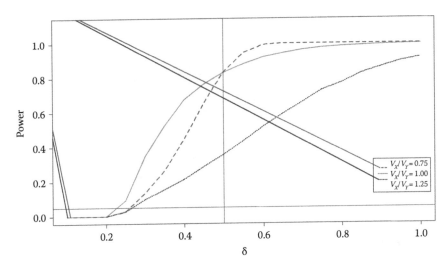

FIGURE 8.1
Empirical power curve versus δ for different V_X/V_Y.

and 1.00. Furthermore, it can be seen that the variance of $\hat{p}_{PB}$ decreases when δ is greater than 0.5.

8.5.5 Numerical Example

A numerical example is used to illustrate the proposed probability-based statistical testing procedure by considering a pharmacokinetic study with parallel design to assess the biosimilarity in variability between an innovator biological product and its follow-on product. Assume that a total of 72 subjects (36 subjects per group) are randomly assigned to receive the innovator product and its follow-on product. The PK parameter AUC is calculated for each of the 72 subjects in the study. The sample variances of AUC are obtained as 8.05 and 10.05 for the innovator product and the follow-on product, respectively. To test their biosimilarity, consider the proposed statistical testing with different biosimilarity limits of δ (i.e., δ = 0.4 and 0.5), and biosimilarity indexes p_0 (i.e., p_0 = 0.60 and 0.70) at the 5% and 10% levels of significance, respectively. The testing results with the corresponding $\hat{p}_{PB}$ are summarized in Table 8.13. As it can be seen in Table 8.6, when the biosimilarity limit δ is 0.4, since only the critical value of 0.7459 at p_0 = 0.60 and α = 0.10 is less than $\hat{p}_{PB}$ of 0.7683, the biosimilarity in variability can only be concluded at p_0 = 0.60 at a 10% statistical significance level. On the other hand, the biosimilarity in variability is concluded at δ = 0.5 at both p_0 of 0.60 and 0.70 at 5% and 10% statistical significance levels because all four critical values at δ = 0.5 are less than $\hat{p}_{PB}$ of 0.8903.

TABLE 8.13

Result of the Example

δ	p_0	$\hat{p}_{PB}$	α	Critical Value	Result
0.4	0.60	0.7683	0.05	0.8288	Non-biosimilarity
			0.10	0.7459	Biosimilarity
	0.70		0.05	0.9278	Non-biosimilarity
			0.10	0.8459	Non-biosimilarity
0.5	0.60	0.8903	0.05	0.7124	Biosimilarity
			0.10	0.6661	Biosimilarity
	0.70		0.05	0.8124	Biosimilarity
			0.10	0.7666	Biosimilarity

8.6 Concluding Remarks

Unlike traditional small-molecule drug products, the characteristic and development of biological products are more complicated and sensitive to many factors. As suggested by Chow et al. (2010a), the assessment of biosimilarity should be based on variability instead of average bioequivalence. In this chapter, the classical Pitman–Morgan's adjusted F-test under a crossover design is introduced. Under a parallel design, an F-type test proposed by Yang et al. (2013) is useful for testing homogeneity of variances of FOBs. Since F-type tests are sensitive to the fundamental distribution assumption, Zhang et al. (2013) suggested the two types of non-parametric methods for comparing variabilities between biosimilar products be used. In the interest of comparing variabilities in biosimilar studies, a pre-study power analysis for sample size calculation can be performed based on the F-type test statistics derived in this chapter under either a crossover design or a parallel group design. It, however, should be noted that statistical tests for comparing variabilities include comparing inter-subject variabilities, comparing intra-subject variabilities, and comparing total variabilities under either a crossover design or a parallel design (with or without replicates). More details regarding sample size calculation in biosimilar studies comparing variabilities are given in the next chapter.

Hsieh et al. (2010), on the other hand, indicated that the probability-based test is more sensitive to the variability and should be employed for assessing biosimilarity in variability between biosimilar products. As indicated by Hsieh et al. (2010), the proposed asymptotic statistical testing procedure based on the probability index can be applied to test hypotheses in Equation 8.9 by using the testing rule described in Equation 8.13. Table 8.8 provides the information for selecting the appropriate sample size for the desirable probability limit δ and probability index p_0 based on the need of the researcher. However, as shown in the simulation study, the empirical size cannot be adequately controlled at a desirable nominal level for all combinations of δ, p_0, and selected sample size. Therefore, in Table 8.12, the combinations of δ and p_0 which can achieve the 5% nominal level for the selected sample sizes and ratios of V_X and V_Y are provided for researcher's reference. The simulation results also show the empirical power increases when δ increases. On the other hand, the smaller ratio of V_X and V_Y will result in the larger power when δ is greater than certain level.

Considering that the study with smaller sample size for assessing biosimilarity of biological products may be employed in general, the exact testing procedure based on the same probability-based criterion may be needed to be developed. In addition, as the assessment of biosimilarity of two biological products should consider the similarity in both average and variability in general, the multiple comparison procedure for comparing the average and variability simultaneously using the separate statistical testing procedures is considered to be conducted for achieving the purpose. An alternative way is to consider an aggregate criterion to integrate the measure for assessment of average and for assessment of variability as one measure, and perform the evaluation of biosimilarity by using a single statistical testing procedure. Further research will be employed for the consideration and topics mentioned earlier.

9

Sample Size for Comparing Variabilities

9.1 Introduction

As indicated in the previous chapter, biosimilar products are variable and very sensitive to small changes (or variations) in environmental factors during the manufacturing process. In a biosimilar study, small variability associated with observed response is an indication that the observed difference in response between biosimilar products is not by chance alone and it is reproducible. In addition, small variability is also an indication of good drug characteristics such as stability and quality of the biosimilar product under investigation. Thus, in addition to the comparison of average responses between a biosimilar (test) product and an innovative (reference) product, it is suggested that the variabilities between the test product and the reference product should also be compared when assessing biosimilarity. The comparison of variabilities of responses between biosimilar products provides valuable information regarding the degree of similarity and how similar is considered highly similar in addition to average biosimilarity.

In practice, the variabilities associated with observed responses are usually classified into two categories: the intra-subject (or within subject) variability and the inter-subject (or between subject) variability. Intra-subject variability refers to the variability observed from repeated measurements from the same subject under the same experimental conditions. On the other hand, inter-subject variability is the variability due to the heterogeneity among subjects. The total variability is simply the sum of the intra-subject and inter-subject variabilities. The identification, elimination, and control of the sources of variabilities are useful for the statistical process of quality control/assurance in the development of biosimilar products. The problem of comparing intra-subject variabilities is well studied by Chinchilli and Esinhart (1996) through an F statistic under a replicated crossover model. A similar idea can be applied to comparing variabilities under a parallel design with and/or without replicates. For comparing intra-subject variabilities and intra-subject coefficients of variation (CV), sample sizes required for achieving a desired power of correct establishment of biosimilarity are derived based on hypotheses testing for similarity. For comparing inter-subject variabilities and total variabilities, sample sizes needed for achieving a desired power (say 80%) at a pre-specified level of significance (say 5%) are derived based on hypotheses testing for non-inferiority and/or equivalence.

In the previous chapter, F-type test statistics and non-parametric methods were derived for comparing variabilities in biosimilar studies under either a crossover design or a parallel design. However, not much details regarding pre-study power analysis for sample size calculation are given. The purpose of this chapter is to derive sample size formulas and/or procedures for comparing variabilities including intra-subject variabilities, inter-subject variabilities, total variabilities, and intra-subject CV in biosimilar studies based on hypotheses testing for non-inferiority or equivalence under either a repeated crossover design or a parallel group design with or without replicates. The comparison of variabilities between treatment groups will provide valuable information regarding the degree of similarity, which may be useful in addressing the question "How similar is considered highly similar?"

The remainder of this chapter is organized as follows. In the next three sections, formulas for sample size calculation for comparing intra-subject variabilities, inter-subject variabilities, and total variabilities under a parallel design with replicates and a replicated crossover design are derived. Section 9.5 provides formulas for sample size calculation for comparing intra-subject CVs. Some practical issues are discussed in the last section of this chapter.

9.2 Comparing Intra-subject Variability

To assess intra-subject variability, replicates from the same subject are necessarily obtained. Thus, in practice, a simple parallel design with replicates or a standard 2 × 2 crossover design with replicates is often considered. In this section, sample size calculation for comparing intra-subject variability of responses between drug products under a parallel design with replicates and a replicated crossover design is considered.

9.2.1 Parallel Design with Replicates

Consider a biosimilar study utilizing a parallel group design with replicates, which is illustrated in Figure 9.1. Qualified subjects are randomly assigned to receive either a biosimilar (test) product or an innovative (reference) product. At the end of the treatment duration and after a sufficient length of washout, subjects will receive the same treatment under similar experimental conditions. The replicates obtained from the same subject provide an independent estimate of the intra-subject variability of the test treatment under study.

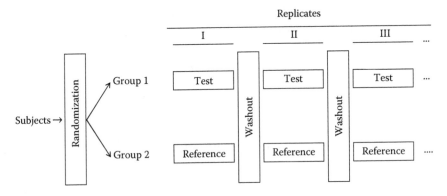

FIGURE 9.1
Parallel design with replicates.

Let y_{ijk} be the observation of the kth replicate ($k = 1, \ldots, m$) of the jth subject ($j = 1, \ldots, n_i$) from the ith treatment ($i = T, R$). Consider the following statistical model under a parallel group design:

$$y_{ijk} = \mu_i + S_{ij} + \epsilon_{ijk}, \qquad (9.1)$$

where
  μ_i is the drug effect
  S_{ij} is the random effect due to the jth subject in the ith group
  ϵ_{ijk} is the intra-subject random error under the ith group

For a fixed i, it is assumed that S_{ij} are independent and identically distributed as normal random variables with mean 0 and variance σ_{Bi}^2, and ϵ_{ijk}, $k = 1, \ldots, m$, are independent and identically distributed as a normal random variable with mean 0 and variance σ_{Wi}^2. Under Model 9.1, an unbiased estimator for σ_{Wi}^2 is given by

$$\hat{\sigma}_{Wi}^2 = \frac{1}{n_i(m-1)} \sum_{j=1}^{n_i} \sum_{k=1}^{m} (y_{ijk} - \bar{y}_{ij\cdot})^2, \qquad (9.2)$$

where

$$\bar{y}_{ij\cdot} = \frac{1}{m} \sum_{k=1}^{m} y_{ijk}. \qquad (9.3)$$

It can be verified that $n_i(m-1)\hat{\sigma}_{Wi}^2/\sigma_{Wi}^2$ is distributed as a $\chi_{n_i(m-1)}^2$ random variable. For testing similarity, the following hypotheses are usually considered:

$$H_0 : \frac{\sigma_{WT}^2}{\sigma_{WR}^2} \geq \delta \quad \text{or} \quad \frac{\sigma_{WT}^2}{\sigma_{WR}^2} \leq \frac{1}{\delta} \quad \text{versus} \quad H_a : \frac{1}{\delta} < \frac{\sigma_{WT}^2}{\sigma_{WR}^2} < \delta,$$

where $\delta > 1$ is the similarity limit. The aforementioned hypotheses can be decomposed into the following two one-sided hypotheses:

$$H_{01}: \frac{\sigma_{WT}}{\sigma_{WR}} \geq \sqrt{\delta} \quad \text{versus} \quad H_{a1}: \frac{\sigma_{WT}}{\sigma_{WR}} < \sqrt{\delta},$$

and

$$H_{02}: \frac{\sigma_{WT}}{\sigma_{WR}} \leq \frac{1}{\sqrt{\delta}} \quad \text{versus} \quad H_{a2}: \frac{\sigma_{WT}}{\sigma_{WR}} > \frac{1}{\sqrt{\delta}}. \tag{9.4}$$

These two one-sided hypotheses can be tested by the following two test statistics:

$$T_1 = \frac{\hat{\sigma}_{WT}}{\sqrt{\delta}\hat{\sigma}_{WR}} \quad \text{and} \quad T_2 = \frac{\sqrt{\delta}\hat{\sigma}_{WT}}{\hat{\sigma}_{WR}}.$$

We then reject the null hypothesis and conclude similarity at the α level of significance if

$$T_1 < F_{1-\alpha, n_T(m-1), n_R(m-1)} \quad \text{and} \quad T_2 > F_{1-\alpha, n_T(m-1), n_R(m-1)}.$$

Assuming that $n = n_1 = n_2$, under the alternative hypothesis that $\sigma_{WT}^2 = \sigma_{WR}^2$, the power of the test can be approximated by

$$1 - \beta = P\left(\frac{F_{\alpha, n(m-1), n(m-1)}}{\delta} < \frac{\hat{\sigma}_{WT}^2}{\hat{\sigma}_{WR}^2} < \delta F_{1-\alpha, n(m-1), n(m-1)} \right)$$

$$= P\left(\frac{1}{F_{\alpha, n(m-1), n(m-1)}\delta} < \frac{\hat{\sigma}_{WT}^2}{\hat{\sigma}_{WR}^2} < \delta F_{1-\alpha, n(m-1), n(m-1)} \right)$$

$$= 1 - 2P\left(\frac{\hat{\sigma}_{WT}^2}{\hat{\sigma}_{WR}^2} > \delta F_{1-\alpha, n(m-1), n(m-1)} \right)$$

$$= 1 - 2P\left(F_{n(m-1), n(m-1)} > \delta F_{1-\alpha, n(m-1), n(m-1)} \right).$$

Thus, the sample size required for achieving a desired power of $1 - \beta$ can be obtained by solving the following equation for n:

$$\delta = \frac{F_{\beta/2, n(m-1), n(m-1)}}{F_{1-\alpha, n(m-1), n(m-1)}}.$$

Note that under the alternative hypothesis, it is also possible that $\sigma_{WT}^2 \neq \sigma_{WR}^2$. In this case, without loss of generality, we assume that $\sigma_{WT}^2 / \sigma_{WR}^2 = r \in (1, \delta)$. Thus, the power of the aforementioned test can be approximated by

$$1 - \beta = P\left(\frac{F_{\alpha, n(m-1), n(m-1)}}{\delta} < \frac{\hat{\sigma}_{WT}^2}{\hat{\sigma}_{WR}^2} < \delta F_{1-\alpha, n(m-1), n(m-1)} \right)$$

$$\approx P\left(\frac{\hat{\sigma}_{WT}^2}{\hat{\sigma}_{WR}^2} < \delta F_{1-\alpha, n(m-1), n(m-1)} \right)$$

$$= P\left(\frac{\hat{\sigma}_{WT}^2}{r \hat{\sigma}_{WR}^2} > \frac{\delta}{r} F_{1-\alpha, n(m-1), n(m-1)} \right)$$

$$= P\left(F_{n(m-1), n(m-1)} > \frac{\delta}{r} F_{1-\alpha, n(m-1), n(m-1)} \right).$$

Hence, the sample size required for achieving the desired power of $1 - \beta$ can be obtained by solving the following equation for n:

$$\frac{\delta}{r} = \frac{F_{\beta, n(m-1), n(m-1)}}{F_{1-\alpha, n(m-1), n(m-1)}}.$$

9.2.1.1 Example

Consider a two-arm parallel trial with three replicates ($m = 3$) comparing intra-subject variabilities of a biosimilar (test) product and an innovative (reference) product. Based on a pilot study, the standard deviation of the test product is estimated to be about 30% ($\sigma_{WT} = 0.30$), whereas the standard deviation for the reference product is about 45% ($\sigma_{WR} = 0.45$). Suppose that the investigator is interested in selecting a sample size for establishing similarity between the test and reference product at the 5% ($\alpha = 0.05$) level of significance with an 80% ($\beta = 0.20$) power. Thus, by the aforementioned formula, the sample size required can be obtained by solving

$$\frac{(0.20)^2}{(0.45)^2} = \frac{F_{0.80, 2n, 2n}}{F_{0.025, 2n, 2n}},$$

which leads to $n = 25$. Hence, a total of 50 subjects (25 subjects per arm) are needed in order to achieve the desired power for establishing similarity in intra-subject variability between treatment groups.

9.2.2 Replicated Crossover Design

Consider a $2 \times 2m$ crossover design comparing two biosimilar products with m replicates, which is illustrated in Figure 9.2. A $2 \times 2m$ crossover design is a design that repeats a 2×2 crossover design m times. Qualified subjects are randomly assigned to receive either sequence 1 or sequence 2 of treatments. A sufficient length of washout is applied between dosing periods. Similar to the parallel design with replicates described in the previous subsection, the replicates obtained from the same subject provide independent estimates of the intra-subject variability of the test treatments under study.

Let n_i be the number of subjects assigned to the ith sequence and y_{ijkl} be the response from the jth subject in the ith sequence under the lth replicate of the kth drug ($k = T, R$). The following mixed effects model is usually considered for data from a $2 \times 2m$ crossover trial:

$$y_{ijkl} = \mu_k + \gamma_{ikl} + S_{ijk} + \epsilon_{ijkl}, \qquad (9.5)$$

where

μ_k is the mean response of the kth drug
γ_{ikl} is the fixed effect of the lth replicate under the kth drug in the ith sequence with constraint

$$\sum_{i=1}^{2} \sum_{l=1}^{m} \gamma_{ikl} = 0,$$

and S_{ijT} and S_{ijR} are the subject random effects of the jth subject in the ith sequence. (S_{ijT}, S_{ijR})'s are assumed independent, identically distributed (i.i.d.) bivariate normal random vectors with mean $(0,0)'$. As S_{ijT} and S_{ijR} are two

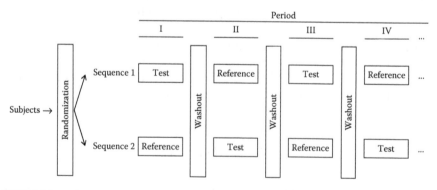

FIGURE 9.2
Replicated $2 \times 2m$ crossover design. *Note:* A $2 \times 2m$ crossover design is a design that repeats 2×2 crossover design m times.

observations taken from the same subject, they are not independent of each other. The following covariance matrix between S_{ijT} and S_{ijR} is usually assumed to describe their relationship:

$$\Sigma_B = \begin{pmatrix} \sigma_{BT}^2 & \rho\sigma_{BT}\sigma_{BR} \\ \rho\sigma_{BT}\sigma_{BR} & \sigma_{BR}^2 \end{pmatrix}.$$

ϵ_{ijkl} are assumed i.i.d. as $N(0,\sigma_{Wk}^2)$. It is also assumed that $(S_{ijT}, S_{ijR})'$ and ϵ_{ijkl} are independent. In order to obtain estimators for intra-subject variances, a new random variable z_{ijkl} is defined by an orthogonal transformation as $z_{ijk} = P'y_{ijk}$, where

$$y'_{ijk} = (y_{ijk1}, y_{ijk2}, \dots, y_{ijkm}),$$

$$z'_{ijk} = (z_{ijk1}, z_{ijk2}, \dots, z_{ijkm}),$$

and P is an $m \times m$ orthogonal matrix with the first column given by $(1,1,\dots,1)'/\sqrt{m}$. It can be verified that for a fixed I and any $l > 1$, z_{ijkl} are i.i.d. normal random variables with variance σ_{Wk}^2. Therefore, σ_{Wk}^2 can be estimated by

$$\hat{\sigma}_{Wk}^2 = \frac{1}{(n_1 + n_2 - 2)(m-1)} \sum_{l=2}^{m} \sum_{i=1}^{2} \sum_{j=1}^{n_i} (z_{ijkl} - \bar{z}_{i \cdot kl})^2$$

and

$$\bar{z}_{i \cdot kl} = \frac{1}{n_i} \sum_{j=1}^{n_i} z_{ijkl}.$$

It should be noted that $\hat{\sigma}_{Wk}^2/\sigma_{Wk}^2$ is χ^2 distributed with $d = (n_1 + n_2 - 2)(m - 1)$ degrees of freedom, and $\hat{\sigma}_{WT}^2$ and $\hat{\sigma}_{WR}^2$ are mutually independent. More details can be found in Chinchilli and Esinhart (1996). Thus, the null hypotheses of dissimilarity in Equation 9.4 would be rejected and similarity would be concluded at the α level of significance if

$$\frac{\hat{\sigma}_{WT}^2}{\delta\hat{\sigma}_{WR}^2} < F_{1-\alpha,d,d} \quad \text{and} \quad \frac{\widehat{\delta\sigma}_{WT}^2}{\hat{\sigma}_{WR}^2} > F_{\alpha,d,d}.$$

Hence, assuming that $n = n_1 = n_2$, the sample size required for achieving the power of $1 - \beta$ can be obtained by solving the following equation:

$$\frac{\delta\sigma_{WT}^2}{\sigma_{WR}^2} = \frac{F_{\frac{\beta}{2},(2n-2)(m-1),(2n-2)(m-1)}}{F_{1-\alpha,(2n-2)(m-1),(2n-2)(m-1)}}.$$

Note that more details can be found in Lee et al. (2002).

9.3 Comparing Inter-subject Variability

For comparing inter-subject variabilities, since an estimator for inter-subject variability can only be obtained under a replicated design and it usually can be expressed as a linear combination of various components estimates whose sampling distributions are relatively difficult to derive. Howe (1974), Graybill and Wang (1980), and Hyslop et al. (2000) developed several methods for estimation of inter-subject variabilities. One important assumption for these methods is that the variance component estimators involved in the estimation must be independent of one another. Lee et al. (2002) generalized these methods for the situation where some variance components are actually dependent on one another. The sample size formulas introduced in this section are mostly based on the methods by Lee et al. (2002).

9.3.1 Parallel Design with Replicates

Under Model 9.1, define

$$s_{Bi}^2 = \frac{1}{n_i - 1} \sum_{j=1}^{n_i} (\bar{y}_{ij\cdot} - \bar{y}_{i\cdot\cdot})^2, \tag{9.6}$$

where

$$\bar{y}_{i\cdot\cdot} = \frac{1}{n_i} \sum_{j=1}^{n_i} \bar{y}_{ij\cdot}.$$

and $\bar{y}_{ij\cdot}$ is given in Equation 9.3. Note that $E(s_{Bi}^2) = \sigma_{Bi}^2 + (\sigma_{Wi}^2/m)$. Therefore,

$$\hat{\sigma}_{Bi}^2 = s_{Bi}^2 - \frac{1}{m} \hat{\sigma}_{Wi}^2$$

are unbiased estimators for the inter-subject variabilities, where $\hat{\sigma}_{Wi}^2$ is defined in Equation 9.2.

Similarly, consider the following hypotheses for establishment of similarity in variability:

$$H_0 : \frac{\sigma_{BT}^2}{\sigma_{BR}^2} \notin \left(\frac{1}{\delta}, \delta\right) \quad \text{versus} \quad H_a : \frac{\sigma_{BT}^2}{\sigma_{BR}^2} \in \left(\frac{1}{\delta}, \delta\right),$$

where $\delta > 1$ is the similarity limit. The aforementioned hypotheses can be decomposed into the following two one-sided hypotheses:

$$H_{01} : \sigma_{BT}^2 - \delta\sigma_{BR}^2 \geq 0 \quad \text{versus} \quad H_{a1} : \sigma_{BT}^2 - \delta\sigma_{BR}^2 < 0,$$

$$H_{02} : \sigma_{BT}^2 - \delta\sigma_{BR}^2 \geq 0 \quad \text{versus} \quad H_{a2} : \sigma_{BT}^2 - \delta\sigma_{BR}^2 < 0.$$

Similarity in inter-subject variability between two drug products can be established if both of the aforementioned two hypotheses are rejected at the α level of significance. The test can be performed by calculating a $(1 - \alpha) \times 100\%$ upper confidence bound for $\eta_1 = \sigma_{BT}^2 - \delta\sigma_{BR}^2$ and a $(1 - \alpha) \times 100\%$ lower confidence bound for $\eta_2 = \delta\sigma_{BT}^2 - \sigma_{BR}^2$ by the modified large sample (MLS) method (Hsylop et al., 2000). The upper and lower $(1 - \alpha) \times 100\%$ confidence bounds are given by

$$\hat{\eta}_{1U} = \hat{\eta}_1 + \sqrt{\Delta_U} \quad \text{and} \quad \hat{\eta}_{2L} = \hat{\eta}_2 + \sqrt{\Delta_L},$$

where

$$\Delta_U = s_{BT}^4 \left(1 - \frac{n_T - 1}{\chi_{1-\alpha, n_T - 1}^2}\right)^2 + \delta^2 s_{BR}^4 \left(1 - \frac{n_R - 1}{\chi_{\alpha, n_R - 1}^2}\right)^2$$

$$+ \frac{\delta^2 \hat{\sigma}_{WT}^4}{m^2} \left(1 - \frac{n_T(m-1)}{\chi_{\alpha, n_T(m-1)}^2}\right)^2 + \frac{\hat{\sigma}_{WR}^4}{m^2} \left(1 - \frac{n_R(m-1)}{\chi_{1-\alpha, n_R(m-1)}^2}\right)^2,$$

and

$$\Delta_L = \delta^2 s_{BT}^4 \left(1 - \frac{n_T - 1}{\chi_{\alpha, n_T - 1}^2}\right)^2 + s_{BR}^4 \left(1 - \frac{n_R - 1}{\chi_{1-\alpha, n_R - 1}^2}\right)^2$$

$$+ \frac{\delta^2 \hat{\sigma}_{WT}^4}{m^2} \left(1 - \frac{n_T(m-1)}{\chi_{1-\alpha, n_T(m-1)}^2}\right)^2 + \frac{\hat{\sigma}_{WR}^4}{m^2} \left(1 - \frac{n_R(m-1)}{\chi_{\alpha, n_R(m-1)}^2}\right)^2.$$

Thus, we would reject the null hypothesis H_{01} at the α level of significance if $\hat{\eta}_{1U} < 0$. Under the assumption that $n = n_T = n_R$, using a similar argument, the power for testing H_{01} can be approximated by

$$1 - \Phi\left(z_\alpha - \frac{\sqrt{n}(\sigma_{BT}^2 - \delta\sigma_{BR}^2)}{\sigma^*}\right),$$

where

$$\sigma^* = 2\left[\left(\sigma_{BT}^2 + \frac{\sigma_{WT}^2}{m}\right)^2 + \delta^2\left(\sigma_{BR}^2 + \frac{\sigma_{WR}^2}{m}\right)^2 + \frac{\sigma_{WT}^4}{m^2(m-1)} + \frac{\delta^2\sigma_{WR}^4}{m^2(m-1)}\right].$$

As a result, the sample size needed in order to achieve the power of $1 - \beta$ at the α level of significance can be obtained by solving

$$z_\alpha - \frac{\sqrt{n}(\sigma_{BT}^2 - \delta\sigma_{BR}^2)}{\sigma^*} = -z_\beta.$$

This gives

$$n = \frac{\sigma^{*2}(z_\alpha + z_\beta)^2}{(\sigma_{BT}^2 - \delta\sigma_{BR}^2)^2}.$$

9.3.1.1 Example

Consider a two-arm parallel trial with three replicates ($m = 3$) for each subject. Suppose that the investigator is interested in comparing the inter-subject variabilities between a test product and a reference product. Based on a pilot study, the standard deviation for the test product is estimated to be about 35% ($\sigma_{BT}^2 = 0.35$), whereas the standard deviation for the reference product is about 45% ($\sigma_{BR} = 0.45$). It is also estimated that $\sigma_{WR} = 0.20$ and $\sigma_{WT} = 0.25$. It follows that

$$\sigma^{*2} = 2\left[\left(0.35^2 + \frac{0.25^2}{3}\right)^2 + \left(0.45^2 + \frac{0.20^2}{3}\right)^2 + \frac{0.25^4}{3^2(3-1)} + \frac{0.20^4}{3^2(3-1)}\right]$$

$$= 0.126.$$

Thus, the sample size required for achieving an 80% power for establishing similarity at the 5% level of significance is given by

$$n = \frac{\sigma^{*2}(z_\alpha + z_\beta)^2}{(\sigma_{BT}^2 - \delta\sigma_{BR}^2)^2} = \frac{0.126(1.65 + 0.84)^2}{(0.35^2 - 0.5^20.45^2)^2}$$

$$\approx 154.$$

Thus, a total of 308 subjects (154 subjects per arm) are needed in order to achieve the desired power for establishing similarity in inter-subject variability between treatment groups.

9.3.2 Replicated Crossover Design

Similarly, under Model 9.5, let $n = n_1 + n_2$; the inter-subject variabilities can be estimated by

$$\hat{\sigma}_{BT}^2 = s_{BT}^2 - \frac{1}{m}\hat{\sigma}_{WT}^2 \quad \text{and} \quad \hat{\sigma}_{BR}^2 = s_{BR}^2 - \frac{1}{m}\hat{\sigma}_{WR}^2,$$

where

$$s_{BT}^2 = \frac{1}{n-2}\sum_{i=1}^{2}\sum_{j=1}^{n_i}(\bar{y}_{ijT\cdot} - \bar{y}_{i\cdot T\cdot})^2,$$

$$s_{BR}^2 = \frac{1}{n-2}\sum_{i=1}^{2}\sum_{j=1}^{n_i}(\bar{y}_{ijR\cdot} - \bar{y}_{i\cdot R\cdot})^2,$$

and

$$\bar{y}_{i\cdot k\cdot} = \frac{1}{n_i}\sum_{j=1}^{n_i}\bar{y}_{ijk\cdot\cdot}.$$

For testing non-inferiority and superiority, similarly, consider the following hypotheses:

$$H_0 : \eta \geq 0 \quad \text{vs.} \quad H_a : \eta < 0,$$

where $\eta = \sigma_{BT}^2 - \delta\sigma_{BR}^2$. For a given significance level of α, let $n_s = n_1 + n_2 - 2$, an approximate $(1-\alpha) \times 100\%$th upper confidence bound for η can be calculated as $\hat{\eta}_U = \hat{\eta} + \sqrt{\Delta_U}$, where

$$\Delta_U = \hat{\lambda}_1^2\left(1 - \frac{n_s - 1}{\chi_{1-\alpha/2,n_s-1}^2}\right)^2 + \hat{\lambda}_2^2\left(1 - \frac{n_s - 1}{\chi_{\alpha/2,n_s-1}^2}\right)^2$$

$$+ \frac{\hat{\sigma}_{WT}^4}{m^2}\left(1 - \frac{n_s(m-1)}{\chi_{1-\alpha/2,n_s(m-1)}^2}\right)^2 + \frac{\hat{\sigma}_{WR}^4}{m^2}\left(1 - \frac{n_s(m-1)}{\chi_{\alpha/2,n_s(m-1)}^2}\right)^2,$$

and

$$\hat{\lambda}_i = \frac{s_{BT}^2 - \delta s_{BR}^2 \pm \sqrt{(s_{BT}^2 + \delta s_{BR}^2)^2 - 4\delta s_{BTR}^4}}{2}.$$

Thus, the null hypothesis is rejected at the α level of significance if $\hat{\eta}_u < 0$. On the other hand, under the alternative hypothesis, the power of the aforementioned test can be approximated by

$$\Phi\left(-z_\alpha - \frac{\sqrt{n_s}(\sigma_{BT}^2 - \delta\sigma_{BR}^2)}{\sigma^*}\right),$$

where

$$\sigma^* = 2\left[\left(\sigma_{BT}^2 + \frac{\sigma_{WT}^2}{m}\right)^2 + \delta^2\left(\sigma_{BR}^2 + \frac{\sigma_{WR}^2}{m}\right)^2 - 2\delta\rho^2\sigma_{BT}^2\sigma_{BR}^2 + \frac{\sigma_{WT}^4}{m^2(m-1)} + \frac{\delta^2\sigma_{WR}^4}{m^2(m-1)}\right].$$

Hence, the sample size needed in order to achieve the power of $1 - \beta$ at the α level of significance is given by

$$n = \frac{\sigma^{*2}(z_\alpha + z_\beta)^2}{(\sigma_{BT}^2 - \delta\sigma_{BR}^2)^2} + 2.$$

9.4 Comparing Total Variability

In practice, in addition to the intra-subject and inter-subject variabilities, the total variability is also of interest to the investigator. The total variability is defined as the sum of the intra-subject and inter-subject variabilities. As the total variability is observable even in an experiment without replicates, in this section, both replicated and non-replicated designs are discussed.

9.4.1 Parallel Design without Replicates

Consider a parallel design without replicates. In this case, Model 9.1 reduces to

$$y_{ij} = \mu_i + \epsilon_{ij}, \tag{9.7}$$

where ϵ_{ij} are assumed to be i.i.d. as $N(0, \sigma_{Ti}^2)$. In this case, the total variability can be estimated by

$$\hat{\sigma}_{Ti}^2 = \frac{1}{n_i - 1}\sum_{j=1}^{n_i}(y_{ij} - \bar{y}_{i\cdot})^2,$$

where

$$\bar{y}_{i\cdot} = \frac{1}{n_i}\sum_{j=1}^{n_i}y_{ij}.$$

Similar to Equation 9.4, the following two one-sided hypotheses are commonly considered for testing similarity in total variability between drug products:

$$H_{01} : \frac{\sigma_{TT}}{\sigma_{TR}} \geq \sqrt{\delta} \quad \text{versus} \quad H_{a1} : \frac{\sigma_{TT}}{\sigma_{TR}} < \sqrt{\delta}$$

and

$$H_{02} : \frac{\sigma_{TT}}{\sigma_{TR}} \leq \frac{1}{\sqrt{\delta}} \quad \text{versus} \quad H_{a2} : \frac{\sigma_{TT}}{\sigma_{TR}} > \frac{1}{\sqrt{\delta}}. \tag{9.8}$$

Thus, for a given significance level α, the null hypothesis of dissimilarity is rejected and the alternative hypothesis of similarity is accepted if

$$\frac{\hat{\sigma}_{TT}^2}{\delta \hat{\sigma}_{TR}^2} < F_{1-\alpha, n_T, n_R} \quad \text{and} \quad \frac{\delta \hat{\sigma}_{TT}^2}{\hat{\sigma}_{TR}^2} > F_{\alpha, n_T, n_R}.$$

On the other hand, under the alternative hypothesis of similarity, a conservative approximation to the power is given by

$$1 - 2P \left(F_{n-1, n-1} > \frac{\delta \hat{\sigma}_{TT}^2}{\sigma_{TR}^2} F_{1-\alpha, n-1, n-1} \right).$$

Hence, the sample size needed for achieving the power of $1 - \beta$ can be obtained by solving the following equation:

$$\frac{\delta \hat{\sigma}_{TT}^2}{\sigma_{TR}^2} = \frac{F_{\beta/2, n-1, n-1}}{F_{1-\alpha, n-1, n-1}}.$$

9.4.2 Parallel Design with Replicates

Under Model 9.7, the total variabilities can be estimated by

$$\hat{\sigma}_{Ti}^2 = s_{Bi}^2 + \frac{m}{m-1} \hat{\sigma}_{Wi}^2,$$

where
s_{Bi}^2 is defined in Equation 9.6
$\hat{\sigma}_{Wi}^2$ is given in Equation 9.2

Let $\eta = \sigma_{TT}^2 - \delta \sigma_{TR}^2$. Then, a natural estimator is given by

$$\hat{\eta} = \hat{\sigma}_{TT}^2 - \delta \hat{\sigma}_{TR}^2.$$

For testing similarity, the hypotheses of interest given in Equation 9.8, we reject the null hypothesis and conclude similarity at the α level of significance if both hypotheses in Equation 9.8 are rejected with significance level α. The test can be performed by calculating a $(1-\alpha) \times 100\%$ upper confidence bound for $\eta_1 = \sigma_{TT}^2 - \delta\sigma_{TR}^2$ and a $(1-\alpha) \times 100\%$ lower confidence bound for $\eta_2 = \delta\sigma_{TT}^2 - \sigma_{TR}^2$ by the MLS method. For example, the $(1-\alpha) \times 100\%$ lower confidence bound for η_1 is given by

$$\hat{\eta}_{1u} = \hat{\eta}_1 + \sqrt{\Delta_u},$$

where

$$\Delta_u = s_{BT}^4\left(1-\frac{n_T-1}{\chi_{1-\alpha,n_T-1}^2}\right)^2 + \delta^2 s_{BR}^4\left(1-\frac{n_R-1}{\chi_{\alpha,n_R-1}^2}\right)^2$$

$$+ \frac{(m-1)^2\hat{\sigma}_{WT}^4}{m^2}\left(1-\frac{n_T(m-1)}{\chi_{\alpha,n_T(m-1)}^2}\right)^2 + \frac{\delta^2(m-1)^2\hat{\sigma}_{WR}^4}{m^2}\left(1-\frac{n_R(m-1)}{\chi_{1-\alpha,n_R(m-1)}^2}\right)^2.$$

Thus, the null hypothesis is rejected at the α level of significance if $\hat{\eta}_{1u} < 0$. The power of the aforementioned test can be approximated by

$$\Phi\left(-z_\alpha - \frac{\sqrt{n}(\sigma_{TT}^2 - \delta\sigma_{TR}^2)}{\sigma^*}\right),$$

where

$$\sigma^* = 2\left[\left(\sigma_{BT}^2 + \frac{\sigma_{WT}^2}{m}\right)^2 + \delta^2\left(\sigma_{BR}^2 + \delta^2\frac{\sigma_{WR}^2}{m}\right)^2 + \frac{(m-1)\sigma_{WT}^4}{m^2} + \frac{(m-1)\sigma_{WR}^4}{m^2}\right].$$

Hence, the sample size needed in order to achieve the power of $1-\beta$ at the α level of significance is given by

$$n = \frac{\sigma^{*2}(z_\alpha + z_\beta)^2}{(\sigma_{TT}^2 + \delta\sigma_{TR}^2)^2}.$$

9.4.3 Standard 2 × 2 Crossover Design

Under the standard 2 × 2 crossover design, the notation defined in Model 9.5 can still be used. However, the subscript 1 is omitted as no replicate exists. Under Model 9.5, the total variability can be estimated by

$$\hat{\sigma}_{TT}^2 = \frac{1}{n_1+n_2-2}\sum_{i=1}^{2}\sum_{j=1}^{n_i}(y_{ijT} - \bar{y}_{i\cdot T})^2,$$

and

$$\hat{\sigma}_{TR}^2 = \frac{1}{n_1 + n_2 - 2} \sum_{i=1}^{2} \sum_{j=1}^{n_i} (y_{ijR} - \bar{y}_{i \cdot R})^2,$$

where

$$\bar{y}_{i \cdot k} = \frac{1}{n_i} \sum_{j=1}^{n_i} y_{ijk}, \quad k = T \text{ or } R.$$

For testing non-inferiority/superiority, similarly, consider the following hypotheses:

$$H_0 : \eta \geq 0 \quad \text{versus} \quad H_a : \eta < 0,$$

where $\eta = \sigma_{TT}^2 - \delta \sigma_{TR}^2$. For a given significance level of α, an approximate $(1 - \alpha) \times 100\%$ upper confidence bound for η can be calculated as $\hat{\eta}_u = \hat{\eta} + \sqrt{\Delta_u}$, where

$$\Delta_u = \hat{\lambda}_1^2 \left(\frac{n_1 + n_2 - 2}{\chi_{\alpha, n_1 + n_2 - 2}^2} - 1 \right)^2 + \hat{\lambda}_2^2 \left(\frac{n_1 + n_2 - 2}{\chi_{1-\alpha, n_1 + n_2 - 2}^2} - 1 \right)^2,$$

and

$$\hat{\lambda}_i = \frac{\hat{\sigma}_{TT}^2 - \delta^2 \hat{\sigma}_{TR}^2 \pm \sqrt{(\hat{\sigma}_{TT}^2 + \delta^2 \hat{\sigma}_{TR}^2)^2 - 4\delta^2 \hat{\sigma}_{BTR}^4}}{2}.$$

Thus, the null hypothesis is rejected at the α level of significance if $\hat{\eta}_u < 0$. On the other hand, under the alternative hypothesis, the power of the aforementioned test can be approximated by

$$\Phi \left(-z_\alpha - \frac{\sqrt{n}(\sigma_{TT}^2 - \delta \sigma_{TR}^2)}{\sigma^*} \right),$$

where

$$\sigma^* = 2(\sigma_{TT}^4 + \delta^2 \sigma_{TR}^4 - 2\delta \rho^2 \sigma_{TT}^2 \sigma_{TR}^2).$$

Hence, the sample size needed in order to achieve the power of $1 - \beta$ at the α level of significance is given by

$$n = \frac{\sigma^{*2}(z_\alpha + z_\beta)^2}{(\sigma_{TT}^2 - \delta \sigma_{TR}^2)^2} + 2.$$

9.4.4 Replicated 2 × 2m Crossover Design

Under Model 9.5, the total variabilities can be estimated by

$$\hat{\sigma}_{Tk}^2 = s_{Bk}^2 + \frac{m-1}{m}\hat{\sigma}_{Wk}^2, \quad k = T,R,$$

where σ_{Wk}^2 and s_{Bk}^2 are as defined earlier. Similarly, for testing non-inferiority and superiority, consider the following hypotheses:

$$H_0 : \eta \geq 0 \quad \text{versus} \quad H_a : \eta < 0,$$

where $\eta = \sigma_{TT}^2 - \delta\sigma_{TR}^2$. For a given significance level of α, let $n_s = n_1 + n_2 - 2$, an approximate $(1 - \alpha) \times 100\%$th upper confidence bound for η can be calculated as $\hat{\eta}_U = \hat{\eta} + \sqrt{\Delta_U}$, where

$$\Delta_U = \hat{\lambda}_1^2 \left(1 - \frac{n_s - 1}{\chi_{\alpha,n_s-1}^2}\right)^2 + \hat{\lambda}_2^2 \left(1 - \frac{n_s - 1}{\chi_{1-\alpha,n_s-1}^2}\right)^2$$

$$+ \frac{(m-1)\hat{\sigma}_{WT}^4}{m^2}\left(1 - \frac{n_s(m-1)}{\chi_{1-\alpha,n_s(m-1)}^2}\right)^2 + \frac{(m-1)\hat{\sigma}_{WR}^4}{m^2}\left(1 - \frac{n_s(m-1)}{\chi_{\alpha,n_s(m-1)}^2}\right)^2,$$

and

$$\hat{\lambda}_i = \frac{s_{BT}^2 - \delta s_{BR}^2 \pm \sqrt{(s_{BT}^2 + \delta s_{BR}^2)^2 - 4\delta s_{BTR}^4}}{2}.$$

Thus, the null hypothesis is rejected at the α level of significance if $\hat{\eta}_U < 0$. On the other hand, under the alternative hypothesis, the power of the aforementioned test can be approximated by

$$\Phi\left(-z_\alpha - \frac{\sqrt{n_s}(\sigma_{TT}^2 - \delta\sigma_{TR}^2)}{\sigma^*}\right),$$

where

$$\sigma^* = 2\left[\left(\sigma_{BT}^2 + \frac{\sigma_{WT}^2}{m}\right)^2 + \delta^2\left(\sigma_{BR}^2 + \frac{\sigma_{WR}^2}{m}\right)^2 - 2\delta\rho^2\sigma_{BT}^2\sigma_{BR}^2\right.$$

$$\left. + \frac{(m-1)\sigma_{WT}^4}{m^2} + \frac{\delta^2(m-1)\sigma_{WR}^4}{m^2}\right].$$

Hence, the sample size needed in order to achieve the power of $1 - \beta$ at the α level of significance is given by

$$n = \frac{\sigma^{*2}(z_\alpha + z_\beta)^2}{(\sigma_{TT}^2 - \delta\sigma_{TR}^2)^2} + 2.$$

9.5 Comparing Intra-subject CVs

In addition to comparing intra-subject variabilities, it is often of interest to study the intra-subject CV, which is a relative standard deviation adjusted for mean. By definition of CV, the problem of comparing CVs is reduced to the problem of comparing intra-subject variabilities if the test product and the reference product have identical mean. On the other hand, if the intra-subject variability of the test product is the same as that of the reference product, the problem of comparing CVs becomes the problem of comparing means between treatment groups. Statistically, comparing intra-subject CVs reduces a two-dimensional comparison (comparing means and comparing intra-subject variabilities) to a one-dimensional comparison.

In recent years, the use of intra-subject CV has become increasingly popular. For example, the FDA defines highly variable drug products based on their intra-subject CVs. That is, a drug product is considered a highly variable drug if its intra-subject CV is greater than 30%. The intra-subject CV is also used as a measure for reproducibility of blood levels of a given drug product when the drug product is repeatedly administered at different dosing periods. In practice, two methods are commonly employed for comparing intra-subject CVs. One is referred to as the conditional random effects model proposed by Chow and Tse (1990) and the other one is called the simple random effects model proposed by Quan and Shih (1996). In this section, the method based on the simple random effects model is introduced.

Under Model 9.5, an estimator of the intra-subject CV can be obtained as

$$\widehat{CV}_i = \frac{\hat{\sigma}_{Wi}}{\hat{\mu}_i},$$

where

$$\hat{\mu}_i = \frac{1}{mn_i} \sum_{j=1}^{n_i} \sum_{k=1}^{m} y_{ijk}.$$

By Taylor's expansion, it follows that

$$\widehat{CV}_i - CV_i = \frac{\hat{\sigma}_{Wi}}{\hat{\mu}_i} - \frac{\sigma_{Wi}}{\mu_i}$$

$$\approx \frac{1}{2\mu_i \sigma_{Wi}} (\hat{\sigma}_{Wi}^2 - \sigma_{Wi}^2) - \frac{\sigma_{Wi}}{\mu_i^2} (\hat{\mu}_i - \mu_i).$$

Hence, by the central limit theorem, $\widehat{CV}_i$ is asymptotically distributed as a normal random variable with mean CV_i and variance σ_i^{*2}/n_i, where

$$\hat{\sigma}_i^{*2} = \frac{\sigma_{Wi}^2}{2m\mu_i^2} + \frac{\sigma_{Wi}^4}{\mu_i^4} = \frac{1}{2m}CV_i^2 + CV_i^4.$$

An intuitive estimator of σ_i^{*2} is given by

$$\hat{\sigma}_i^{*2} = \frac{1}{2m}\widehat{CV}_i^2 + \widehat{CV}_i^4.$$

For testing similarity, the following hypotheses are usually considered:

$$H_0 : |CV_T - CV_R| \geq \delta \quad \text{versus} \quad H_a : |CV_T - CV_R| < \delta.$$

The two drug products are concluded to be similar to each other if the null hypothesis is rejected at the α level of significance if

$$\frac{\widehat{CV}_T - \widehat{CV}_R + \delta}{\sqrt{\sigma_T^{*2}/n_T + \sigma_R^{*2}/n_R}} > z_\alpha \quad \text{and} \quad \frac{\widehat{CV}_T - \widehat{CV}_R - \delta}{\sqrt{\sigma_T^{*2}/n_T + \sigma_R^{*2}/n_R}} < -z_\alpha.$$

Under the alternative hypothesis that $|CV_T - CV_R| < \delta$, the power of the aforementioned test is approximately

$$2\Phi\left(\frac{\delta - |CV_T - CV_R|}{\sqrt{\sigma_T^{*2}/n_T + \sigma_R^{*2}/n_R}} - z_\alpha\right) - 1.$$

Hence, under the assumption that $n = n_1 = n_2$, the sample size needed in order to achieve $1 - \beta$ at the α level of significance can be obtained by solving

$$\frac{\delta - |CV_T - CV_R|}{\sqrt{\sigma_T^{*2}/n_T + \sigma_R^{*2}/n_R}} - z_\alpha = z_{\beta/2}.$$

This gives

$$n = \frac{(z_\alpha + z_{\beta/2})^2(\sigma_R^{*2} + \sigma_T^{*2})}{(\delta - |CV_T - CV_R|)^2}.$$

9.6 Concluding Remarks

For assessment of average bioequivalence or biosimilarity, a one-size-fits-all criterion of (80%, 125%) is adopted based on log-transformed data. For assessment of equivalence or similarity in variability including intra-subject variability, inter-subject variability, and total variability as described in this chapter, a one-size-fits-all criterion of $(\delta, 1/\delta)$, where $0 < \delta < 1$, is considered. In practice, $\delta = 1/2$ or $\delta = 2/3$ are often considered. In order to address the degree of similarity and the question "How similar is considered highly similar?" disaggregated criteria by comparing average responses first and then the variability in responses is suggested. However, further research is needed in order to have a better understanding of the statistical properties of the proposed disaggregated criteria. To provide a better understanding of sample sizes required for comparing variabilities, Table 9.1 gives a summary of formulas for sample size calculation for achieving an 80% power for establishment of similarity in variability (including intra-subject variability, inter-subject variability, total variability, and intra-subject CV) between a biosimilar (test) product and an innovative (reference) product under a parallel design with replicates and a replicated crossover design.

For comparing intra-subject variabilities and/or intra-subject CVs between drug products, replicates from the same subject are essential regardless of whether the study design is a parallel group design or a crossover design. In clinical research, data are often log-transformed before the analysis. It should be noted that the intra-subject standard deviation of log-transformed data is approximately equal to the intra-subject CV of the untransformed (raw) data. As a result, it is suggested that intra-subject variability be used

TABLE 9.1

Sample Size Formulas for Comparing Variabilities

Comparison	Parallel Design with Replicates	Replicated 2 × 2m Crossover Design
Intra-subject	$\dfrac{\delta}{r} = \dfrac{F_{\beta,n(m-1),n(m-1)}}{F_{1-\alpha,n(m-1),n(m-1)}}$	$\dfrac{\delta \sigma_{WT}^2}{\sigma_{WR}^2} = \dfrac{F_{\beta/2,(2n-2)(m-1),(2n-2)(m-1)}}{F_{1-\alpha,(2n-2)(m-1),(2n-2)(m-1)}}$
Inter-subject	$n = \dfrac{\sigma^{*2}(z_\alpha + z_\beta)^2}{(\sigma_{BT}^2 - \delta\sigma_{BR}^2)}$	$N = \dfrac{\sigma^{*2}(z_\alpha + tcz_\beta)^2}{(\sigma_{BT}^2 - \delta\sigma_{BR}^2)} + 2$
Total	$n = \dfrac{\sigma^{*2}(z_\alpha + z_\beta)^2}{(\sigma_{TT}^2 - \delta\sigma_{TR}^2)}$	$N = \dfrac{\sigma^{*2}(z_\alpha + z_\beta)^2}{(\sigma_{TT}^2 - \delta\sigma_{TR}^2)} + 2$
Intra-subject CVs	$n = \dfrac{(z_\alpha + z_{\beta/2})^2(\sigma_R^{*2} + \sigma_T^{*2})}{(\delta - |CV_T - CV_R|)^2}$	$n = \dfrac{(z_\alpha + z_{\beta/2})^2(\sigma_R^{*2} + \sigma_T^{*2})}{(\delta - |CV_T - CV_R|)^2}$

Note: δ, similarity limit; $r = (\sigma_{WT}^2/\sigma_{WR}^2) \in (1, \delta)$; $N = n_1 + n_2$; $n = n_1 = n_2$; m, number of replicate.

when analyzing log-transformed data, while the intra-subject CV be considered when analyzing untransformed data.

As indicated earlier, comparing intra-subject variabilities and/or intra-subject CVs requires replicates from the same subjects. This is a limitation for parallel design, which is considered the design of choice for the assessment of biosimilarity of biosimilar products. To overcome this problem, alternatively, it is suggested that the comparison between total variabilities of the test product and the reference product be performed under the assumption that the difference in intra-subject variabilities is within an acceptable range.

For assessment of inter-subject variability and/or total variability, Chow and Tse (1991) indicated that the usual analysis of variance models could lead to negative estimates of the variance components, especially the inter-subject variance component. In addition, the sum of the best estimates of the intra-subject variance and the inter-subject variance may not lead to the best estimate for the total variance. Chow and Shao (1988) proposed an estimation procedure for variance components that will not only avoid negative estimates but also provide a better estimate as compared to the maximum likelihood estimates. For estimation of total variance, Chow and Tse (1991) proposed a method as an alternative to the sum of estimates of individual variance components. These ideas could be applied to provide a better estimate of sample sizes for studies comparing variabilities between drug products.

In recent years, the assessment of reproducibility in terms of intra-subject variability or intra-subject CV in clinical research has received much attention. Shao and Chow (2002) defined reproducibility of a study drug as a collective term that encompasses consistency, similarity, and stability (control) within therapeutic index (or window) of a subject's clinical status (e.g., clinical response of some primary study endpoint, blood levels, or blood concentration–time curve) when the study drug is repeatedly administered at different dosing periods under the same experimental conditions. Reproducibility of clinical results observed from a clinical study can be quantitated through the evaluation of the so-called reproducibility probability, which will be further discussed in Chapter 11.

In biosimilar studies, one of the controversial issues is that what if we pass biosimilarity assessment based on the analysis of average responses but detect that there is a significant difference in variability of the responses (intra-subject variability, inter-subject variability, or total variability). In this case, it is a concern whether the heterogeneity of the variabilities (intra-subject variability, inter-subject variability, or total variability) will post any safety concern in real practice as biosimilar products are known to be sensitive to a small change or variation in environmental factors during the manufacturing process. Thus, it is of particular interest to study the potential impact of the heterogeneity of the variabilities on the assessment of biosimilarity and especially interchangeability (in terms of the concepts of switching and alternating) if possible.

10

Impact of Variability on Biosimilarity Limits for Assessing Follow-on Biologics

10.1 Introduction

As mentioned in the previous chapters, in a typical bioequivalence study for generic approval, the test product is said to be average bioequivalent with the reference product if the 90% confidence interval of the ratio of geometric means of the primary pharmacokinetic (PK) responses such as AUC and C_{max} is within the bioequivalence limits of 80% and 125% (FDA, 2001, 2003). This one-size-fits-all ABE criterion ignores the variability associated with the responses although the number of subjects required for concluding ABE with a desired power depends upon the magnitude of the within-subject variability of the product. One of the major criticisms is that the one-size-fits-all ABE criterion may penalize good products with smaller variability in the sense that they may fail to pass the one-size-fits-all ABE criterion if the intra-subject variability of the reference product is large. To overcome the problem, it is suggested to widen the bioequivalence limits for products with large variability in order to increase the probability of passing for those drug products with smaller variability.

Since mid-1990s, the FDA considers drug products with a within-subject coefficient of variation (CV) of 30% or more as *highly variable drugs* (Shah et al., 1996). The assessment of bioequivalence for highly variable drugs has attracted much attention since then (see, e.g., Boddy et al., 1995; Tothfalusi et al., 2001, 2009; Tothfalusi and Endrenyi, 2003; Endrenyi and Tothfalusi, 2009). Most discussions are directed to (1) proposal of more flexible bioequivalence limits, e.g., bioequivalence limits adjusted for intra-subject variability and/or therapeutic index, and (2) increase the probability of success for the development of highly variable drug products by widening the bioequivalence limits. For these purposes, Haidar et al. (2008) proposed the use of the so-called reference scaled average bioequivalence criterion (SABE). This proposal was subsequently adopted by the FDA as standards for bioequivalence assessment of highly variable drug products.

For assessment of biosimilarity of biosimilar products or follow-on biologics, large variability is likely to occur during the manufacturing process of biological products than that of the traditional small-molecule drug products. This large variability may be due to variability in the biologic mechanisms, inputs, and relatively large number of complex steps in the process (Roger, 2006; Roger and Mikhail, 2007; Woodcock, 2007; Chow and Liu, 2010). Thus, some researchers consider that biosimilar products are highly variable drug products and recommend that the assessment of biosimilarity should take variability into consideration whenever possible. As a result, biosimilarity assessment based on the SABE is recommended (Hsieh et al., 2010).

In this chapter, we focus on the assessment of average biosimilarity of follow-on biologics based on some clinical endpoints from parallel group designs. In the next section, the relationship between variability and biosimilarity limit is studied given that power and all other parameters fixed. Based on this relationship, several scaled biosimilarity limits are proposed in Section 10.3. The properties of the proposed biosimilarity limits for assessing biosimilar products are studied and compared in the subsequent section. Conclusions and discussions are presented in the last section.

10.2 Relationship between Variability and Biosimilarity Limits

In this section, we start with the average biosimilarity and explore the impact of variability on biosimilarity limits given that other parameters (e.g., power of $1 - \beta$, type I error of α, sample size, and true treatment effect) are fixed. The relationship can help in addressing the questions of quantitative standard for what constitutes highly variable drugs; and what biosimilarity limits are appropriate for highly variable biologics. As indicated in the previous chapters, several different criteria for assessing average bioequivalence (ABE) or biosimilarity have been proposed in the literature. For simplicity, in this section, we will focus on the moment-based criteria as described later.

Consider a parallel design of the study employed for evaluating the ABE of the test product with the reference product. Let T and R be the parameters of interest with means of μ_T and μ_R, respectively. For example, in a typical BE study with primary PK responses and ABE limit of (80%, 125%), the interval hypothesis for testing the ABE of two products can be expressed as

$$H_0 : \frac{\mu_T}{\mu_R} \leq 80\% \quad \text{or} \quad \frac{\mu_T}{\mu_R} \geq 125\% \quad \text{vs.} \quad H_\alpha : 80\% < \frac{\mu_T}{\mu_R} < 125\%.$$

Since the natural log transformation of PK response usually follows the normal distribution, the hypothesis can be re-expressed in terms of difference as

$$H_0: \ln(\mu_T) - \ln(\mu_R) \leq -0.2231 \quad \text{or} \quad \ln(\mu_T) - \ln(\mu_R) \geq 0.2231$$

$$\text{vs.} \quad H_\alpha: -0.2231 < \ln(\mu_T) - \ln(\mu_R) < 0.2231.$$

However, in the assessment of FOB, a clinical trial is required where the parameters of interest are clinical endpoints that are often assumed to be normally distributed. Therefore, without loss of generality, here we focus on the interval hypothesis expressed using mean difference as follows:

$$H_0: \mu_T - \mu_R \leq \theta_L \quad \text{or} \quad \mu_T - \mu_R \geq \theta_U \quad \text{vs.} \quad H_\alpha: \theta_L < \mu_T - \mu_R < \theta_U, \quad (10.1)$$

where (θ_L, θ_U) is the average biosimilarity limit. Adopting the concept used in the non-inferiority trials, the FOB is expected to obtain similar fraction of effect, μ_R, as observed in the reference drug. We therefore choose to form the biosimilarity limit as $\theta = \lambda \times \mu_R$, $0 \leq \lambda \leq 1$, e.g., $\pm 20\% \times \mu_R$. In particular, if symmetric limits on either direction are desired for biosimilarity, we will employ $\theta = \theta_U = -\theta_L$ for rest of the discussions.

Let us denote independent samples of T_i and R_j to be the observations of T and R with $i = 1, \ldots, n_T$ and $j = 1, \ldots, n_R$. Without loss of generality, assume T_i and R_j are independent samples from $N(\mu_T, V_T)$ and $N(\mu_R, V_R)$, respectively. Then the $100(1 - 2\alpha)\%$ confidence interval based on the parallel design for $\mu_T - \mu_R$ can be expressed as

$$\left[(\bar{T} - \bar{R}) - Z_{1-\alpha} \sqrt{\frac{V_T}{n_T} + \frac{V_R}{n_R}}, \; (\bar{T} - \bar{R}) + Z_{1-\alpha} \sqrt{\frac{V_T}{n_T} + \frac{V_R}{n_R}} \right],$$

where $\bar{T}$ and $\bar{R}$ are the unbiased estimators of μ_T and μ_R, and $Z_{1-\alpha}$ the $(1 - \alpha)$ percentile of standard normal distribution. The ABE of the test and reference products will be concluded at the significance level of α if the aforementioned confidence interval lies entirely within (θ_L, θ_U). Thus, the probability of concluding ABE can be expressed as

$$P\left(\theta_L \leq (\bar{T} - \bar{R}) - Z_{1-\alpha} \sqrt{\frac{V_T}{n_T} + \frac{V_R}{n_R}} \quad \text{and} \quad (\bar{T} - \bar{R}) + Z_{1-\alpha} \sqrt{\frac{V_T}{n_T} + \frac{V_R}{n_R}} \leq \theta_U \right)$$

$$= P\left(\theta_L + Z_{1-\alpha} \sqrt{\frac{V_T}{n_T} + \frac{V_R}{n_R}} \leq (\bar{T} - \bar{R}) \leq \theta_U - Z_{1-\alpha} \sqrt{\frac{V_T}{n_T} + \frac{V_R}{n_R}} \right). \quad (10.2)$$

In particular, if $\theta = \theta_U = -\theta_L$ (i.e., symmetric limits on either direction), $n_T = an_R$, $V_T = bV_R$, and $C = \sqrt{(1/n_R + b/an_R)} \times |\mu_R|$, the aforementioned equation can be expressed as

$$P\left(-\left[\theta - Z_{1-\alpha}\sqrt{\left(\frac{1}{n_R} + \frac{b}{an_R}\right)} \times V_R\right] \leq (\bar{T} - \bar{R}) \leq \theta - Z_{1-\alpha}\sqrt{\left(\frac{1}{n_R} + \frac{b}{an_R}\right)} \times V_R\right)$$

$$= P\left(-\left[\theta - Z_{1-\alpha}\sqrt{\left(\frac{1}{n_R} + \frac{b}{an_R}\right)} \times |\mu_R| \times CV_R\right] \leq (\bar{T} - \bar{R})\right.$$

$$\left. \leq \theta - Z_{1-\alpha}\sqrt{\left(\frac{1}{n_R} + \frac{b}{an_R}\right)} \times |\mu_R| \times CV_R\right)$$

$$= \Phi\left(\frac{\theta - Z_{1-\alpha} \times C \times CV_R - (\mu_T - \mu_R)}{C \times CV_R}\right) - \Phi\left(\frac{-[\theta - Z_{1-\alpha} \times C \times CV_R] - (\mu_T - \mu_R)}{C \times CV_R}\right).$$

Since the power of the test is defined as correctly concluding ABE when $\mu_T - \mu_R$ is 0 or close to 0 (within the biosimilarity limit), we can obtain the required biosimilarity limit (θ) to achieve desired power and type I error, given the variability as measured by CV by solving the equation

$$\Phi\left(\frac{\theta - Z_{1-\alpha} \times C \times CV_R - (\mu_T - \mu_R)}{C \times CV_R}\right) - \Phi\left(\frac{-[\theta - Z_{1-\alpha} \times C \times CV_R] - (\mu_T - \mu_R)}{C \times CV_R}\right)$$

$$= 1 - \beta. \tag{10.3}$$

Figure 10.1 visually illustrated the relationship between θ and CV obtained from the numerical solution of the aforementioned equation under various scenarios. From the plot, an approximate linear pattern between the margin θ and CV is observed, which motivates us to approximate Expression 10.2 using the first order of Taylor expansion around $\mu_T - \mu_R$ as follows:

$$2 \times \Phi\left(\frac{\theta - Z_{1-\alpha} \times C \times CV_R - (\mu_T - \mu_R)}{C \times CV_R}\right) - 1 + o(\mu_T - \mu_R)$$

$$= 1 - \beta.$$

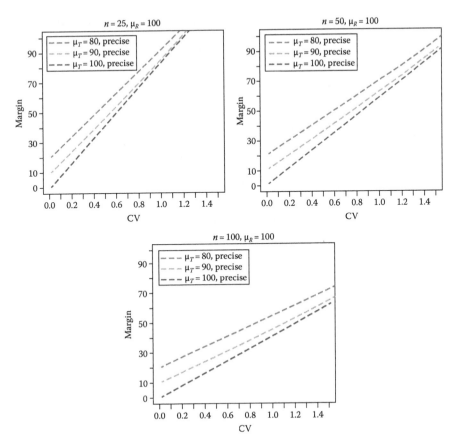

FIGURE 10.1
Relationship between the margin and CV obtained from the numerical solution of Equation 10.3: $n_T = n_R$, $V_T = V_R$, and $\alpha = 0.05$, $\beta = 0.2$.

Solving the equation, we get

$$\theta = \left(Z_{1-\alpha} + Z_{1-(\beta/2)}\right) \times C \times CV_R + \left(\mu_T - \mu_R\right) + o\left(\mu_T - \mu_R\right).$$

Therefore, when $\mu_T - \mu_R$ is close to 0, the closed form of relationship between θ and CV can be approximated as

$$\theta = \left(Z_{1-\alpha} + Z_{1-(\beta/2)}\right) \times C \times CV_R.$$

When $\mu_T - \mu_R$ is largely deviated from 0 (e.g., outside of the biosimilarity limit), the probability of concluding biosimilarity in Expression 10.2 will be mainly obtained by one side of the interval:

$$P\left(-\left[\theta - Z_{1-\alpha}\sqrt{(V_T/n_T)+(V_R/n_R)}\right] \leq (\bar{T}-\bar{R}) \leq \theta - Z_{1-\alpha}\sqrt{(V_T/n_T)+(V_R/n_R)}\right)$$

$$\approx \Phi\left(\frac{\theta - Z_{1-\alpha}\sqrt{(V_T/n_T)+(V_R/n_R)} - (\mu_T - \mu_R)}{(V_T/n_T)+(V_R/n_R)}\right) \quad \text{if } \mu_T - \mu_R \gg 0$$

or $P\left(-\left[\theta - Z_{1-\alpha}\sqrt{(V_T/n_T)+(V_R/n_R)}\right] \leq (\bar{T}-\bar{R}) \leq \theta - Z_{1-\alpha}\sqrt{(V_T/n_T)+(V_R/n_R)}\right)$

$$\approx 1 - \Phi\left(\frac{-\left[\theta - Z_{1-\alpha}\sqrt{(V_T/n_T)+(V_R/n_R)}\right] - (\mu_T - \mu_R)}{\sqrt{(V_T/n_T)+(V_R/n_R)}}\right) \quad \text{if } \mu_T - \mu_R \ll 0.$$

$$(10.4)$$

Under this situation, we get

$$\theta = \left(Z_{1-\alpha} + Z_{1-\beta}\right)\sqrt{\frac{V_T}{n_T} + \frac{V_R}{n_R}} + |\mu_T - \mu_R|$$

$$= \left(Z_{1-\alpha} + Z_{1-\beta}\right)\sqrt{\left(\frac{1}{n_R} + \frac{b}{an_R}\right)} \times |\mu_R| \times CV_R + |\mu_T - \mu_R|. \qquad (10.5)$$

Expressions 10.4 and 10.5 provide us some closed form of relationship between biosimilarity limit (θ) and variability as measured by CV, approximately. In Figure 10.2, we compare the approximation obtained from Expressions 10.4 and 10.5 with the exact numerical solutions. It turns out that the approximation is close to the precise numerical solution. When $\mu_T = \mu_R$, the solid and dotted purple lines are overlapped. The precise numerical solution and the approximation from those closed forms are off slightly as CV goes beyond 1. But the difference decreases as the sample size increases. So when the sample size reaches 100, they are almost overlapped again. This suggests that the relationship provided in closed form in Expressions 10.4 and 10.5 approximates the real precise relationship very well, and they are much easier to use. Therefore, they will be utilized in our following discussions about scaled biosimilarity limits.

Another observation from Expressions 10.4 and 10.5 is that the required margin is linearly related to the CV, given the fixed choice of type I error, desired power, and sample size. In a traditional PK bioequivalence study

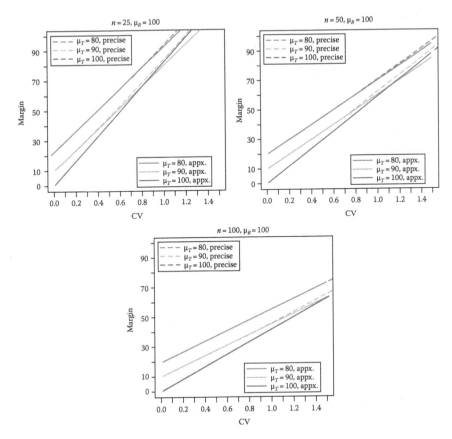

FIGURE 10.2
Comparison of the relationship between the margin and CV obtained from the numerical solution of Equation 10.3 and from the approximations of Equations 10.4 and 10.5: $n_T = n_R$, $V_T = V_R$, and $\alpha = 0.05$, $\beta = 0.2$.

where sample size is generally less (e.g., n from 18 to 24), the margin of $\pm 20\% \times \mu_R$ will provide enough power for $CV \leq 30\%$, which is consistent with current generally accepted criteria. In the FOB assessment where a clinical study is planned, the sample size per group usually can go up to fifty or hundreds per group. With the larger sample sizes, a fixed margin of $\pm 20\% \times \mu_R$ can provide enough power for CV up to 40%. However, when CV is even larger than 40%, which is common in biological products, scaled margins need to be applied to account for the large variability of the reference drug itself.

In the next section, several scaled margins are proposed based on the literature or the relationship derived.

10.3 Scaled Biosimilarity Margins

Zhang et al. (2013) proposed the following margins aim to have the following properties:

1. Continuous.
2. When CV is small, the margin is fixed and consistent with current regulatory standards.
3. When CV is large, the adjusted margin becomes wider but shall not be too wide to properly control the consumer's risk.

These margins are described in the following sections.

10.3.1 Fixed Cutoff Linear Scaled Margin

The fixed cutoff linear scaled margin can be expressed as follows:

$$\theta = \begin{cases} \theta_0, & \text{if } CV \le CV_0 \\ \dfrac{CV}{CV_0} \times \theta_0, & \text{if } CV > CV_0 \end{cases} \tag{10.6}$$

where CV_0 is the chosen cutoff for high-variability drug definition (e.g., 30% or 40%), and θ_0 is the fixed margin commonly accepted (e.g., a margin of ±20% of μ_R).

Note that $CV = \sqrt{V}/\mu$ are actually two components. Therefore, $CV > CV_0$ does not necessarily mean larger variability. It could also imply small means. However, in a trial of evaluating FOB, the CV reflects the inner property of the reference drug and is expected to remain constant. Therefore, it is a fine quantitative for defining high-variable drugs and to be used in the scaled margin adjustment. It should be noted that the margin given in Equation 10.6 is similar to the SABE described in the literature, which is illustrated in Figure 10.3.

As we can see, the slope of the scaled margin is decided by two points: $CV = 0$ and $CV = CV_0$. When CV is close to 0, which means no variability around mean, the margin should be small and near 0 too. When $CV = CV_0$, the margin equals the fixed margin so the continuity can be reserved.

However, this proposed margin tends to become wider when the CV is really high. For example, take $CV_0 = 0.3$ and $\theta_0 = \pm 20\%$ of μ_R. When true $CV = 1.2$, the scaled margin will be $\pm 80\% {}^* \mu_R$ for $\mu_T - \mu_R$. With this more than half of the treatment effect difference, usually it is not advisable to conclude biosimilarity. Therefore, in our next proposal, we try to slow down the magnitude of the slope by taking the square root of the original slope (Figure 10.4).

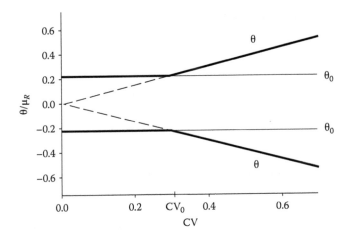

FIGURE 10.3
Fixed cutoff linear scaled margin for $CV_0 = 30\%$ and $\theta_0 = 20\%$ of μ_R.

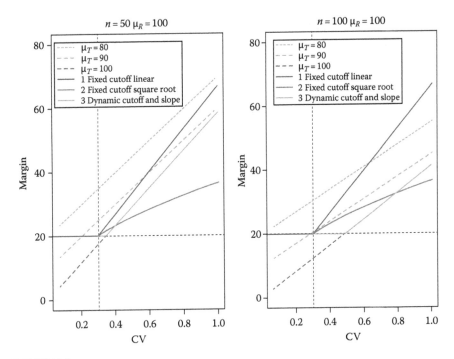

FIGURE 10.4
Proposed margins versus required margins.

10.3.2 Fixed Cutoff Square Root Scaled Margin

Unlike the fixed cutoff linear margin, the fixed cutoff square root scaled margin is given as follows:

$$\theta = \begin{cases} \theta_0, & \text{if } CV \le CV_0 \\ \sqrt{\dfrac{CV}{CV_0}} \times \theta_0, & \text{if } CV > CV_0 \end{cases} \tag{10.7}$$

where again CV_0 is the chosen cutoff for high-variability drug definition, and θ_0 is the fixed margin commonly accepted.

In the two proposals described earlier, the adjustment is based on some pre-specified CV_0 and θ_0. However, unlike BE studies where primary endpoints are typically PK responses, endpoints from clinical studies vary a lot for different disease areas. It is not practical to define a uniform cutoff for highly variable drug definition, as what has been done in BE studies.

10.3.3 Dynamic Cutoff Scaled Margin

Here, utilizing the relationship derived in the first part of the chapter, a third scaled margin with dynamic cutoff of CV is proposed as follows:

$$\theta = \begin{cases} \theta_0, & \text{if } CV \le CV_0 \\ (Z_{1-\alpha} + Z_{1-(\beta/2)}) \times \sqrt{\dfrac{2}{n_R}} \times \mu_R \times CV, & \text{if } CV > CV_0 \end{cases} \tag{10.8}$$

where θ_0 is the fixed margin commonly accepted (e.g., a margin of $\pm 20\%$ of μ_R) and

$$CV_0 = \frac{\theta_0}{\mu_R} \times \frac{1}{(Z_{1-\alpha} + Z_{1-(\beta/2)}) \times \sqrt{2/n_R}}.$$

As it can be seen, the high-variable drug cutoff CV_0 also depends on the sample size. Bearing in mind that a study with large enough sample size can always get small standard error no matter how big the inner variability of the reference drug is, a fixed CV_0 for high-variable drug and thus a wider margin will make it easier for a study with large sample size to achieve biosimilarity, by benefiting from the large sample size used.

By using the proposed CV_0 mentioned earlier, the $(CV/CV_0 \times \theta_0)$ results in the scaled margin as shown in Expression 10.8. This expression is roughly similar to the required margin for given power as derived in Formula 10.4 because when $n_T = n_R = n$ and $V_T = V_R$

$$\theta = \left(Z_{1-\alpha} + Z_{1-(\beta/2)}\right)\sqrt{\frac{V_T}{n_T} + \frac{V_R}{n_R}} = \left(Z_{1-\alpha} + Z_{1-(\beta/2)}\right)\sqrt{\frac{V_R}{n_R} + \frac{V_R}{n_R}}$$

$$= \left(Z_{1-\alpha} + Z_{1-(\beta/2)}\right)\sqrt{\frac{2}{n_R}} \times \sqrt{V_R} = \left(Z_{1-\alpha} + Z_{1-(\beta/2)}\right)\sqrt{\frac{2}{n_R}} \times \mu_R \times CV_R.$$

10.3.4 Dynamic Cutoff with Factor Scaled Margin

$$\theta = \begin{cases} \theta_0, & \text{if } CV \le CV_0 \\ \left(Z_{1-\alpha} + Z_{1-(\beta/2)}\right) \times \sqrt{\frac{2}{n_R + factor}} \times \mu_R \times CV, & \text{if } CV > CV_0 \end{cases} \tag{10.9}$$

where θ_0 is the fixed margin commonly accepted (e.g., a margin of $\pm 20\%$ of μ_R) and

$$CV_0 = \frac{\theta_0}{\mu_R} \times \frac{1}{\left(Z_{1-\alpha} + Z_{1-(\beta/2)}\right) \times \sqrt{2/(n_R + factor)}}.$$

The thinking behind this proposal is similar to the third scaled margin mentioned earlier, but with a factor (e.g., 48) enforced to define highly variable drug and control scaled margin not to exceed a certain level.

10.3.5 Dynamic Cutoff with Slope Scaled Margin

The scaled margins proposed so far are based on the closed form of relationship between the margin and variability obtained, given power and other parameters. Power is the probability of correctly concluding biosimilarity, given the test drug is truly similar to the reference drug. For a study where test drug is deviated from reference drug, we would like to control the type I error (thus consumer's risk) rather than wanting more power. Therefore, in the following proposal, we also take the adjustment of β into consideration when scaling the margins:

$$\theta = \begin{cases} \theta_0, & \text{if } CV \le CV_0 \\ \max\left(\theta_0, \left(Z_{1-\alpha} + Z_{1-(\tilde{\beta}/2)}\right) \times \sqrt{\frac{2}{n_R}} \times \mu_R \times CV\right), & \text{if } CV > CV_0 \end{cases} \tag{10.10}$$

where θ_0 is the fixed margin commonly accepted (e.g., a margin of $\pm 20\%$ of μ_R) and $CV_0 = \dfrac{\theta_0}{\mu_R} \times \dfrac{1}{\left(Z_{1-\alpha} + Z_{1-(\beta/2)}\right) \times \sqrt{2/n_R}}$

$$\tilde{\beta} = \begin{cases} \beta, & \text{if } |\mu_T - \mu_R| < \theta_0 \\ \min\left(1\dfrac{(1-\alpha-\beta) \times |\mu_T - \mu_R|}{\theta_0} + \beta\right), & \text{if } |\mu_T - \mu_R| \ge \theta_0 \end{cases}.$$

Figure 10.4 compares the first three proposed margins with the required margins, given power is 80%. As we can see, the blue line (fixed cutoff linear scaled margin) got inflated and outbound the required margin when $\mu_T = \mu_R = 100$ (the purple dotted line) when CV is large. On the other hand, the fixed cutoff square root scaled margin (red solid line) gives us a smaller margin than actually needed. The dynamic cutoff and slope scaled margin overlapped with the purple dotted line when CV is larger than the cutoff, which suggests that it gives the same margin as required for achieving the desired power. When CV is small (smaller than the cutoff), it uses the commonly accepted margin (e.g., $\pm 20\%$ of μ_R).

10.4 Simulations

To compare the performances of the proposed scaled margins and unscaled margin, we carried out the simulations under different scenarios with

- $\alpha = 0.05$ and $\beta = 0.2$ (i.e., power of 80%)
- Sample size: 50, 100 per group
- $\mu_R = 100$; and $\mu_T = 50$ to 100 by 5
- CV = 0.1 to 1 by 0.05
- $\theta_0 = 20\%$ of μ_R
- $CV_0 = 30\%$ used in the two fixed cutoff margins
- *factor* = 48 used in the dynamic cutoff with factor scaled margin

The results from 5000 iterations are illustrated in Figures 10.5 and 10.6.

As shown in the left column of Figure 10.5, when we have equal means between reference and test sample, the power to detect the biosimilarity will drop substantially for unscaled margin with the increase of CV, while all the proposed scaled margins show improved power in different levels. The fixed cutoff linear scaled margin (FCLM) improves power the most at sample sizes of 50 and 100. The fixed cutoff square root scaled margin (FCSRM) improves the power to a lesser degree than the fixed cutoff linear scaled margin. It provides 80% power when CV = 0.75 with sample size 100, but only less than 40% with sample size 50. Both the dynamic cutoff (DCM) and dynamic cutoff and scope scaled (DCSM) margins provide around 80% power for both sample sizes. The dynamic cutoff with factor scaled margin (DCFM) is a little bit less powerful than the DCM and DCSM, with power maintained around 60% (Figure 10.7).

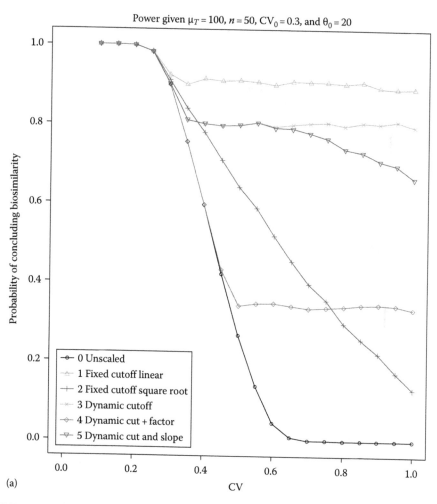

(a)

FIGURE 10.5

Probability of concluding biosimilarity given various CVs. (a) $\mu_T = 100$ and $n = 50$.

(*continued*)

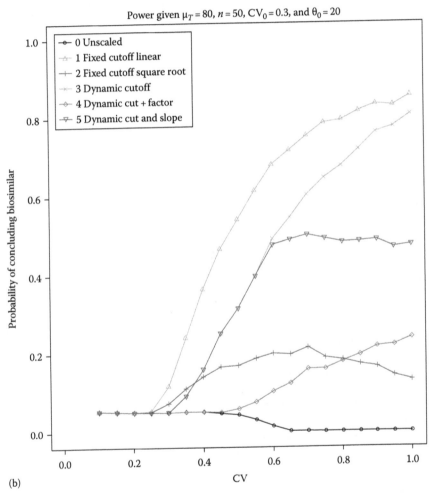

FIGURE 10.5 (continued)
Probability of concluding biosimilarity given various CVs. (b) $\mu_T = 80$ and $n = 50$.

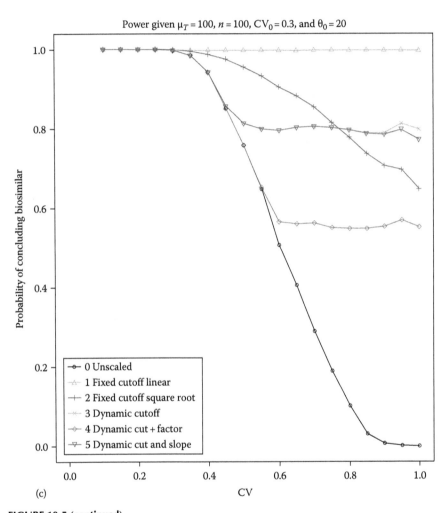

FIGURE 10.5 (continued)
Probability of concluding biosimilarity given various CVs. (c) $\mu_T = 100$ and $n = 100$.

(*continued*)

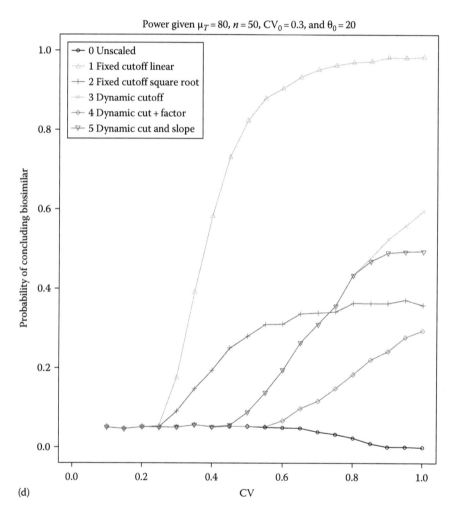

(d)

FIGURE 10.5 (continued)
Probability of concluding biosimilarity given various CVs. (d) $\mu_T = 80$ and $n = 50$.

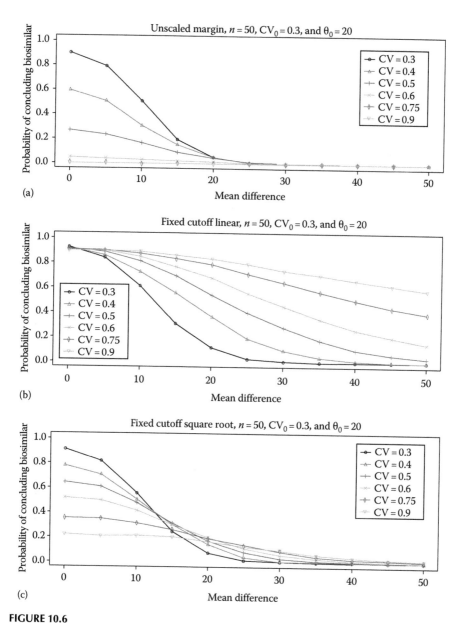

FIGURE 10.6
(a–f) Probability of concluding biosimilarity given various mean differences ($n = 50$).

(continued)

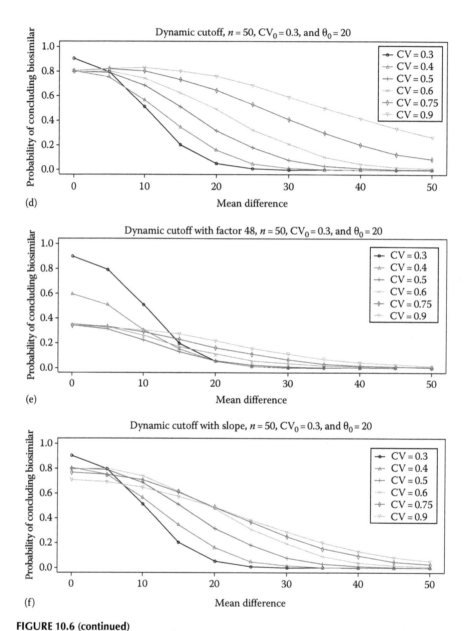

FIGURE 10.6 (continued)
(a–f) Probability of concluding biosimilarity given various mean differences ($n=50$).

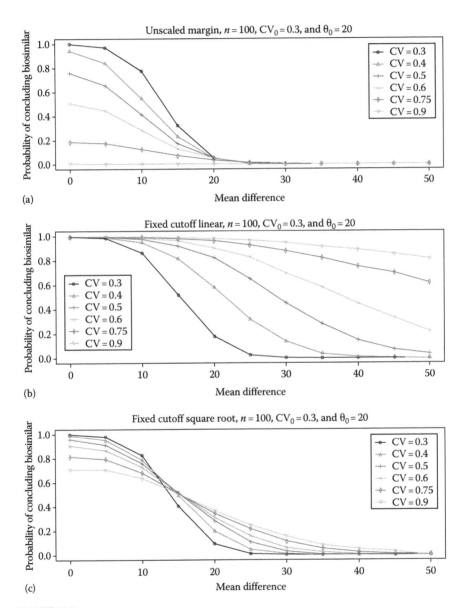

FIGURE 10.7
(a–f) Probability of concluding biosimilarity given various mean differences ($n = 100$).

(continued)

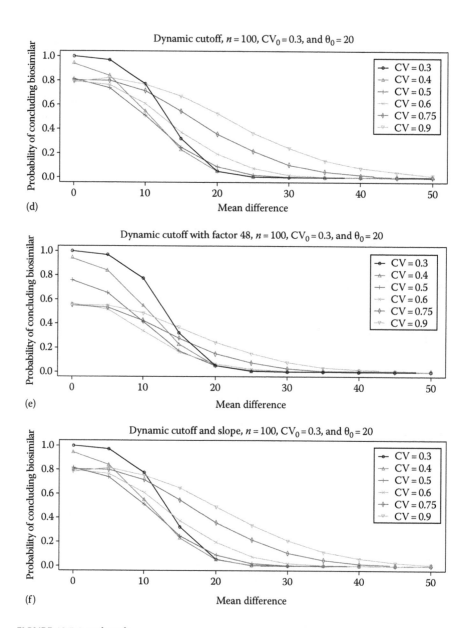

FIGURE 10.7 (continued)
(a–f) Probability of concluding biosimilarity given various mean differences ($n = 100$).

Figure 10.5d is for mean difference at 20, which reflects the performance of the scaled margins with respect to type I error. From the graph, the unscaled margin controls the type I error at the very low level for all various CVs, while all the proposed scaled margins inflate the type I error to a certain level. The FCLM results in the unreasonable type I error. The DCFM inflates at a much lesser degree only when CV is greater than 60%.

In the other set of plots (Figure 10.6), the probability of concluding biosimilarity was plotted against mean difference of $\mu_T - \mu_R$, under sample sizes of 50 and 100, and CV = 0.3, 0.4, 0.5, 0.6, 0.75, and 0.9. The results are consistent with Figure 10.5. All the proposed scaled margins improve the power compared to the unscaled margin, but inflate the type I error to different degrees. The dynamic cutoff and the dynamic cutoff and slope scaled margins are very comparable. The dynamic cutoff with factor shows the most desired pattern.

10.5 Discussions

In the evaluation of bioequivalence for small-molecular drugs, there is scientific justification for defining wider bioequivalence limits for highly variable drugs, and regulatory agencies are moving toward this direction. Given that large variability is often more likely to occur for biological products than for the traditional small-molecular drug products, evaluation of biosimilarity for highly variable biological products shall take this into consideration as well. In this chapter, we showed that to maintain desired power with reasonable sample size, biosimilarity margins should take variability into consideration when assessing ABE in FOBs. For this purpose, five scaled margins were proposed and their performances were evaluated. From simulations, it turns out it is hard to reach the ideal situation when the margin is power efficient and well controlling the type I error rate (i.e., consumer's risk) simultaneously. The dynamic scaled margins perform relatively better than the other two fixed scaled margins in balancing power and type I error, especially when sample size is 100. This is because the scaled margin well reflects the theoretically derived relationship between variability and required margins to achieve the given power. Therefore, the scaled margins, especially the one with empirical factors, are those that we will further explore and recommend to be used in evaluating FOBs.

In addition, in the small-molecular drugs world, a within-subject CV of 30% or more had become a generally accepted quantitative standard for what constitutes highly variable drugs. This standard may not apply to clinical trials for assessing FOBs given the following:

The endpoints in the traditional BE study are uniform (AUC or C_{max} of PK). For assessing FOBs, most likely, a clinical trial is needed where the clinical endpoints really vary from indication to indication.

The traditional BE study is intended to be a small study with about 25 subjects at the most, while clinical trial size could vary from dozens to hundreds.

Therefore, the choice of definition for the highly variable biological drugs should be further considered.

11

Drug Interchangeability

11.1 Introduction

In the United States, for traditional chemical (small-molecule) drug products, when an innovative (brand-name) drug product is going off patent, pharmaceutical and/or generic companies may file an abbreviated new drug application (ANDA) for the approval of generic copies of the brand-name drug product. In 1984, the U.S. Food and Drug Administration (FDA) was authorized to approve generic drug products under the *Drug Price Competition and Patent Term Restoration Act*, which is known as the *Hatch–Waxman Act*. For the approval of small-molecule generic drug products, the FDA requires that evidence of the *average* bioavailability be provided in terms of the rate and extent of drug absorption. As indicated earlier, the assessment of bioequivalence as a surrogate endpoint for the quantitative evaluation of drug safety and efficacy is based on the *Fundamental Bioequivalence Assumption*. It states that if two drug products are shown to be bioequivalent in terms of average bioavailability, then it is assumed that they will reach the same therapeutic effect or that they are therapeutically equivalent and hence can be used *interchangeably*. Under the Fundamental Bioequivalence Assumption, regulatory requirements, study design, criteria, and statistical methods for assessment of bioequivalence have been well established (see, e.g., Schuirmann, 1987; EMA, 2001; FDA, 2001, 2003; WHO, 2005; Chow and Liu, 2008).

As the patents of a number of biological products are due to expire in the next few years, the subsequent production of biosimilar products has attracted much attention within the pharmaceutical/biotechnology industry as biosimilar manufacturers strive to obtain part of an already large and rapidly growing market. The potential opportunity for price reduction be provided the originator biological products remains to be determined, as the advantage of a slightly cheaper price may be outweighed by the hypothetical increased risk of side-effects from biosimilar molecules that are not exact copies of their originators. Thus, it is a great concern whether the approved biosimilar products can be used interchangeably and safely.

In the next section, the concepts of population and individual bioequivalence (IBE) for addressing drug interchangeability in terms of prescribability and switchability for small-molecule drug products are reviewed. Section 11.3 focuses on the definition, interpretation, and assessment of interchangeability in terms of the concepts of switching and alternating for biosimilars as described in the BPCI Act. Several study designs for addressing switching, alternating, and/or switching/alternating are summarized in Section 11.4. A general unified approach using the biosimilarity index for the assessment of biosimilarity and interchangeability, which are derived based on the concept of reproducibility probability, is proposed and discussed in Section 11.5. Brief concluding remarks are given in the last section.

11.2 Population and Individual Bioequivalence

As indicated earlier, when a generic drug is claimed to be bioequivalent to a brand-name drug, it is assumed that they are therapeutically equivalent. A generic drug can be generally used as a substitution of the brand-name drug if it has been shown to be bioequivalent to the brand-name drug. The FDA does not indicate that two generic copies of the same brand-name drug can be used interchangeably even though they are bioequivalent to the same brand-name drug. In practice, bioequivalence between generic copies of a brand-name drug is not required. However, as more generic drug products become available, it is a concern whether the approved generic drug products have mutually the same quality and therapeutic effect even if each of them is bioequivalent to the brand-name drug product, and whether they can be used safely and interchangeably. The concept of drug interchangeability for small-molecule drug products involves drug prescribability and drug switchability. To evaluate whether generic drug products can be used safely and interchangeably, the FDA suggested that population bioequivalence (PBE) and IBE be assessed for addressing drug prescribability and drug switchability of approved generic drug products, respectively (FDA, 2001, 2003).

11.2.1 Population Bioequivalence

Drug prescribability is referred to as the physician's choice for prescribing an appropriate drug for his/her patients between the brand-name drug and its generic copies. To address drug prescribability, the FDA recommended that PBE be assessed. In addition to the average of bioavailability, PBE focuses on the variability of bioavailability. As indicated in Section 2.3, the 2001 FDA guidance recommends the following criterion be used for assessing PBE:

$$\theta_P = \frac{(\delta^2 + \sigma_{TT}^2 - \sigma_{TR}^2)}{\max\{\sigma_{T0}^2, \sigma_{TR}^2\}},$$

where $\delta = \mu_T - \mu_R, \sigma_{TT}^2, \sigma_{TR}^2$ are the total variances for the test product and the reference product, respectively, and σ_{T0}^2 is the scale parameter specified by the regulatory agency or the sponsor. PBE can be claimed if the one-sided 95% upper confidence bound for θ_P is less than a pre-specified bioequivalence limit. In view of the previously mentioned PBE criterion, PBE can be claimed if the null hypothesis in

$$H_0 : \lambda \geq 0 \quad \text{versus} \quad H_a : \lambda < 0$$

is rejected at the 5% level of significance and the observed geometric means ratio (GMR) is within the limits of 80% and 125%, where

$$\lambda = \delta^2 + \sigma_{TT}^2 - \sigma_{TR}^2 - \theta_{PBE} \max(\sigma_{TR}^2, \sigma_0^2),$$

and θ_{PBE} is a constant specified in the 2001 FDA draft guidance. Under a 2×2 crossover design, the one-sided 95% upper confidence bound for θ_P can be obtained under the following model:

$$y_{ijk} = \mu + F_l + P_j + Q_k + S_{ikl} + \epsilon_{ijk}, \tag{11.1}$$

where
μ is the overall mean
P_j is the fixed effect of the jth period
Q_k is the fixed effect of the kth sequence
F_l is the fixed effect of the lth drug product
S_{ijk} is the random effect of the ith subject in the kth sequence under the lth drug product
ϵ_{ijk}'s are independent random errors distributed as $N(0, \sigma_{Wl}^2)$

It is assumed that S_{ijk}'s and ϵ_{ijk}'s are mutually independent. It can be verified that $(S_{ikT}, S_{ikR}), i = 1, 2, \ldots, n_k; k = 1, 2,$ are independent and identically distributed bivariate normal random vectors with mean 0 and an unknown covariance matrix

$$\begin{pmatrix} \sigma_{BT}^2 & \rho\sigma_{BT}\sigma_{BR} \\ \rho\sigma_{BT}\sigma_{BR} & \sigma_{BR}^2 \end{pmatrix},$$

where σ_{Bl}^2 denotes the between-subject variability for the lth drug product and ρ is the correlation coefficient between the variations of the two formulations. Thus, we have

$$\sigma_{TT}^2 = \sigma_{BT}^2 + \sigma_{WT}^2 \quad \text{and} \quad \sigma_{TR}^2 = \sigma_{BR}^2 + \sigma_{WR}^2.$$

Under the Model 11.1, unbiased estimators for δ, σ_{TT}^2, and σ_{TR}^2 can be obtained as follows:

$$\hat{\delta} = \frac{\bar{y}_{11} - \bar{y}_{12} - \bar{y}_{21} + \bar{y}_{22}}{2} \sim N\left(\delta, \frac{\sigma_{1,1}^2}{4}\left(\frac{1}{n_1} + \frac{1}{n_2}\right)\right),$$

where $\bar{y}_{jk}$ is the sample mean of the observations in the kth sequence at the jth period and $\sigma_{1,1}^2$ is $\sigma_{a,b}^2 = \sigma_D^2 + a\sigma_{WT}^2 + b\sigma_{WR}^2$ with $a = 1$ and $b = 1$. Commonly considered unbiased estimators for σ_{TT}^2 and σ_{TR}^2 are given by

$$\hat{\sigma}_{TT}^2 = \frac{1}{n_1 + n_2 - 2}\left[\sum_{i=1}^{n_1}(y_{i11} - \bar{y}_{11})^2 + \sum_{i=1}^{n_2}(y_{i22} - \bar{y}_{22})^2\right]$$

$$\sim \frac{\sigma_{TT}^2 \lambda_{n_1+n_2-2}^2}{n_1 + n_2 - 2}$$

and

$$\hat{\sigma}_{TR}^2 = \frac{1}{n_1 + n_2 - 2}\left[\sum_{i=1}^{n_1}(y_{i21} - \bar{y}_{21})^2 + \sum_{i=1}^{n_2}(y_{i12} - \bar{y}_{12})^2\right]$$

$$\sim \frac{\sigma_{TR}^2 \lambda_{n_1+n_2-2}^2}{n_1 + n_2 - 2}$$

According to Chow et al. (2002), the following approximate 95% upper confidence bound for λ when $\sigma_{TR}^2 \geq \sigma_0^2$ can be obtained:

$$\hat{\lambda}_U = \hat{\delta}^2 + \hat{\sigma}_{TT}^2 - (1 + \theta_{PBE})\hat{\sigma}_{TR}^2 + t_{0.05, n_1 + n_2 - 2}\sqrt{V},$$

where V is an estimated variance of $\hat{\delta}^2 + \hat{\sigma}_{TT}^2 - (1 + \theta_{PBE})\hat{\sigma}_{TR}^2$ of the form

$$V = (2\hat{\delta}, 1, -(1 + \theta_{PBE}))C(2\hat{\delta}, 1, -(1 + \theta_{PBE}))'$$

and C is an estimated variance-covariance matrix of $(\hat{\delta}, \hat{\sigma}_{TT}^2, \hat{\sigma}_{TR}^2)$. Since $\hat{\delta}$ and $(\hat{\sigma}_{TT}^2, \hat{\sigma}_{TR}^2)$ are independent, C is given by

$$C = \begin{pmatrix} \dfrac{\sigma_{1,1}^2}{4}\left(\dfrac{1}{n_1}+\dfrac{1}{n_2}\right) & (0,0) \\ (0,0)' & \dfrac{(n_1-1)C_1}{(n_1+n_2-2)^2}+\dfrac{(n_2-1)C_2}{(n_1+n_2-2)^2} \end{pmatrix},$$

where C_1 is the sample covariance matrix of $((y_{i11}-\bar{y}_{11})^2,(y_{i21}-\bar{y}_{21})^2), i=1,2,...,n_1$, and C_2 is the sample covariance matrix of $((y_{i22}-\bar{y}_{22})^2),(y_{i12}-\bar{y}_{12})^2), i=1,2,...,n_2$. On the other hand, when $\sigma_{TR}^2 < \sigma_0^2$, the upper confidence bound for λ should be modified as follows:

$$\hat{\lambda}_U = \hat{\delta}^2 + \hat{\sigma}_{TT}^2 - (1+\theta_{PBE})\hat{\sigma}_0^2 + t_{0.05, n_1+n_2-2}\sqrt{V_0},$$

where

$$V_0 = (2\hat{\delta}, 1, -1)C(2\hat{\delta}, 1, -1)'.$$

11.2.2 Individual Bioequivalence

Drug switchability is referred to as the switch from a drug (e.g., a brand-name drug or its generic copies) to another (e.g., a generic copy) within the same patient whose concentration of the drug has been titrated to a steady, efficacious, and safe level. To address drug switchability, the FDA suggested that IBE be assessed under replicated crossover designs such as a replicated 2×2 crossover design, i.e., (TRTR, RTRT), or a 2×3 two-sequence dual design, i.e., (TRT, RTR). In addition to comparison of means, IBE focuses on the variability of bioavailability and variability due to subject-by-drug interaction. Recall, the 2001 FDA guidance recommended that the following criterion be used for assessing IBE:

$$\theta_I = \frac{(\delta^2 + \sigma_D^2 + \sigma_{WT}^2 - \sigma_{WR}^2)}{\max\{\sigma_{W0}^2, \sigma_{WR}^2\}},$$

where $\delta = \mu_T - \mu_R, \sigma_{WT}^2, \sigma_{WR}^2, \sigma_D^2$ are the true difference between the means, the intra-subject variabilities of the test product and the reference product, and the variance component due to subject-by-formulation interaction between drug products, respectively. σ_{W0}^2 is a scale parameter specified by the regulatory agency or the sponsor. In view of the IBE criterion mentioned earlier, IBE can be claimed if the null hypothesis in

$$H_0 : \gamma \geq 0 \quad \text{versus} \quad H_a : \gamma < 0$$

is rejected at the 5% level of significance and the observed GMR is within the limits of 80% and 125%, where

$$\gamma = \delta^2 + \sigma_D^2 + \sigma_{WT}^2 - \sigma_{WR}^2 - \theta_{IBE} \max\left(\sigma_{WR}^2, \sigma_{W0}^2\right)$$

and θ_{IBE} is a constant specified in the 2001 FDA draft guidance.

For the assessment of IBE, FDA recommends that a replicated 2×2 crossover design, i.e., (TRTR, RTRT) or (RTRT, TRTR), be used. Under the 2×2 replicated crossover design, the one-sided 95% upper confidence bound for θ_I can be obtained under the following statistical model:

$$y_{ijk} = \mu + F_l + W_{ljk} + S_{ikl} + \epsilon_{ijk}, \tag{11.2}$$

where
  μ is the overall mean
  F_l is the fixed effect of the lth drug product
  W_{ljk}'s are fixed period, sequence, and interaction effects
  S_{ijk} is the random effect of the ith subject in the kth sequence under the lth drug product
  ϵ_{ijk}'s are independent random errors distributed as $N(0,\sigma_{Wl}^2)$

It is assumed that S_{ijk}'s and ϵ_{ijk}'s are mutually independent. Under Model 11.2, and σ_D^2 is given by

$$\sigma_D^2 = \sigma_{BT}^2 + \sigma_{BR}^2 - 2\rho\sigma_{BT}\sigma_{BR},$$

which is the variance of $S_{ikT} - S_{ikR}$. Note that σ_D^2 is usually referred to as the variance component due to the subject-by-drug interaction. It can be verified that when $\sigma_{WR}^2 \geq \sigma_{W0}^2$, the linearized criterion γ can be decomposed as follows:

$$\gamma = \delta^2 + \sigma_{0.5,0.5}^2 + 0.5\sigma_{WT}^2 - (1.5 + \theta_{IBE})\sigma_{WR}^2.$$

Now, under Model 11.2, for subject i in sequence k, let x_{ilk} and z_{ilk} be the average and the difference, respectively, of the observations from drug product l, and let $\bar{x}_{lk}$ and $\bar{z}_{lk}$ be respectively the sample means based on

x_{ilk}'s and z_{ilk}'s. Thus, under Model 10.2, unbiased estimators for δ, $\sigma^2_{0.5,0.5}$, and σ^2_{WR} can be obtained as follows:

$$\hat{\delta} = \frac{\bar{x}_{T1} - \bar{x}_{R1} + \bar{x}_{T2} - \bar{x}_{R2}}{2} \sim N\left(\delta, \frac{\sigma^2_{0.5,0.5}}{4}\left(\frac{1}{n_1} + \frac{1}{n_2}\right)\right),$$

$$\hat{\sigma}^2_{0.5,0.5} = \frac{(n_1 - 1)s^2_{d1} + (n_2 - 1)s^2_{d2}}{n_1 + n_2 - 2} \sim \frac{\sigma^2_{0.5,0.5}\lambda^2_{n_1+n_2-2}}{n_1 + n_2 - 2},$$

where s^2_{dk} is the sample variance based on $x_{iTk} - x_{iRk}$, $i = 1, 2, ..., n_k$; an unbiased estimator of σ^2_{WT} is given by

$$\hat{\sigma}^2_{WT} = \frac{(n_1 - 1)s^2_{T1} + (n_2 - 1)s^2_{T2}}{n_1 + n_2 - 2} \sim \frac{\sigma^2_{WT}\lambda^2_{n_1+n_2-2}}{n_1 + n_2 - 2},$$

where s^2_{Tk} is the sample variance based on z_{iTk}, $i = 1, 2, ..., n_k$. An unbiased estimator of σ^2_{WR} is given by

$$\hat{\sigma}^2_{WR} = \frac{(n_1 - 1)s^2_{R1} + (n_2 - 1)s^2_{R2}}{n_1 + n_2 - 2} \sim \frac{\sigma^2_{WR}\lambda^2_{n_1+n_2-2}}{n_1 + n_2 - 2},$$

where s^2_{Rk} is the sample variance based on z_{iRk}, $i = 1, 2, ..., n_k$. Furthermore, since $\hat{\delta}$, $\hat{\sigma}^2_{0.5,0.5}$, $\hat{\sigma}^2_{WT}$, and $\hat{\sigma}^2_{WR}$ are independent, when $\sigma^2_{WR} \geq \sigma^2_{W0}$, an approximate 95% confidence upper bound for γ can be obtained as follows:

$$\hat{\gamma}_U = \hat{\delta}^2 + \hat{\sigma}^2_{0.5,0.5} + 0.5\hat{\sigma}^2_{WT} - (1.5 + \theta_{IBE})\hat{\sigma}^2_{WR} + \sqrt{U},$$

where U is the sum of the following four quantities:

$$\left[\left(\left|\hat{\delta}\right| + t_{0.05,n_1+n_2-2}\frac{\hat{\sigma}_{0.5,0.5}}{2}\sqrt{\frac{1}{n_1} + \frac{1}{n_2}}\right)^2 - \hat{\delta}^2\right]^2,$$

$$\hat{\sigma}^4_{0.5,0.5}\left(\frac{n_1 + n_2 - 2}{\lambda^2_{0.05,n_1+n_2-2,}} - 1\right)^2,$$

$$0.5^2\hat{\sigma}^4_{WT}\left(\frac{n_1 + n_2 - 2}{\lambda^2_{0.05,n_1+n_2-2,}} - 1\right)^2,$$

and

$$(1.5 + \theta_{IBE})^2\hat{\sigma}^4_{WR}\left(\frac{n_1 + n_2 - 2}{\lambda^2_{0.05,n_1+n_2-2}} - 1\right)^2.$$

When $\hat{\sigma}^2_{WR} < \hat{\sigma}^2_{W0}$, an approximate 95% confidence upper bound for γ is given by

$$\hat{\gamma}_u = \hat{\delta}^2 + \hat{\sigma}^2_{0.5,0.5} + 0.5\hat{\sigma}^2_{WT} - 1.5\hat{\sigma}^2_{WR} - \theta_{IPE}\sigma^2_{W0} + \sqrt{U_0},$$

where U_0 is the sum as U except that the four quantities should be replaced by

$$1.5^2\hat{\sigma}^4_{WR}\left(\frac{n_1 + n_2 - 2}{\lambda^2_{0.05,\,n_1+n_2-2}} - 1\right)^2.$$

11.2.3 Remarks

Both criteria for PBE and IBE are aggregated moment-based criteria, which involve several variance components including the inter-subject and intra-subject variabilities. Since the criteria are non-linear functions of the direct drug effect, inter-subject and intra-subject variabilities for the test product and the reference product, and the variability due to subject-by-drug interaction (for the IBE criterion), a typical approach is to linearize the criteria and then apply the method of modified large sample (MLS) or extended MLS for obtaining an approximate 95% upper confidence bound of the linearized criteria (see, e.g., Hyslop et al., 2000; Lee et al., 2004). The key is to decompose the linearized criteria into several components and obtain independent and unbiased estimators of these components for obtaining a valid approximate upper confidence bound.

Alternatively, one may consider the method of generalized pivotal quantity (GPQ) to assess PBE and/or IBE (see, e.g., Chiu et al., 2013). The idea of GPQ is briefly described later. Suppose that Y is a random variable whose distribution depends on a vector of unknown parameters, $\zeta = (\theta, \eta)$, where θ is a parameter of interest and η is a vector of nuisance parameters. Let y be a random sample from Y and $\hat{y}$ be the observed value of Y. Furthermore, let $R = R(\hat{y}; y, \zeta)$ be a function of $\hat{y}$, y, and ζ. The random quantity R is referred to as a GPQ, which satisfies the following two conditions:

1. The distribution of R does not depend on any unknown parameters.
2. The observed value of R, say $r = R(\hat{y}; y, \zeta)$, is free of the vector of nuisance parameters η.

In other words, r is only a function of $(\hat{y}, \theta)$. Thus, a $(1 - \alpha) \times 100\%$ generalized upper confidence limit for θ is given by $R_{1-\alpha}$, which is the $100(1 - \alpha)$th percentile of the distribution of R. The percentiles of can be analytically estimated using a Monte Carlo algorithm.

11.3 Interchangeability for Biosimilar Products

As indicated in the Public Health Act subsection 351(k)(3), the term *interchangeable* or *interchangeability* in reference to a biological product that is shown to meet the standards described in subsection (k)(4) (i.e., interchangeability) means that the biological product may be substituted for the reference product without the intervention of the health care provider who prescribed the reference product. Along this line, in what follows, the definition and basic concepts of interchangeability (in terms of switching and alternating) are given.

11.3.1 Definition and Basic Concepts

As indicated in the Public Health Act subsection 351(k)(3), a biological product is considered to be interchangeable with the reference product if (1) the biological product is biosimilar to the reference product; and (2) it can be expected to produce the same clinical result in *any given patient*. In addition, for a biological product that is administered more than once to an individual, the risk in terms of safety or diminished efficacy of alternating or switching between the use of the biological product and the reference product is not greater than the risk of using the reference product without such alternation or switch.

Thus, there is a clear *distinction* between biosimilarity and interchangeability. In other words, biosimilarity does not imply interchangeability which is much more stringent. Intuitively, if a test product is judged to be interchangeable with the reference product, then it may be substituted, even alternated, without a possible intervention, or even notification, of the health care provider. However, the interchangeability is expected to produce the *same* clinical result in *any given patient*, which can be interpreted as that the same clinical result can be expected in *every single patient*. In reality, conceivably, lawsuits may be filed if adverse effects are recorded in a patient after switching from one product to another.

It should be noted that when FDA declares the biosimilarity of two drug products, it may not be assumed that they are interchangeable. Therefore, labels ought to state whether for a follow-on biologic which is biosimilar to a reference product, interchangeability has or has not been established. However, payers and physicians may, in some cases, switch products even if interchangeability has not been established.

11.3.2 Switching and Alternating

Unlike drug interchangeability (in terms of prescribability and switchability) (Chow and Liu, 2008), the FDA has slight perception of drug interchangeability for biosimilars. From the FDA's perspectives, interchangeability includes the concept of switching and alternating between an innovative biological products (R) and its follow-on biologic (T). The concept of switching is referred to as not only the switch from "R to T" or "T to R" (narrow sense of switchability) but also "T to T" and "R to R" (broader sense of switchability). Note that "T to T" could indicate a switch from an approved biosimilar product to another approved biosimilar product, while "R to R" could be a switch from an innovative biological product to itself (e.g., from a different batch or made at a different location). As a result, in order to assess switching, biosimilarity for "R to T," "T to R," "T to T," and "R to R" needs to be assessed based on some biosimilarity criteria under a valid study design. The BPCI Act indicates that the risk in terms of safety or diminished efficacy of switching between the use of the biological product and the reference product should not be greater than the risk of using the reference product without such a switch. This suggests that the risk of switching between T_i, $i = 1, \ldots, K$, where K is the number of approved biosimilars, and R should not be greater than the risk of switching between R and R.

On the other hand, the concept of alternating (in the sense that it only involves one test product T and one reference product R) is referred to as either a switch from T to R and then switch back to T (i.e., "T to R to T") or the switch from R to T and then switch back to R (i.e., "R to T to R"). Thus, the difference between "the switch from T to R" then "the switch from R to T" and "the switch from R to T" then "the switch from T to R" needs to be assessed for addressing the concept of alternating. The BPCI Act also indicates that the risk in terms of safety or diminished efficacy of alternating between use of the biological product and the reference product should not be greater than the risk of using the reference product without such alternating. In practice, however, it should be noted that there may be more than one test product on the market. Thus, several switches are possible, e.g., R to T_1 to T_2 to R to T_2, etc., which will make the assessment of alternation even more complicated if it is not impossible.

Thus, in practice, it is very difficult, if not impossible, to assess drug interchangeability of approved biosimilar products especially when there are multiple T's and R's in the marketplace. As stated in the BPCI Act, the relative risk between switching/alternating and without switching/alternating must be evaluated. However, little or no discussion about the criteria for assessment of the relative risk was mentioned in the BPCI Act. In the recent FDA draft guidances on the demonstration of biosimilarity of follow-on biologics, little or no discussion was mentioned either regarding the criteria, study design, and statistical methods for the assessment of drug interchangeability in terms of switching and alternating. Thus, detailed regulatory guidances regarding the assessment of drug interchangeability in terms of switching and/or alternating need to be developed.

For assessing drug interchangeability, an appropriate study design should be chosen in order to address (1) the risk in terms of safety or diminished efficacy of alternating or switching between the uses of the biosimilar product and the reference product, (2) the risk of using the reference product without such alternation or switch, and (3) the relative risk between switching/alternating and without switching/alternating.

In order to assess switching, an appropriate study design should allow the assessment of biosimilarity for "R to T," "T to R," "T to T," and "R to R" so that we can evaluate the risk of switching between use of the biological product and the reference product and the risk of using the reference product without such a switch. In this case, the Balaam's 4 × 2 crossover design, i.e., (*TT, RR, TR, RT*) may be useful. Under a Balaam's design, the risk of switching from "T to T," "R to R," "T to R" and "R to T" can be assessed. Consequently, the relative risk between the switching and without switching can be assessed.

11.3.3 Remarks

With small-molecule drug products, bioequivalence generally reflects therapeutic equivalence. Drug prescribability, switching, and alternating are generally considered reasonable. With biological products, however, variations are often larger (other than pharmacokinetic factors may be sensitive to small changes in conditions). Thus, often only parallel-group design rather than crossover kinetic studies can be performed. It should be noted that very often, with follow-on biologics, biosimilarity does *not* reflect therapeutic comparability. Therefore, switching and alternating should be pursued only with substantial caution, provided that clear regulatory guidances about criteria, design and analysis are available.

11.4 Study Designs for Interchangeability

For assessment of bioequivalence for chemical drug products, a standard two-sequence, two-period (2 × 2) crossover design is often considered, except for drug products with relatively long half-lives. Since most biosimilar products have relatively long half-lives, it is suggested that a parallel-group design should be considered. However, parallel-group design does not provide independent estimates of variance components such as inter- and intra-subject variabilities and variability due to subject-by-product interaction. Thus, it is a major challenge for assessing biosimilarity (especially for assessing drug interchangeability) under parallel-group designs since each subject will receive the same product once.

As indicated in the BPCI Act, for a biological product that is administered more than once to an individual, the risk in terms of safety or diminished efficacy of alternating or switching between use of the biological product and the reference product is not greater than the risk of using the reference product without such alternation or switch. Thus, for assessing drug interchangeability, an appropriate study design should be chosen in order to address (1) the risk in terms of safety or diminished efficacy of alternating or switching between use of the biological product and the reference product, (2) the risk of using the reference product without such alternation or switch, and (3) the relative risk between switching/alternating and without switching/alternating. In this section, several useful designs for addressing switching and alternation of biosimilar products are discussed.

11.4.1 Designs for Switching

Consider the broader sense of switchability. In this case, the concept of switching includes (1) switch from "R to T," (2) switch from "T to R," (3) switch from "T to T," and (4) switch to "R to R." Thus, in order to assess interchangeability of switching, a valid study design should be able to assess biosimilarity between "R and T," "T and R," "T and T," and "R and R" based on some biosimilarity criteria. For this purpose, the following study designs are useful.

11.4.1.1 Balaam Design

Balaam design is a 4 × 2 crossover design, denoted by (*TT, RR, TR, RT*). Under a 4 × 2 Balaam's design, qualified subjects will be randomly assigned to receive one of the four sequences of treatments: *TT, RR, TR,* and *RT.* For example, subjects in sequence 1 of *TT* will receive the test (biosimilar) product first and then cross-overed to receive the reference (innovative biological) product after a sufficient length of washout (see Figure 11.1). In practice, a Balaam design is considered the combination of a parallel design (the first two sequences) and a crossover design (sequences #3 and #4). The purpose

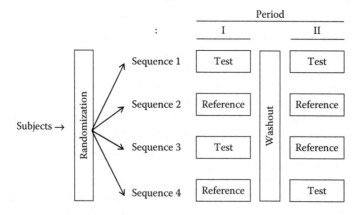

FIGURE 11.1
Balaam design. *Note:* Balaam design is a 4 × 2 crossover design.

of the part of parallel design is to obtain independent estimates of intra-subject variabilities for the test product and the reference product. In the interest of assigning more subjects to the crossover phase, an unequal treatment assignment is usually employed. For example, we may consider a $1:2$ allocation to the parallel phase and the crossover phase. In this case, for a sample size of $N = 24$, 8 subjects will be assigned to the parallel phase and 16 subjects will be assigned to the crossover phase. As a result, four subjects will be assigned to sequences #1 and #2, while eight subjects will be assigned to sequences #3 and #4, assuming that there is a 1:1 ratio treatment allocation within each phase.

As it can be seen from Figure 11.1, the first sequence provides not only independent estimate of the intra-subject variability of the test product but also the assessment for "switch from T to T," while the second sequence provides independent estimate of the intra-subject variability of the reference product and compares difference between "R and R." The other two sequences assess similarity for "switch from T to R" and "switch from R to T," respectively. Under the 4×2 Balaam design, the following comparisons are usually assessed:

1. Comparisons by sequence
2. Comparisons by period
3. T vs. R based on sequences #3 and #4—this is equivalent to a typical 2×2 crossover design
4. T vs. R given T based on sequences #1 and #3
5. R vs. T given R based on sequences #2 and #4
6. The comparison between (1) and (3) for assessment of treatment-by-period interaction

It should be noted that the interpretations of the comparisons mentioned earlier are different. More information regarding statistical methods for data analysis of Balaam design can be found in Chow and Liu (2008).

11.4.1.2 Two-Stage Design

Alternatively, a two-stage crossover design described in Figure 11.2 may be useful for addressing interchangeability of switching. Under the two-stage design, qualified subjects are randomly assigned to receive either the test product or the reference product at the first stage. At the second stage, after a sufficient length of washout, subjects are randomly assigned to receive either the test product or the reference product with either equal or unequal ratio of treatment allocation. At the end of the study, the two-stage design will lead to four sequences of treatments, i.e., TT, TR, RT, and RR, similar to those in Balaam's design.

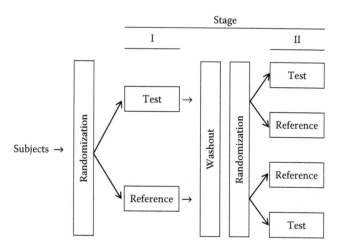

FIGURE 11.2
Two-stage design. *Note:* Stage 2 is nested within stage 1.

Note that the previously mentioned two-stage design that consists of a parallel phase (stage 1) and a crossover phase (stage 2) is similar to a placebo-challenging design proposed by Chow et al. (2000). As a result, statistical methods proposed by Chow et al. (2000) are useful for a valid analysis of data collected from a two-stage design described earlier. Under the two-stage design, similarly, the comparisons (1)–(6) can also be made based on the methods proposed by Chow et al. (2000).

11.4.2 Designs for Alternating

For addressing the concept of alternating, an appropriate study design should allow the assessment of differences between "R to T" and "T to R" for alternating of "R to T to R" to determine whether the drug effect has returned to the baseline after the second switch.

For this purpose, the following study designs are useful.

11.4.2.1 Two-Sequence Dual Design

Two-sequence dual design is a 2×3 higher-order crossover design consisting of two dual sequences, namely *TRT* and *RTR* (Figure 11.3). Under the two-sequence dual design, qualified subjects will be randomly assigned to receive either the sequence of *TRT* or the sequence of *RTR*. Of course, there is a sufficient length of washout between dosing periods. Under the two-sequence dual design, we will be able to evaluate the relative risk of alternating between use of the biological product and the reference product and the risk of using the reference product without such alternating.

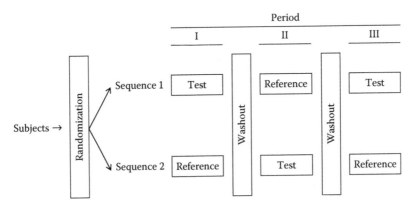

FIGURE 11.3
Two-sequence dual design. *Note:* Two-sequence dual design is a 2 × 3 crossover design.

Note that expected values of the sequence-by-period means, analysis of variance table, and statistical methods (e.g., the assessment of average biosimilarity, inference on carry-over effect, and the assessment of intra-subject variabilities) for analysis of data collected from a two-sequence dual design are given in Chow and Liu (2008). In case there are missing data (i.e., incomplete data), statistical methods proposed by Chow and Shao (1997) are useful.

11.4.2.2 Williams' Design

For a broader sense of alternation involving more than two biologics, e.g., two biosimilars T_1 and T_2 and one innovative product R, there are six possible sequences: $(R\ T_2\ T_1)$, $(T_1\ R\ T_2)$, $(T_2\ T_1\ R)$, $(T_1\ T_2\ R)$, $(T_2\ R\ T_1)$, and $(R\ T_1\ T_2)$. In this case, a 6 × 3 Williams' design for comparing three products is useful (see, also, Chow and Liu, 2008). A William design is a variance-balanced design, which consists of six sequences and three periods. Under the 6 × 3 Williams' design, qualified subjects are randomly assigned to receive one of the six sequences. Within each sequence, a sufficient length of wash is applied between dosing periods (see also Figure 11.4).

Detailed information regarding (1) construction of a William design, (2) analysis of variance table, and (3) statistical methods for analysis of data collected from a 6 × 3 William design adjusted for carry-over effects, in the absence of unequal carry-over effects, and adjusted for drug effect can be found in Chow and Liu (2008).

11.4.3 Designs for Switching/Alternating

In the previous two sub-sections, useful study designs for addressing switching and alternating of drug interchangeability are discussed, respectively. In practice, however, it is of interest to have a study design which can address both switching and alternating. In this case, an intuitive study design is to

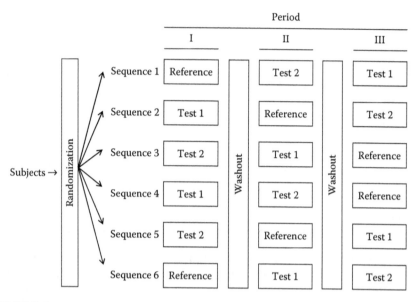

FIGURE 11.4

William design for comparing three treatments. *Note:* Test 1 and Test 2 are two different biosimilar products and Reference is the reference (innovative) product.

combine a switching design with an alternating design. Along this line, in this section, several useful designs for addressing both switching and alternating of drug interchangeability are introduced.

11.4.3.1 Modified Balaam Design

As indicated earlier, Balaam's design is useful for addressing switching, while a two-sequence dual design is appropriate for addressing alternating. In the interest of addressing both switching and alternating in a single trial, we may combine the two study designs as follows: (*TT, RR, TRT, RTR*), which consists of a parallel design (the first two sequences) and a two-sequence dual design (the last two sequences). We will refer to this design as a modified Balaam design, which is illustrated in Figure 11.5.

As it can be seen from Figure 11.5, data collected from the first two dosing periods (which are identical to the Balaam design) can be used to address switching, while data collected from sequences #3 and #4 can be used to assess the relative risks of alternating.

11.4.3.2 Complete Design

It can be seen that the modified Balaam's design is not a balanced design in terms of the number of dosing periods. In the interest of balance in dosing periods, it is suggested the modified Balaam's design be further modified

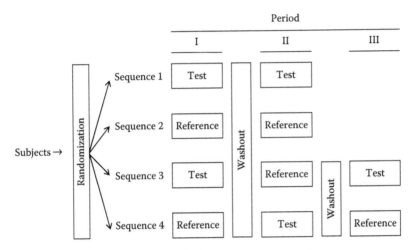

FIGURE 11.5
Modified Balaam design for addressing switching/alternation of interchangeability. *Note:*
Sequence #3 and #4 is a two-sequence dual design.

as (*TTT, RRR, TRT, RTR*). We will refer to this design as a complete design.
The difference between the complete design and the modified Balaam
design is that the treatments are repeated at the third dosing period for
sequences #1 and #2. Data collected from sequence #1 will provide a more
accurate and reliable assessment of intra-subject variability, while data collected from sequence #2 are useful in establishing the baseline for the reference product (Figure 11.6).

Note that statistical methods for analysis of data collected from the complete design are similar to those under the modified Balaam's design.

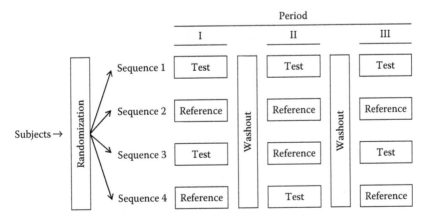

FIGURE 11.6
Complete design for addressing switching/alternation of interchangeability.

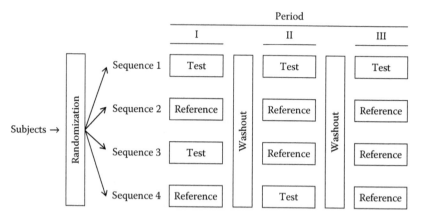

FIGURE 11.7
Alternative design for addressing interchangeability. *Note*: Sequences #3 and #4 is an extra-reference design.

11.4.3.3 Alternative Designs

For assessment of IBE under a replicated design, Chow et al. (2002) indicated that the optimal design among 2×3 crossover designs is the so-called extra-reference design, which is given by (TRR, RTR) (Figure 11.7). Thus, an alternative design is to combine a parallel design (TTT, RRR) and a 2×3 extra-reference design for addressing both switching and alternating. The resultant study design is then given by (TTT, RRR, RTR, TRR).

11.4.3.4 Adaptive Designs

In recent years, the use of adaptive design methods in clinical research has become very popular due to their flexibility and efficiency for identifying any (or optimal) clinical benefits of the test treatment under investigation (see, e.g., Chow and Chang, 2011). Similar ideas can be applied for assessment of biosimilarity and interchangeability of biosimilar products. For example, a two-stage adaptive design that combines two independent studies into a single trial may be useful. Some adaptations (modifications or changes) can be implemented at the end of the first stage after the review of accumulated data collected from the first stage. More information regarding various adaptive trial designs can be found in Chow and Chang (2011).

11.4.4 Bridging Studies

Under certain assumptions such as (1) in vitro testing is predictive of in vivo testing; in other words, there is a correlation between in vitro testing and in vivo testing (IVIVC); (2) animal model is predictive of human model; or (3) biomarker such as PK/PD marker or genomic marker is predictive of clinical outcomes, bridging studies may be useful by providing totality-of-the-evidence for assessment of biosimilarity and for evaluation of the relative risks of switching and/or alternating for addressing interchangeability.

For example, Chow et al. (2010) derived statistical methods for assessment of average biosimilarity using biomarker(s) data according to both the moment-based criterion and the probability-based criterion under a parallel-group design assuming that the biomarker (or biomarkers) is predictive of clinical outcomes for evaluation of safety and efficacy of the follow-on biologics.

11.4.5 Remarks

There is a clear distinction between the concepts for drug interchangeability for generic drugs and for biosimilar products. For drug interchangeability of generic drugs, the FDA suggests focusing on the assessment of the variability due to subject-by-product interaction although its clinical relevance has not yet been fully understood and demonstrated. Alternatively, it is suggested that the assessment of the variability due to subject-by-product adjusted for the intra-subject variability of the reference product be assessed for addressing drug interchangeability of small-molecule generics. This new criterion is currently being studied by Endrenyi et al. (2013).

Under an appropriate study design for switching or alternating or switching/alternating, statistical methods for assessment of biosimilarity between products could be based on testing for average bioequivalence (similarity) or testing for PBE (similarity) or IBE (similarity). It should be noted that FDA recommended a replicated crossover design such as (TRTR, RTRT) or (TRT, RTR) be employed for assessment of IBE (similarity).

11.5 Statistical Methods

In practice, switching and alternating can be assessed only after the biosimilar products under study have been shown to be highly similar to the innovative biological drug product. Based on a parallel idea for the development the biosimilarity index as described in Chapter 6, a general approach for the development of a switching index (SI) and/or alternating index (AI) for addressing switching and/or alternating can be obtained.

11.5.1 Totality Biosimilarity Index

As indicated in Chapter 6, for a given criterion for biosimilarity and under a valid study design, the biosimilarity index for a given functional area or domain can be obtained by the following steps:

Step 1: Assess the average biosimilarity based on a given criterion, e.g., (80%, 125%) based on log-transformed data.

Step 2: Calculate the local biosimilarity index (i.e., reproducibility) based on the observed ratio and variability.

Step 3: Claim local biosimilarity if the 95% confidence lower bound of p is larger than p_0, a pre-specified number, where p_0 can be obtained based on an estimate of reproducibility probability for a study comparing a reference product to itself (the reference product), i.e., an R–R study.

Similar to what was described in Chapter 6, a *totality biosimilarity index* can be derived across all functional areas or domains by the following steps:

Step 1: Obtain $\hat{p}_i$, the biosimilarity index for the ith domain.

Step 2: Define the totality biosimilarity index as $\hat{p}_T = \sum_{i=1}^{K} w_i \hat{p}_i$, where w_i is the weight for the ith domain, where $i = 1, 2, ..., K$ (the number of domains or functional areas).

Step 3: Claim biosimilarity if the 95% confidence lower bound of p_T is greater than a pre-specified value p_{T_0}, which can be determined based on an estimate of totality biosimilarity index for studies comparing a reference product to itself (the reference product).

The totality biosimilarity index, described earlier, has the advantages that (1) it is robust with respect to the selected study endpoint, biosimilarity criterion, and study design; (2) it takes variability into consideration (one of the major criticisms in the assessment of average bioequivalence); (3) it allows the definition and assessment of the degree of similarity (in other words, it provides a partial answer to the question "how similar is considered similar?"), and (4) the use of the biosimilarity index or totality biosimilarity index will reflect the sensitivity of heterogeneity in variance.

11.5.2 Switching Index

A similar idea can be applied to developing an SI under an appropriate study design such as a 4×2 Balaam's crossover design described earlier. Thus, biosimilarity for "R to T," "T to R," "T to T," and "R to R" needs to be assessed for addressing the issue of switching.

Define $\hat{p}_{Ti}$, the totality biosimilarity index for the ith switch, where $i = 1$ (switch from R to R), 2 (switch from T to T), 3 (switch from R to T), and 4 (switch from T to R). As a result, the SI can be obtained as follows:

Step 1: Obtain $\hat{p}_{Ti}$, $i = 1, ..., 4$.

Step 2: Define the switching index as $SI = \min_i\{p_{Ti}\}$, $i = 1, ..., 4$, which is the largest order of the biosimilarity indices.

Step 3: Claim switchability if the 95% confidence lower bound of p_S is larger than a pre-specified value p_{S0}.

Let $P_{T_1}, P_{T_2}, \ldots, P_{T_4}$ be a random sample from a continuous distribution with probability density function $f(p)$ and cumulative distribution function $F(p)$, and let $P_{T_{(1)}}, P_{T_{(2)}}, \ldots, P_{T_{(4)}}$ be the order statistics obtained from the sample mentioned earlier. Thus, the probability density function of the defined switching index $SI = P_{T_{(4)}}$ is given by

$$f_{SI}(p) = \frac{4!}{3!}(F(p))^0(1 - F(p))^3 f(p) = 4(1 - F(p))^3 f(p),$$

and the expected value and the variance of SI can be given by

$$\mu_{SI} = E(SI) = 4 \int p(1 - F(p))^3 f(p)dp$$

and

$$\mathrm{Var}(SI) = E(SI^2) - (\mu_{SI})^2,$$

where $E(SI^2) = \int p^2(1 - F(p))^3 f(p)dp$ is denoted as the second raw moment of SI.

With a given distribution function $F(p)$, the expected value and the variance of order statistics could be derived (see David and Nagaraja, 2003). However, the population distribution may be unknown or difficult to determine. Several results of non-parametric bounds for the moments of order statistics have been provided. David (1981) summarized the distribution-free bounds on the expected values of the order statistics when the observations $p_{T_1}, p_{T_2}, \ldots, p_{T_4}$ are i.i.d. from a population with expectation μ and variance σ^2. The earliest result provided in Gumbel (1954) and Hartley and David (1954) concerns the minimum,

$$\mu_{SI} \le \mu + \sigma(n - 1)(2n - 1)^{-1/2} = \mu + 1.1339\sigma, \tag{11.3}$$

where sample size $n = 4$ here.

However, the observations may be dependent and/or from different distributions. It could be obtained, as in Arnold and Groeneveld (1979), that the bound in Equation 11.3 becomes

$$\mu - \sigma(n - 1)^{1/2} \le \mu_{SI} \le \mu,$$

which yields

$$\mu - 1.73205\sigma \le \mu_{SI} \le \mu, \tag{11.4}$$

when independence cannot be assumed. On the other hand, for the variance of order statistics, the upper bound derived by Papadatos (1995) can be used. That is,

$$\mathrm{Var}(SI) < n\sigma^2 = 4\sigma^2. \tag{11.5}$$

In order to obtain the estimates of the expectation and variance of SI, the sample mean and sample variance of the observations $p_{T_1}, p_{T_2}, \ldots, p_{T_4}$ could be used to replace μ and σ^2, respectively, in the bound Equation 11.4 or 11.5 of μ_{SI} and the bound Equation 11.5 of $Var(SI)$.

As a result, the 95% confidence low bound of SI can be obtained. We then claim switching if the 95% confidence low bound for SI is greater than p_{S_0}.

11.5.3 Alternating Index

A similar idea can be applied in order to develop an AI under an appropriate study design. Under the modified Balaam's crossover design of (TT, RR, TRT, RTR), biosimilarity for "R to T to R" and "T to R to T" needs to be assessed for the evaluation of alternating. For example, the assessment of differences between "R to T" and "T to R" for alternating of "R to T to R" needs to be evaluated in order to determine whether the drug effect has returned to the baseline after the second switch.

Define p_{Ti} as the totality biosimilarity index for the ith switch, where $i = 1$ (switch from R to R), 2 (switch from T to T), 3 (switch from R to T), or 4 (switch from T to R). As a result, the AI can be obtained as follows:

> *Step 1*: Obtain $\hat{p}_{Ti}$, $i = 1, \ldots, 4$.
>
> *Step 2*: Define the range of these indexes, $AI = \max_i\{\hat{p}_{Ti}\} - \min_i\{\hat{p}_{Ti}\}$, $i = 1, \ldots, 4$, as the AI.
>
> *Step 3*: Claim alternation if the 95% confidence lower bound of AI is larger than a pre-specified value p_{A_0}.

The estimates of the expected value and variance of AI could be similarly obtained following the process of the confidence lower bound for SI. Suppose that $P_{T_1}, P_{T_2}, \ldots, P_{T_4}$ is a random sample from a continuous distribution with a probability density function $f(p)$ and cumulative distribution function $F(p)$, and $P_{T_{(1)}}, P_{T_{(2)}}, \ldots, P_{T_{(4)}}$ are the order statistics obtained from the sample mentioned earlier. Thus, the joint density function of $\max_i\{\hat{p}_{Ti}\}$ and $\min_i\{\hat{p}_{Ti}\}$ denoted by $f_{(1,4)}(p_{T_{(1)}}, p_{T_{(4)}},)$ is given by

$$f_{(1,4)}(p_{T_{(1)}}, p_{T_{(4)}},) = \frac{4!}{2!} f(p_{T_{(1)}}) f(p_{T_{(1)}}) \left[F(p_{T_{(1)}}) - F(p_{T_{(1)}}) \right]^2$$

$$= 12 f(p_{T_{(1)}}) f(p_{T_{(1)}}) \left[F(p_{T_{(1)}}) - F(p_{T_{(1)}}) \right]^2.$$

The expected value and the variance of AI can be given by

$$\mu_{AI} = E(AI) = 12 \int \int (p_{T_{(1)}} - p_{T_{(1)}}) f(p_{T_{(1)}}) f(p_{T_{(1)}}) \left[F(p_{T_{(1)}}) - F(p_{T_{(1)}}) \right]^2 dp_{T_{(1)}} dp_{T_{(4)}}$$

and

$$\mathrm{Var}(AI) = E(AI^2) - (\mu_{AI})^2,$$

where

$$E(SI^2) = 12 \int \int (p_{T_{(1)}} - p_{T_{(1)}})^2 f(p_{T_{(1)}}) f(p_{T_{(1)}}) \left[F(p_{T_{(1)}}) - F(p_{T_{(1)}}) \right]^2 dp_{T_{(1)}} dp_{T_{(4)}}$$

is denoted as the second moment of the sample range.

Based on the results of dependent distribution-free samples in Arnold and Groeneveld (1979), the bound on the expected value for the range of order statistics is given by

$$\mu_{AI} = E \max_i \{p_{Ti}\} - E \min_i \{p_{Ti}\}$$

$$\leq \sigma \left\{ \frac{n(n - k_2 + 1 + k_1)}{(n - k_2 + 1)k_1} \right\}^{1/2} = 2.82\sigma,$$

where $k_1 = 1$ and $k_2 = 4$ denote the orders of the difference. On the other hand, the upper bound for the variance of AI could be obtained by

$$\mathrm{Var}(AI) = \mathrm{Var}(P_{T_{(1)}}) + \mathrm{Var}(P_{T_{(4)}}) + 2\mathrm{Cov}(P_{T_{(1)}}, P_{T_{(4)}})$$

$$< \mathrm{Var}(P_{T_{(1)}}) + \mathrm{Var}(P_{T_{(4)}}) + 2\mathrm{Var}(P_{T_{(1)}})^{1/2} \mathrm{Var}(P_{T_{(4)}})^{1/2},$$

$$< n\sigma^2 + n\sigma^2 + 2n\sigma^2 = 16\sigma^2,$$

which is derived based on Cauchy–Schwarz inequality (Casella and Berger, 2002) and the result for the upper bound of the variance of order statistics (Papadatos, 1995). We could estimate μ and σ^2 by the sample mean and sample variance in order to construct the confidence lower bound for AI. Thus, we then claim switching if the 95% confidence lower bound for AI is greater than p_{A0}. Therefore, we may claim interchangeability if both switching and alternating are concluded.

11.5.4 Remarks

The above biosimilarity index (totality biosimilarity index) for assessment of biosimilarity and SI and/or AI for assessment of interchangeability are developed based on reproducibility probability. Hence, they are probability-based indices. In practice, we may consider moment-based indices for assessment of biosimilarity and interchangeability. For example, we may consider

$$\hat{z}_d = \frac{\hat{\mu}_T - \hat{\mu}_R}{\hat{\sigma}_d}$$

a standardized score for measuring the distance between the test (T) and the reference (R) products. In this case, the biosimilarity index can be defined as $BI = \hat{z}_d$ or $BI = \Phi(\hat{z}_d)$.

11.6 Concluding Remarks

The concept of drug interchangeability in terms of prescribability and switchability for small-molecule drug products is similar but different from that for large-molecule biological products. Thus, the usual methods for addressing drug interchangeability through the assessment of population/IBE cannot be directly applied for the assessment of drug interchangeability for biosimilar products.

Based on the totality biosimilarity index for the assessment of biosimilarity, the SI and AI for addressing drug interchangeability of biosimilar products can be obtained under an appropriate switching design and alternating design, respectively. The proposed switching/alternating indices have the advantages that (1) they can be applied regardless of the criteria for biosimilarity and study design used; (2) the assessment is made based on the relative difference with the reference product; (3) they can address the commonly asked questions concerning how similar is considered highly similar, the degree of similarity, and interchangeability in terms of switching and alternating; and most importantly, (4) the proposed method is in compliance with current regulatory thinking.

It should, however, be noted that the proposed totality biosimilarity index and/or switching/alternating indices depend upon the selection of weights in each domain for achieving the totality-of-the-evidence for the assessment of biosimilarity and/or interchangeability.

12

Issues on Immunogenicity Studies

12.1 Introduction

As indicated earlier, the U.S. BPCI Act defines a biosimilar product as a product that is highly similar to an innovative biological product notwithstanding minor differences in clinically inactive components and there are no clinically meaningful differences in terms of *safety*, purity, and potency. Thus, safety is a great concern when assessing biosimilarity of biosimilar products. Since the issue of immunogenicity is one of the fundamental differences between small-molecule drug products and biological products, when to conduct immunogenicity testing for the evaluation of immunotoxicity has become an important issue in biosimilar studies.

The U.S. FDA defines drug immunogenicity as the ability of a drug to induce an immune response. The clinical consequences of immunogenicity include the potential loss of efficacy and possible alteration of the safety profile. As indicated in the 2002 FDA guidance on *Immunotoxicology Evaluation of Investigational New Drugs*, in general, drugs can be grouped into two major classes with respect to potential immunogenicity. These two classes are (1) polypeptides or proteins with molecular weights larger than or equal to 10,000, and (2) low-molecular weight compounds (less than 1000). Smaller peptides or proteins in the 5000–10,000 range may also be immunogenic, although immune responses to these drugs may be fairly weak. On the other hand, De Weck (1974) indicated that immunogenicity is unpredictable for compounds in the 1000–5000 range.

In recent years, the number of biological/biotechnology-derived proteins used as therapeutic agents has been steadily increasing. These products may induce an unwanted immune response in treated patients, which can be influenced by various factors, including patient-related or disease-related factors and product-related factors. Unwanted immune reactions inducing anti-drug antibodies (ADA) may neutralize drug efficacy or cause allergic reactions and other severe side effects, representing a major issue in the development of therapeutic proteins. Thus, proteins developed as vaccines have to be designed, manufactured, and formulated to induce the best protective immune response possible, directed primarily against specific epitopes and not against non-relevant portions like protein scaffolds or carrier molecules.

In the next section, regulatory requirements from the European Medicines Agency (EMA), the U.S. Food and Drug Administration (FDA), and the International Conference on Harmonization (ICH) for the assessment of immunotoxicity (e.g., immunogenicity) during the development of biosimilar products are briefly described. Section 12.3 provides some insight regarding assay development/validation for distinguishing neutralizing from non-neutralizing antibodies. Basic design considerations, data collection and analysis, and interpretation for immunogenicity studies are given in Section 12.4. Section 12.5 discusses sample size calculations/justifications for immunogenicity studies with extremely low incidence rates (immune responses) based on precision analysis for achieving certain statistical assurance (inference) to detect a clinically meaningful immune response. Also included in this section is a proposed statistical procedure for data safety monitoring during the conduct of immunogenicity studies. Some concluding remarks are given in the last section of the chapter.

12.2 Regulatory Requirements

In this section, regulatory requirements from the EMA, the FDA, and the ICH for the evaluation of immunotoxicity (immunogenicity) of biosimilar products are briefly described.

12.2.1 European Medicines Agency

In 2007, the Committee for Medicinal Products for Human Use (CHMP) of the EMA released a guideline on *Immunogenicity Assessment of Biotechnology-Derived Therapeutic Proteins* to assist sponsors in the evaluation of drug effects on the immune system. The guideline intends to cover proteins and polypeptides, their derivatives, and products of which they are components such as conjugates. These proteins and polypeptides are produced from recombinant or non-recombinant cell-culture expression systems. The guideline provides general principles on (1) risk factors for developing an immune response against a therapeutic protein, (2) predictivity of non-clinical models, (3) development of assays for humoral and cellular immune response, (4) potential clinical consequences of immunogenicity, (5) clinical safety, and (6) risk management plan.

The most commonly seen risk factors for developing an immune response include patient-related, disease-related, and product-related risk factors. Patient-related risk factors include age and genetic factors such as certain allelic loci, gene polymorphisms for cytokines, and gene defects which could alter the immune response to a therapeutic protein. Disease-related risk factors are referred to as a patient's underlying disease itself such as an autoimmune disease, chronic infections, or advanced metastatic disease. Product-related risk factors include the protein structure, formulation, aggregation, excipients, and impurities. These factors definitely could impact immunogenicity (EMA, 2007).

For predictivity of non-clinical models, therapeutic proteins are different in various species. Thus, the evaluation of immunogenicity in animal models is generally *not* predictive of human models. As most therapeutic proteins induce unwanted immune responses that may be caused by more than one single risk factor, it is important to adopt or develop adequate screening and/or confirmatory assays for an accurate and reliable assessment of the immune response against a therapeutic protein.

Potential clinical consequences of immunogenicity include the possible loss of efficacy and the alteration of the safety profile. For example, neutralizing antibodies which interfere with biological activity by binding to or near the active site, or by induction of conformational changes, could induce loss of efficacy. However, loss of efficacy and alteration of the safety profile are not necessarily linked. Safety issues such as infusion-related reactions can occur even when there is no loss of efficacy. In addition, antibodies developing against therapeutic proteins can cross-react with an endogenous protein in cases where the/endogenous protein is still produced.

For clinical safety, the 2007 EMA guidance recommends the following principles: pre-authorization of signal detection in clinical setting, the evaluation of the impact of both neutralizing and non-neutralizing antibodies on the pharmacokinetics of the product, and methodology development for assessing the comparability of immunogenicity between biosimilar products and a reference product. As indicated by the 2007 EMA guidance, studies should be carefully planned and data should be systematically collected from a *sufficiently large* number of patients to characterize the variability in antibody response.

The 2007 EMA guidance also emphasizes that the risk of immunogenicity should be addressed in a risk management plan according to the principles outlined in the guidance. The risk management plan should take into account risks identified during product development and potential risks that may occur in the post-marketing setting.

12.2.2 United States Food and Drug Administration

In 2002, the FDA published a guidance entitled *Immunotoxicology Evaluation of Investigational New Drugs* to assist sponsors in the evaluation of the drug effects on the immune system. The guidance makes recommendations on (1) the parameters that should be routinely assessed in toxicology studies to determine effects of a drug on the immune function, (2) when additional immunogenicity studies should be conducted, and (3) when additional mechanistic information could help to characterize the significance of a given drug's effect on the immune system.

The 2002 FDA guidance indicated that assessment of potential adverse effects on the immune system is an important component of the overall evaluation of drug toxicity. In practice, there are two major concerns associated with drug immunogenicity: drug allergenicity (which is referred to as either protein allergens or small-molecular weight drugs that become allergens when bound to proteins) and the ability of antidrug immune responses to alter the biological activities of the drug (e.g., PK, PD, and/or toxicities), (see, e.g., Schellekens, 2003). Evaluation of protein drugs for allergenic potential is difficult in non-clinical toxicology. As indicated by the FDA, although immunogenicity is an important property of protein allergens, not all protein immunogens are allergens (see also Kimber et al., 1999). In practice, evidence of immunotoxicity can be observed in standard non-clinical toxicology studies, but in some cases additional studies are important. Observation of immune system effects may also suggest that more follow-up studies should be considered.

It should be noted that the 2002 FDA guidance is intended for drug products and not for biological products. The FDA encourages that sponsors of biological products should refer to the principles outlined in the ICH guidance (ICH, 1997), which is briefly described later.

12.2.3 International Conference on Harmonization

In 1997, ICH published a guideline on *Preclinical Safety Evaluation of Biotechnology-Derived Pharmaceuticals* to assist sponsors in preclinical safety evaluation of biotechnology-derived pharmaceuticals (ICH, 1997). The primary goal is to assist sponsors in improving the quality and consistency of the preclinical safety data which support the development of biopharmaceuticals. This guidance is intended primarily to recommend a basic framework for the preclinical safety evaluation of biotechnology-derived pharmaceuticals such as active substances including proteins and peptides, their derivatives, and products of which they are components. These biotechnology-derived pharmaceuticals include, but are not limited to, cytokines, plasminogen activators, recombinant plasma factors, growth factors, fusion proteins, enzymes, receptors, hormones, and monoclonal antibodies.

As indicated in the 1997 ICH guideline, many biotechnology-derived pharmaceuticals intended for humans are immunogenic in animals. Thus, antibody responses such as titer, number of responding animals, neutralizing or non-neutralizing, should be characterized. In addition, these responses should be correlated with any pharmacological and/or toxicological changes. Specifically, the effects of antibody formation on pharmacokinetic/pharmacodynamic parameters, incidence and/or severity of adverse effects, complement activation, or the emergence of new toxic effects should be considered when interpreting the data. The 1997 ICH guideline also pointed out that special attention should also be paid to the evaluation of possible pathological changes related to immune complex formation and deposition.

The detection of antibodies is important in the evaluation of pre-clinical safety of biotechnology-derived pharmaceuticals. It, however, should be noted that, as indicated by the 1997 ICH guideline, the detection of antibodies should not be the only criterion for the early termination of a pre-clinical safety study unless the immune response neutralizes the pharmacological and/or toxicological effects of the biopharmaceutical in the majority of the animals under study. In most cases, the immune response to biopharmaceuticals is expected to be variable (similar observations were seen in humans). Furthermore, in many cases, the induction of antibody formation in animals is found *not* to be predictive of antibody formation in humans. This is because humans may develop serum antibodies against humanized proteins, and frequently the therapeutic response persists in their presence. The occurrence of severe anaphylactic responses to recombinant proteins is rare in humans. In this regard, such pre-clinical safety studies are considered of little value for the routine evaluation of these types of products.

The 1997 ICH guideline also pointed out that the assessment of potential immunogenicity is an important aspect for the immunotoxicological evaluation of biotechnology-derived pharmaceuticals, which are intended to stimulate or suppress the immune system. Thus, biotechnology-derived pharmaceuticals may affect not only humoral but also cell-mediated immunity. In addition, inflammatory reactions at the injection site may be indicative of a stimulatory response. It should also be noted that the expression of surface antigens on target cells may be altered, which has implications for autoimmune potential. To clarify these issues, immunotoxicological testing strategies may require screening studies followed by mechanistic studies.

12.3 Assay Development/Validation

In immunogenicity studies, it is essential to adopt an appropriate strategy for the development of adequate screening and confirmatory assays to measure an immune response against a therapeutic protein. Assays must be capable of distinguishing neutralizing from non-neutralizing antibodies, and to be used in pivotal clinical trials as well as in post-authorization studies to be validated.

12.3.1 Assay Development

As indicated in the 2007 EMA guidance, unwanted immunogenicity induced by biological products could include humoral and cellular immune responses. It is therefore very important to select and/or develop assays and assay strategies for the assessment of such immune responses. In practice, most effort is usually directed to antibody detection and characterization because this is technically feasible and often related to clinical safety and efficacy. However, cell-mediated responses could play an important role and their assessment may be considered by applicants on a case-by-case basis.

12.3.1.1 Screening Assays

A screening assay should be capable of detecting antibodies induced against the biological product in all antibody positive samples/patients. This implies that detection of some false positive results is inevitable as absolute screening-assay specificity is normally unattainable and false negative results must be avoided. The desirable characteristics of screening assays are sensitivity, specificity, precision, reproducibility, and robustness.

12.3.1.2 Assays for Confirming the Presence of Antibodies

These assays are necessary for the elimination of false positive samples/patients following the initial screen. Various approaches can be adopted for this purpose but it is necessary to select assays taking account of the limitations and characteristics of the screening assay(s). To confirm specificity, it is not normally sufficient or appropriate to simply repeat the screening assay in its original form.

12.3.1.3 Assays for Dissecting the Specificity of Antibodies

Assays which provide information concerning the specificity of the antibodies detected may be useful in some cases. These data contribute to the confirmation of the specificity of the immune response.

12.3.1.4 Neutralization Assays

Assessing the neutralizing capacity of antibodies usually requires the use of bioassays. An assay must be selected or developed which responds well to the biological product. Bioassays used for measuring the potency of biological products, e.g., for lot release purposes, can often be adapted to assess neutralizing antibodies. However, they frequently require refining if they are to perform optimally for measuring the neutralizing capacity of antibodies. If neutralizing cell-based assays are not feasible/available, competitive binding assays or other alternatives may be suitable. However, when these are used, it must be demonstrated that they reflect neutralizing capacity/potential in an appropriate manner.

12.3.2 Assay Validation

Assay validation is an ongoing process throughout product development. Assays used for the pivotal clinical trials need to be validated for their intended purpose. Validation studies must be conducted to establish that the assays show appropriately linear, concentration-dependent responses to relevant analytes as well as appropriate accuracy, precision, sensitivity, specificity, and robustness. For pivotal clinical trials, the use of a central laboratory to perform the assays may be helpful to avoid inter-laboratory variability. In the post-approval setting, it is also important to consider inter-laboratory variability.

The 2007 EMA guidance indicated that assays must also be validated to show that matrix effects caused by reagents or substances present in samples do not adversely affect the obtained results. This is normally addressed by "recovery" investigations conducted by observing the effects of such substances present in the matrix on the response obtained in their absence. This needs to be investigated for the full range of dilutions of samples, which are to be used in assays, and, at least in some cases, limits the dilutions, which can be validly assessed.

It should be noted that the residual biological product present in patients' blood can complex with induced antibody and hence reduce the amount of antibody detectable by assays. This may affect assays differently, depending on the assay, assay format or type, and the antibody characteristics. If this occurs, it may be circumvented/resolved by using a number of approaches, e.g., by dissociating the immune complexes with acid, removing excess biological by solid-phase adsorption, use of long incubation times, and/or using an assay which allows sufficient sample dilution to avoid this problem. Such approaches must themselves be validated for effectiveness and adopted on a case-by-case basis according to needs. In some cases this problem can be overcome by appropriate spacing of the timing between the administration of the product and the sampling for antibody assessment, i.e., allowing time for the product to be cleared from the circulation before sampling. However, the latter approach must not significantly compromise the detection of antibodies or the treatment of the patient.

If antibodies are detected in patients undergoing therapy, these need to be characterized to establish their clinical significance. This normally involves an immunological and/or biological assessment of antibody characteristics and the investigation of effects of the antibodies (or other induced immune responses) on the product. Some of this can be addressed by non-antibody assays as part of in vitro studies, but it may also require clinical assessment of the patients receiving therapy.

12.4 Design for Immunogenicity Studies

Most biological/biotechnology-derived proteins induce an unwanted immune response that may be triggered by more than a single factor. This immunological response is complex and could contribute to potential adverse responses. The consequences of an immune reaction to a therapeutic protein range from the transient appearance of antibodies without any clinical significance to severe life-threatening conditions. Potential clinical consequences of an unwanted immune response are a loss of efficacy of the therapeutic protein, serious general immune effects such as anaphylaxis, and, for therapeutic proteins used for substitution, a potential cross-reactivity with the endogenous counterpart in case it is still produced. Thus, immunogenicity studies need to be carefully and prospectively designed to ensure that all essential procedures are in place before the commencement of clinical assessment. Basic design considerations for an immunogenicity study are described later followed by the identification of risk factors, selection and assessment of assays, data collection and analysis, and the interpretation of analysis results.

12.4.1 Basic Design Considerations

As indicated in the 2007 EMA guidance on the immunogenicity assessment of biotechnology-derived therapeutic proteins, immunogenicity studies should be carefully planned and data should be systematically collected from a *sufficiently large* number of *patients* to characterize the *variability* in antibody response. Some basic design considerations regarding immunogenicity studies are briefly described later.

12.4.1.1 Patient Population

The patient population should be representative of the target population intended for clinical practice. A homogenous patient population should be chosen whenever possible. Due to expected differential susceptibility, immunogenicity data from healthy volunteers may not be suitable. For most biosimilar products, immunogenicity is studied in previously unexposed patients. Children should be studied separately.

12.4.1.2 Randomization

The 2007 EMA guidance suggests that if applicable, stratified randomization by age should be employed.

12.4.1.3 Washout

For immunogenicity studies, it is suggested that a sufficient washout period for previous treatments potentially influencing the immune response should be included. The washout should take into account not only elimination but also the reversal of the pharmacodynamic effect, where appropriate.

12.4.1.4 Variability in Antibody Response

For the comparative evaluation of immunogenicity between a biosimilar product and a reference product, inter-product and intra-product variabilities are inevitable. Inter-product variability is referred to as the variability due to similar biological medicinal products or products in the same class, while intra-product variability is the variability due to different versions of the product, indications or different patient populations for a given product. Variations of the production process have been reported to alter considerably their immunogenic properties. The assessment of inter-product and intra-product variabilities is useful in detecting signals of immunogenicity. For example, if intra-product comparative immunogenicity is analyzed when changes in production have been made, a population should be chosen in an indication where differences can best be detected (i.e., due to susceptibility to immunogenicity).

12.4.1.5 Sample Size

Since the immune response is expected to be low, a large sample size may be required for achieving a desired power for detecting a relatively small difference of clinically importance if such a difference truly exists at a pre-specified level of significance. In practice, a large sample size may not be feasible. Alternatively, Chow and Chiu (2013) proposed to select/justify a sample size based on the concept of precision analysis in conjunction with a sensitivity analysis. More details are provided in the next section of this chapter.

12.4.1.6 Surrogate Endpoints

In some cases, surrogate endpoints such as pharmacodynamic parameters may be used to assess immunogenicity. In this case, as indicated by the 2007 EMA guidance, surrogate endpoints should correlate with clinically relevant endpoints and have to be *fully* justified.

12.4.2 Risk Factors

Many factors may influence the immunogenicity of therapeutic proteins. They can be considered to be patient-related, disease-related, or product-related. Patient-related factors that might predispose an individual to an immune response include the underlying disease, genetic background, immune status, including immunomodulating therapy, and the dosing schedule. Product-related factors also influence the likelihood of an immune response, e.g., the manufacturing process, formulation, and stability characteristics. Although data on possible unwanted immune reactions to therapeutic proteins are required before marketing authorization, problems may still be encountered in the post-authorization period. In the marketing authorization application, the applicant should include a summary of the investigations of immunogenicity in the respective overview sections with full cross-reference to the data in the relevant modules. Depending on the immunogenic potential of the therapeutic protein and the rarity of the disease, the extent of immunogenicity data before approval might be limited. Further systematic immunogenicity testing might become necessary after marketing authorization, and may be included in the risk management plan.

The most commonly seen patient-related risk factors are age and genetic factors such as certain allelic loci, gene polymorphisms for cytokines, and gene defects which could alter the immune response to a therapeutic protein. Disease-related risk factors are referred to as a patient's underlying disease itself such as autoimmune disease, chronic infections, or advanced metastatic diseases. In practice, the immune reaction against a therapeutic protein can be reduced when immunosuppressive agents are used concomitantly. As a result, it is expected that concomitant therapies may decrease the risk of an immune response to a therapeutic protein. Thus, the 2007 EMA guidance indicated that if clinical trials are performed in conjunction with immunosuppressants, a claim for the use of the therapeutic protein in monotherapy must be accompanied by adequate clinical data on the immunogenicity profile in monotherapy. Product-related risk factors include the protein structure, formulation, aggregation, excipients, and impurities. These factors could impact on immunogenicity. Thus, it is suggested that careful planning of immunogenicity evaluation should be exercised and data should be systematically collected from a sufficiently *large* number of patients to characterize the *variability* in antibody response.

12.4.3 Selection/Assessment of Assays

This applies to assays used to measure and characterize antibodies and to methods employed for assessing clinical responses to antibodies if they are induced. Much of this needs to be established on a case-by-case basis, taking account of product, patients, and expected clinical parameters. Such studies can provide valuable information concerning significant immunogenicity of biological products, their characteristics and potential clinical consequences. They can be valuable for comparative immunogenicity studies for biosimilar products or following production/process changes introduced for established products. However, unwanted immunogenicity can occur at a level which will not be detected by such studies when conducted at a pre-approval stage, due to the restricted number of patients normally available for study. In view of this, it is often necessary to continue the assessment of unwanted immunogenicity and its clinical significance post-approval, usually as part of pharmacovigilance surveillance. In some cases, post-approval clinical studies may be needed to establish the risk associated with an unwanted immune response

12.4.4 Data Collection and Analysis

The 2007 EMA guidance suggests that in the clinical setting, careful planning of immunogenicity evaluation should include data systematically collected from a sufficient number of patients. For a given product, sampling should preferably be standardized across studies (e.g., sampling at the baseline, under treatment and follow-up samples). The sampling schedule for each product is determined on a case-by-case basis, taking into account also the risks associated with an unwanted immune response to patients. Data on the impact on efficacy and safety should be collected in order to fully understand the clinical consequences of the immune response. Immunogenicity issues should be further addressed in the risk management plan.

12.4.5 Interpretation of Results

For the interpretation of results, the 2007 EMA guidance also indicated that it is essential to establish clear criteria for deciding how samples will be considered positive or negative, and also how positive results will be confirmed. Approaches to these can differ according to assay, etc. and need to be decided accordingly. A common procedure for establishing a positive cut-off for immunoassays is to establish the assay background. A statistical approach should preferably be used to establish the assay cut-off value. Alternatively, real data (e.g., double background value) can be used to determine what will be considered the lowest positive result.

12.5 Sample Size for Immunogenicity Studies

In immunogenicity studies, the incidence rate of immune responses is expected to be low. In this case, the usual pre-study power analysis for sample size calculation for detecting a clinically meaningful difference may not be feasible. Alternatively, we may consider selecting an appropriate sample size based on precision analysis rather than power analysis to provide some statistical inference. In this section, a simple procedure based on precision analysis for selecting an appropriate sample size in immunogenicity studies is introduced. In addition, a strategy for data safety monitoring during the conduct of a given immunogenicity study with extremely low incidence rate, proposed by Chow and Chiu (2013), is discussed.

12.5.1 Sample Size Determination

In clinical trials, a pre-study power analysis for sample size calculations is often performed to ensure that an intended clinical trial will achieve a desired power for correctly detecting a clinically meaningful treatment effect at a pre-specified level of significance. For clinical trials with extremely low incidence rate, sample size calculations based on power analysis may not be feasible. Alternatively, it is suggested that sample size calculations be done based on precision analysis. In this section, pre-study power analysis and precision analysis for sample size calculation are briefly described.

12.5.1.1 Power Analysis

Under a two-sample parallel-group design, let x_{ij} be a binary response (e.g., adverse events, immune responses, or infection rate post-surgery) from the jth subject in the ith group, $j = 1, \ldots, n$, $i = T$ (test), R (reference or control). Then, $\hat{p}_i = 1/n \sum_{i=1}^{n} x_{ij}$ are the incidence rates for the test group and the control group, respectively. Let, $\delta = p_R - p_T$ be the difference in incidence rates between the test group and the control group. For simplicity, consider the following hypotheses for testing equality between p_R and p_T:

$$H_0 : \delta = 0 \quad \text{versus} \quad H_a : \delta \neq 0$$

Thus, under the alternative hypothesis, the power of $1 - \beta$ can be approximately obtained by the following equation (see, e.g., Chow et al., 2007):

$$\Phi\left(\frac{|\hat{\delta}|}{\sqrt{(\hat{p}_R(1-\hat{p}_R)+\hat{p}_T(1-\hat{p}_T))/n}} - Z_{1-\alpha/2}\right),$$

where
 Φ is the cumulative standard normal distribution function
 $Z_{1-\alpha/2}$ is the upper $\alpha/2$th quantile of the standard normal distribution

As a result, the sample size needed for achieving a desired power of $1 - \beta$ at the α level of significance can be obtained by the following equation:

$$n_{power} = \frac{(Z_{1-\alpha/2} + Z_{\beta})^2}{\hat{\delta}^2} \hat{\sigma}^2, \tag{12.1}$$

where
 $\hat{\delta} = \hat{p}_R - \hat{p}_T$
 $\hat{\sigma}^2 = \hat{p}_R(1-\hat{p}_R)+\hat{p}_T(1-\hat{p}_T)$

12.5.1.2 Precision Analysis

On the other hand, the $(1 - \alpha) \times 100\%$ confidence interval (CI) for $\delta = p_R - p_T$, based on large-sample normal approximation, is given by

$$\hat{\delta} \pm Z_{1-\alpha/2} \frac{\hat{\sigma}}{\sqrt{n}},$$

where
 $\hat{\delta} = \hat{p}_R - \hat{p}_T$
 $\hat{\sigma} = \sqrt{\hat{\sigma}_R^2 + \hat{\sigma}_T^2}$
 $\hat{\sigma}_R^2 = \hat{p}_R(1-\hat{p}_R)$
 $\hat{\sigma}_T^2 = \hat{p}_T(1-\hat{p}_T)$
 $Z_{1-\alpha/2}$ is the upper $\alpha/2$th quantile of the standard normal distribution

Denote the half of the width of the CI by $w = Z_{1-\alpha/2}\hat{\sigma}$, which is usually referred to as the *maximum error margin allowed* for a given sample size n. In practice, the maximum error margin allowed represents the precision that one would expect for the selected sample size. The precision analysis for sample size determination is to consider the maximum error margin allowed. In other words, we are confident that the true difference $\delta = p_R - p_T$ would fall within the margin of $w = Z_{1-\alpha/2}\hat{\sigma}$ for a given sample size of n. Thus, the sample size required for achieving the desired precision can be chosen as

$$n_{\text{precision}} = \frac{Z_{1-\alpha/2}^2 \hat{\sigma}^2}{w^2}, \tag{12.2}$$

where $\hat{\sigma}^2 = \hat{p}_R(1-\hat{p}_R) + \hat{p}_T(1-\hat{p}_T)$.

This approach, based on the interest in only the type I error, is to specify precision while estimating the true δ for selecting n. By Equations 12.1 and 12.2, we can also get the relationship between the sample size based on power analysis and precision analysis:

$$R = \frac{n_{\text{power}}}{n_{\text{precision}}} = \left(1 + \frac{Z_\beta}{Z_{1-\alpha/2}}\right)^2 \frac{w^2}{\delta^2}.$$

Thus, R is proportional to $1/\delta^2$ or w^2. Under a fixed power and significance level, the sample size based on power analysis is much larger than the sample size based on precision analysis with extremely low infection rate difference or large allowed error margin.

Without loss of generality, $(1 + Z_\beta/Z_{1-\alpha/2})$ is always much larger than 1 (e.g., if power $1 - \beta = 80\%$ and significance level $\alpha = 5\%$ then $(1 + Z_\beta/Z_{1-\alpha/2})^2 = 2.04$). It means that if $w/\delta > 0.7$, the proposed sample size based on power analysis will be larger than the one based on precision analysis. The sample size determined by power analysis will be large when the difference between the test group and the control group is extremely small. Table 12.1 shows the comparison of sample sizes determined by power analysis and precision analysis. The power is fixed at 80% and the significance level is 5%. When $(\hat{p}_R, \hat{p}_T) = (2\%, 1\%)$, compare the sample sizes calculated by the two methods. The sample sizes determined by precision analysis are much smaller than the sample sizes determined by power analysis.

12.5.1.3 Sensitivity Analysis

$n_{\text{precision}}$ in Equation 12.2 is very sensitive to small changes in p_R and p_T. The following sensitivity analysis evaluates the impact of small deviations from the true incidence rates. The true incidence rates for the reference and

TABLE 12.1

Sample Size Based on Power Analysis and Precision
Analysis

ω		δ		n_{power}	$n_{precision}$	R
0.08$\hat{\sigma}$	1.37%	0.04$\hat{\sigma}$	0.69%	4906	600	8.2
	1.37%	0.05$\hat{\sigma}$	0.86%	3140	600	5.2
	1.37%	0.06$\hat{\sigma}$	1.03%	2180	600	3.6
	1.37%	0.07$\hat{\sigma}$	1.20%	1602	600	2.7
	1.37%	0.08$\hat{\sigma}$	1.37%	1226	600	2.0
0.10$\hat{\sigma}$	1.72%	0.04$\hat{\sigma}$	0.69%	4906	384	12.8
	1.72%	0.05$\hat{\sigma}$	0.86%	3140	384	8.2
	1.72%	0.06$\hat{\sigma}$	1.03%	2180	384	5.7
	1.72%	0.07$\hat{\sigma}$	1.20%	1602	384	4.2
	1.72%	0.08$\hat{\sigma}$	1.37%	1226	384	3.2
0.12$\hat{\sigma}$	2.06%	0.04$\hat{\sigma}$	0.69%	4906	267	18.4
	2.06%	0.05$\hat{\sigma}$	0.86%	3140	267	11.8
	2.06%	0.06$\hat{\sigma}$	1.03%	2180	267	8.2
	2.06%	0.07$\hat{\sigma}$	1.20%	1602	267	6.0
	2.06%	0.08$\hat{\sigma}$	1.37%	1226	267	4.6

control groups have a small shift, then, $p'_R = p_R + \varepsilon_R$ and $p'_T = p_T + \varepsilon_T$. Thus, the required sample size can be chosen as

$$n_s = \frac{Z^2_{1-\alpha/2}\hat{\sigma}'^2}{w^2},$$
(12.3)

where

$$\hat{\sigma}' = \sqrt{\sigma'^2_R + \sigma'^2_T}$$

$$\sigma'^2_R = (\hat{p}_R + \varepsilon_R)(1 - \hat{p}_R - \varepsilon_R)$$

$$\sigma'^2_T = (\hat{p}_T + \varepsilon_T)(1 - \hat{p}_T - \varepsilon_T)$$

$Z_{1-\alpha/2}$ is the upper $(\alpha/2)$th quantile of the standard normal distribution

We let the shift $\varepsilon_R = \varepsilon_T = \varepsilon$. By Formulas 12.2 and 12.3, we can also get the relationship between the sample size based on precision analysis and the sample size adjusted by sensitivity analysis.

$$\frac{n_s}{n_{precision}} = \frac{(p_R + \varepsilon)(1 - p_R - \varepsilon) + (p_T + \varepsilon)(1 - p_T - \varepsilon)}{p_R(1 - p_R) + p_T(1 - p_T)}$$

$$= \frac{p_R + p_T - p_R^2 - p_T^2 - 2(p_R + p_T)\varepsilon + 2\varepsilon - \varepsilon^2}{p_R + p_T - p_R^2 - p_T^2}.$$

Obviously, the aforementioned ratio is independent of $Z_{1-\alpha/2}$ and w. It becomes a ratio of variances before and after shift. Moreover,

$$\frac{n_s}{n_{\text{precision}}} < 1 \quad \text{if } \varepsilon = 0,$$

$$\frac{n_s}{n_{\text{precision}}} > 1 \quad \text{if } \varepsilon = 0,$$

and

$$\frac{n_s}{n_{\text{precision}}} = 1 \quad \text{if } \varepsilon = 0.$$

This means that when $\varepsilon > 0$, the sample size adjusted by sensitivity analysis, n_s, will be smaller than $n_{\text{precision}}$ relying on precision analysis. On the other hand, n_s will be larger than $n_{\text{precision}}$ if $\varepsilon < 0$.

12.5.1.4 Procedure for Sample Size Determination

As indicated earlier, for clinical trials with extremely low incidence rates, sample sizes required for achieving a desired power for detecting a small difference may not be feasible. Sample size justification based on a small difference (absolute change) may not be of practical interest. Alternatively, sample size justification based on relative change is often considered. For example, suppose that the incidence rate for the control group is 2% and the incidence rate for the test group is 1%. The absolute change in infection rate is 1% = 2% − 1%. This small difference may not be of any clinical or practical meaning. However, if we consider relative change, then the difference becomes appealing. In other words, there is a 50% relative reduction in incidence rate from 2% to 1%. In this section, we introduce a procedure based on precision analysis for selecting an appropriate sample size for clinical trials with extremely low incidence rate, which will also take into account relative change.

Suppose that p_R and p_T are incidence rates for the control group and the test group, respectively. Define relative improvement (or % improvement) as follows:

$$\% \text{ Improvement} = \frac{p_R - p_T}{p_R} \times 100\%.$$

Note that when $p_R < p_T$, the aforementioned measure becomes that of % worsening. Based on the precision analysis and considering the relative improvement at the same time, the following step-by-step procedure. for choosing an appropriate sample size is recommended:

Step 1: Determine the maximum allowed error margin. Choose a maximum error margin that one feels comfortable with. In other words, we are 95% confident that the true difference in incidence rates between the two groups is within the maximum error margin.

Step 2: Select the highest % improvement. Since it is expected that the relative improvement in infection rate is somewhere within the range, we may choose the combination of incidence rates which gives the highest % improvement.

Step 3: Select the sample size that reaches statistical significance. We then select the sample size for achieving statistical significance (i.e., those CIs that do not cover 0). In other words, the observed difference is not by chance above zero and is reproducible if we repeat the study under similar experimental conditions.

Note that with a selected sample size (based on the earlier procedure), we can also evaluate the corresponding power. If one feels uncomfortable, one may increase the sample size. In practice, it is suggested that the selected sample size should have at least 50% power at a pre-specified level of significance.

12.5.1.5 Example

A biotechnology company is interested in conducting a clinical trial for evaluating immune responses of one of their products as compared to an innovative product. Suppose that the incidence rate for the control group is extremely low, which is ranging from 1.7% to 2.1% with a mean incidence rate of 1.9%. The sponsor expects that the incidence rate for the test product is about 1.0% and targets for an at least 50% improvement in the immune response rate. Based on a pre-study power analysis for sample size calculation, a total sample size of 6532 (3266 per group) is required for achieving a 90% power for detecting a difference in incidence rate of 0.95% if such a difference truly exists at the 5% level of significance. With this huge sample size, the sponsor cannot afford to support the study, and it may not be of any practical use. Alternatively, based on the suggestions in the preceding sections, we may pursue the following steps to choose an appropriate sample size for the proposed clinical study:

Step 1: Assume that the true incidence rate for the control group is 1.90% and we expect that there is a 50% relative reduction for the test group. In other words, the true incidence rate for the test group is 0.95%. Now suppose that the sponsor is willing to tolerate a 50% error margin. Thus, we choose a maximum error margin allowed to be 50.

Step 2: We then use Table 12.2 to select the combination of (p_R, p_T) with the highest possible % improvement. Table 12.2 suggests that the second column with 53% relative improvement be considered.

TABLE 12.2

95% CIs ($p_R = 1.90\%$) for the Determination of Sample Sizes

p_T % of Improvement	0.85% 55%			0.90% 53%			0.95% 50%			1.00% 47%			1.05% 45%		
n	Lower (%)	Upper (%)	Power	Lower (%)	Upper (%)	Power	Lower (%)	Upper (%)	Power	Lower (%)	Upper (%)	Power	Lower (%)	Upper (%)	Power
200	-1.23	3.33	14.52	-1.30	3.30	13.39	-1.37	3.27	12.35	-1.44	3.24	11.38	-1.51	3.21	10.48
300	-0.81	2.91	19.64	-0.88	2.88	17.97	-0.95	2.85	16.42	-1.01	2.81	14.98	-1.08	2.78	13.66
400	-0.56	2.66	24.71	-0.63	2.63	22.51	-0.69	2.59	20.45	-0.76	2.56	18.55	-0.82	2.52	16.80
500	-0.39	2.49	29.71	-0.46	2.46	26.99	-0.52	2.42	24.46	-0.58	2.38	22.10	-0.64	2.34	19.92
600	-0.27	2.37	34.58	-0.33	2.33	31.40	-0.39	2.29	28.42	-0.45	2.25	25.62	-0.51	2.21	23.03
700	-0.17	2.27	39.30	-0.23	2.23	35.71	-0.29	2.19	32.30	-0.35	2.15	29.10	-0.41	2.11	26.11
800	-0.09	2.19	43.85	-0.15	2.15	39.89	-0.21	2.11	36.11	-0.27	2.07	32.52	-0.33	2.03	29.15
900	-0.02	2.12	48.19	-0.08	2.08	43.93	-0.14	2.04	39.81	-0.20	2.00	35.88	-0.26	1.96	32.16
1000	0.03	2.07	52.32	-0.03	2.03	47.81	-0.09	1.99	43.40	-0.15	1.95	39.16	-0.21	1.91	35.11
1100	0.08	2.02	56.23	0.02	1.98	51.51	-0.04	1.94	46.87	-0.10	1.90	42.35	-0.16	1.86	38.01

(continued)

TABLE 12.2 (continued)

95% CIs ($p_R = 1.90\%$) for the Determination of Sample Sizes

p_T % of Improvement	0.85%			0.90%			0.95%			1.00%			1.05%		
	55%			53%			50%			47%			45%		
n	Lower (%)	Upper (%)	Power	Lower (%)	Upper (%)	Power	Lower (%)	Upper (%)	Power	Lower (%)	Upper (%)	Power	Lower (%)	Upper (%)	Power
1200	0.12	1.98	59.91	0.06	1.94	55.04	0.00	1.90	50.20	−0.06	1.86	45.44	−0.11	1.81	40.84
1300	0.16	1.94	63.35	0.10	1.90	58.39	0.04	1.86	53.40	−0.02	1.82	48.44	−0.08	1.78	43.60
1400	0.19	1.91	66.57	0.13	1.87	61.56	0.07	1.83	56.45	0.02	1.78	51.33	−0.04	1.74	46.28
1500	0.22	1.88	69.56	0.16	1.84	64.55	0.10	1.80	59.37	0.05	1.75	54.12	−0.01	1.71	48.89

Step 3: We then select a sample size that reaches statistical significance. It can be seen from Table 12.2 that $n = 1100$ per group will reach statistical significance (i.e., the observed difference is *not* by chance alone and it is reproducible).

Thus, the total sample size required for the proposed study for achieving the desired precision (i.e., the maximum allowed error margin) and the relative improvement of 53% is 2200 (1100 per group), assuming that the true incidence rate for the control group is 1.9%. With the selected sample size of $N = 2n = 2200$, the corresponding power for correctly detecting a difference of $\delta = p_R - p_T = 1.9\% - 0.9\% = 1.0\%$ is 53.37. Note that the selected sample size does not account for possible dropouts in the proposed study (Table 12.3).

12.5.2 Strategy for Data Safety Monitoring Procedure

For clinical trials with extremely low incidence rate, it will take a large sample to observe a few responses. The time and cost are of a great concern to the sponsor of the trial. In practice, it is then of particular interest to stop the trial early if the test treatment will not achieve the study objectives. In this section, a statistical data safety monitoring procedure, based on the probability statement proposed by Chow and Chiu (2013), is outlined in order to assist the sponsor in making a decision as to whether the trial should stop at the interim.

Assume that an interim look is to be taken when we reach the sample size of $N' = N/2 = n$, where $N = 2n$ is the total sample size for the trial. At the interim, suppose that $p\%$ (where $p = (p_R + p_T)/2$) incidences are expected to be observed from the N' samples. Then one can follow the procedure described later for data safety monitoring (Figure 12.1):

For the purpose of illustration, consider the example described in Section 12.5.1.5. Assume that the incidence rate of the reference group is 1.9% and 0.95% is for the test group. Thus, the blinded expected total incidence rate will be 1.425% and the expected mean is $15.68 \approx 16$. We can also find the 95% upper and lower limits of the expected observed numbers for the entire trial which are (8, 23). If the observed incidence number is 23 ($\hat{\mu} = 23$, which is within the 95% CI) at the interim, one can consider to continue the trial by probability. The expected incidences are shown in Table 12.4 for illustration. For the entire trial, the estimated expected mean and the 95% confidence limits in the reference group are 28 and (16, 40); and they are in the test group 14 and (6, 23) if $\hat{\mu} = \mu_U$. For the possible combination of sample sizes, we provide the probabilities $P\left(\sum_{i=1}^{n} x_{Rj} \mid p_R\right) \times P\left(\sum_{i=1}^{n} x_{Tj} \mid p_T\right)$ for each case in Table 12.5.

12.5.3 Bayesian Approach

As discussed earlier, formulas for sample size calculations were derived based on the concept of frequentists. Information obtained from previous studies or small pilot studies is often used to estimate the parameters

TABLE 12.3

95% CIs ($p_R = 2.00\%$) for the Determination of Sample Sizes

p_T % of Improvement	0.90% 55%			0.95% 53%			1.00% 50%			1.05% 48%			1.10% 45%		
n	Lower (%)	Upper (%)	Power	Lower (%)	Upper (%)	Power	Lower (%)	Upper (%)	Power	Lower (%)	Upper (%)	Power	Lower (%)	Upper (%)	Power
200	-1.24	3.44	14.95	-1.31	3.41	13.83	-1.38	3.38	12.79	-1.45	3.35	11.82	-1.52	3.32	10.92
300	-0.81	3.01	20.28	-0.88	2.98	18.61	-0.94	2.94	17.07	-1.01	2.91	15.63	-1.08	2.88	14.30
400	-0.55	2.75	25.55	-0.62	2.72	23.36	-0.68	2.68	21.32	-0.75	2.65	19.41	-0.81	2.61	17.65
500	-0.38	2.58	30.73	-0.44	2.54	28.05	-0.51	2.51	25.52	-0.57	2.47	23.17	-0.63	2.43	20.98
600	-0.25	2.45	35.78	-0.31	2.41	32.64	-0.37	2.37	29.67	-0.44	2.34	26.89	-0.50	2.30	24.28
700	-0.15	2.35	40.65	-0.21	2.31	37.11	-0.27	2.27	33.74	-0.33	2.23	30.55	-0.39	2.19	27.56

800	−0.07	45.32	2.27	−0.13	41.44	2.23	**−0.19**	**37.71**	**2.19**	−0.25	34.15	2.15	−0.31	30.79	2.11
900	0.00	49.77	2.20	−0.06	45.60	2.16	**−0.12**	**41.55**	**2.12**	−0.18	37.67	2.08	−0.24	33.97	2.04
1000	0.05	53.98	2.15	−0.01	49.58	2.11	**−0.06**	**45.27**	**2.06**	−0.12	41.09	2.02	−0.18	37.08	1.98
1100	0.10	57.94	2.10	0.04	53.37	2.06	**−0.01**	**48.85**	**2.01**	−0.07	44.41	1.97	−0.13	40.12	1.93
1200	0.14	61.66	2.06	0.09	56.97	2.01	**0.03**	**52.27**	**1.97**	−0.03	47.62	1.93	−0.09	43.09	1.89
1300	0.18	65.12	2.02	0.12	60.36	1.98	**0.07**	**55.54**	**1.93**	0.01	50.72	1.89	−0.05	45.97	1.85
1400	0.22	68.34	1.98	0.16	63.56	1.94	**0.10**	**58.65**	**1.90**	0.04	53.69	1.86	−0.01	48.76	1.81
1500	0.25	71.32	1.95	0.19	66.55	1.91	**0.13**	**61.60**	**1.87**	0.07	56.54	1.83	0.02	51.46	1.78

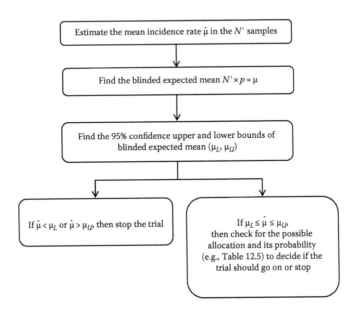

FIGURE 12.1
Flow chart for data safety monitoring.

TABLE 12.4

Expected Incidence Numbers and the Corresponding 95% Confidence Limits in Each Group for *Whole Trail* Intermit the Interim

	Interim	Target	Reference			Test		
	$N' = 1100$	$N = 2200$	$n_R = 1100$			$n_T = 1100$		
Sample Size	Expected Incidence Numbers		Lower	Mean	Upper	Lower	Mean	Upper
Upper	23	47	16	28	40	6	14	23
Mean	16	31	12	21	30	4	10	17
Lower	8	16	8	14	19	3	7	11

required for sample size calculations. In practice, the sample sizes required for achieving a desired precision may be further improved by taking the Bayesian approach into consideration. For the purpose of illustration, a sample size calculation based on precision analysis in conjunction with the Bayesian approach with a non-informative uniform prior is performed, based on the following assumptions:

1. Since the primary endpoint x_{ij} is a binary response, it follows Bernoulli distribution.
2. $p_R > p_T$.
3. Let $\delta_i | \theta, \sigma^2 \sim N(\theta, \sigma^2)$ and $\sigma^2 \sim \text{Uniform}(0,1)$.

TABLE 12.5

Probabilities That Each Sample Size Combination Is Likely to Occur

Incidences		Prob (%)	Incidences		Prob (%)	Incidences		Prob (%)	Incidences		Prob (%)	Incidences		Prob (%)
Reference	Test		Reference	Test		Reference	Test		Reference	Test		Reference	Test	
16	6	1.71	21	6	5.84	26	6	9.17	31	6	10.17	36	6	10.30
16	7	3.00	21	7	10.26	26	7	16.10	31	7	17.87	36	7	18.10
16	8	4.69	21	8	16.05	26	8	25.19	31	8	27.95	36	8	28.31
16	9	6.66	21	9	22.78	26	9	35.76	31	9	39.68	36	9	40.19
16	10	8.73	21	10	29.83	26	10	46.83	31	10	51.96	36	10	52.62
16	11	10.68	21	11	36.53	26	11	57.34	31	11	63.62	36	11	64.44
16	12	12.39	21	12	42.36	26	12	66.50	31	12	73.78	36	12	74.73
16	13	13.76	21	13	47.04	26	13	73.84	31	13	81.93	36	13	82.98
16	14	14.78	21	14	50.53	26	14	79.31	31	14	88.00	36	14	89.13
16	15	15.49	21	15	52.95	26	15	83.11	31	15	92.22	36	15	93.40
16	16	15.95	21	16	54.52	26	16	85.58	31	16	94.96	36	16	96.18
16	17	16.23	21	17	55.49	26	17	87.10	31	17	96.63	36	17	97.87
16	18	16.39	21	18	56.04	26	18	87.97	31	18	97.60	36	18	98.85
16	19	16.48	21	19	56.34	26	19	88.44	31	19	98.13	36	19	99.39
16	20	16.53	21	20	56.50	26	20	88.69	31	20	98.40	36	20	99.67
16	21	16.55	21	21	56.58	26	21	88.81	31	21	98.54	36	21	99.80
16	22	16.56	21	22	56.62	26	22	88.87	31	22	98.60	36	22	99.87
16	23	16.56	21	23	56.63	26	23	88.90	31	23	98.63	36	23	99.90
17	6	2.38	22	6	6.70	27	6	9.52	32	6	10.23	37	6	10.31
17	7	4.18	22	7	11.76	27	7	16.71	32	7	17.96	37	7	18.10

(continued)

TABLE 12.5 (continued)

Probabilities That Each Sample Size Combination Is Likely to Occur

Incidences		Prob	Incidences		Prob	Incidences		Prob	Incidences		Prob	Incidences		Prob
Reference	Test	(%)	Reference	Test	(%)	Reference	Test	(%)	Reference	Test	(%)	Reference	Test	(%)
17	8	6.54	22	8	18.40	27	8	26.14	32	8	28.10	37	8	28.32
17	9	9.29	22	9	26.13	27	9	37.12	32	9	39.90	37	9	40.20
17	10	12.17	22	10	34.21	27	10	48.60	32	10	52.24	37	10	52.64
17	11	14.90	22	11	41.89	27	11	59.52	32	11	63.97	37	11	64.47
17	12	17.27	22	12	48.58	27	12	69.02	32	12	74.18	37	12	74.75
17	13	19.18	22	13	53.95	27	13	76.64	32	13	82.38	37	13	83.01
17	14	20.60	22	14	57.95	27	14	82.32	32	14	88.48	37	14	89.16
17	15	21.59	22	15	60.72	27	15	86.27	32	15	92.72	37	15	93.44
17	16	22.23	22	16	62.53	27	16	88.83	32	16	95.47	37	16	96.21
17	17	22.63	22	17	63.63	27	17	90.40	32	17	97.16	37	17	97.91
17	18	22.85	22	18	64.27	27	18	91.31	32	18	98.13	37	18	98.89
17	19	22.98	22	19	64.62	27	19	91.80	32	19	98.66	37	19	99.43
17	20	23.04	22	20	64.80	27	20	92.06	32	20	98.94	37	20	99.71
17	21	23.07	22	21	64.88	27	21	92.18	32	21	99.08	37	21	99.84
17	22	23.09	22	22	64.93	27	22	92.24	32	22	99.14	37	22	99.91
17	23	23.09	22	23	64.95	27	23	92.27	32	23	99.17	37	23	99.94
18	6	3.17	23	6	7.48	28	6	9.77	33	6	10.26	38	6	10.31
18	7	5.56	23	7	13.13	28	7	17.17	33	7	18.02	38	7	18.11
18	8	8.70	23	8	20.54	28	8	26.85	33	8	28.19	38	8	28.32
18	9	12.35	23	9	29.16	28	9	38.13	33	9	40.03	38	9	40.21
18	10	16.17	23	10	38.19	28	10	49.92	33	10	52.42	38	10	52.65
18	11	19.81	23	11	46.76	28	11	61.13	33	11	64.19	38	11	64.48

N	k	value	N	k	value	N	k	value	N	k	value	N	k	value
18	12	22.97	23	12	54.23	28	12	70.89	33	12	74.43	38	12	74.77
18	13	25.50	23	13	60.22	28	13	78.72	33	13	82.66	38	13	83.03
18	14	27.39	23	14	64.68	28	14	84.56	33	14	88.78	38	14	89.18
18	15	28.71	23	15	67.78	28	15	88.61	33	15	93.03	38	15	93.46
18	16	29.56	23	16	69.79	28	16	91.24	33	16	95.80	38	16	96.23
18	17	30.08	23	17	71.02	28	17	92.85	33	17	97.49	38	17	97.93
18	18	30.38	23	18	71.73	28	18	93.78	33	18	98.47	38	18	98.91
18	19	30.55	23	19	72.12	28	19	94.29	33	19	99.00	38	19	99.45
18	20	30.63	23	20	72.32	28	20	94.55	33	20	99.27	38	20	99.73
18	21	30.67	23	21	72.42	28	21	94.68	33	21	99.41	38	21	99.86
18	22	30.69	23	22	72.47	28	22	94.74	33	22	99.48	38	22	99.93
18	23	30.70	23	23	72.49	28	23	94.77	33	23	99.50	38	23	99.96
19	6	4.03	24	6	8.15	29	6	9.96	34	6	10.28	39	6	10.31
19	7	7.08	24	7	14.32	29	7	17.49	34	7	18.06	39	7	18.11
19	8	11.08	24	8	22.40	29	8	27.36	34	8	28.25	39	8	28.33
19	9	15.73	24	9	31.80	29	9	38.85	34	9	40.11	39	9	40.22
19	10	20.59	24	10	41.64	29	10	50.87	34	10	52.52	39	10	52.66
19	11	25.22	24	11	50.99	29	11	62.29	34	11	64.32	39	11	64.49
19	12	29.24	24	12	59.13	29	12	72.23	34	12	74.58	39	12	74.78
19	13	32.48	24	13	65.66	29	13	80.21	34	13	82.82	39	13	83.04
19	14	34.88	24	14	70.53	29	14	86.16	34	14	88.96	39	14	89.19
19	15	36.55	24	15	73.91	29	15	90.28	34	15	93.22	39	15	93.47
19	16	37.64	24	16	76.11	29	16	92.97	34	16	95.99	39	16	96.24
19	17	38.30	24	17	77.45	29	17	94.61	34	17	97.69	39	17	97.94
19	18	38.69	24	18	78.22	29	18	95.56	34	18	98.67	39	18	98.92
19	19	38.90	24	19	78.65	29	19	96.07	34	19	99.20	39	19	99.46
19	20	39.01	24	20	78.87	29	20	96.34	34	20	99.48	39	20	99.74

(continued)

TABLE 12.5 (continued)

Probabilities That Each Sample Size Combination Is Likely to Occur

Incidences			Incidences			Incidences			Incidences			Incidences		
Reference	Test	Prob (%)	Reference	Test	Prob (%)	Reference	Test	Prob (%)	Reference	Test	Prob (%)	Reference	Test	Prob (%)
19	21	39.06	24	21	78.98	29	21	96.47	34	21	99.62	39	21	99.87
19	22	39.08	24	22	79.03	29	22	96.54	34	22	99.68	39	22	99.94
19	23	39.10	24	23	79.05	29	23	96.56	34	23	99.71	39	23	99.97
20	6	4.94	25	6	8.72	30	6	10.09	35	6	10.30	40	6	10.31
20	7	8.67	25	7	15.31	30	7	17.72	35	7	18.08	40	7	18.11
20	8	13.57	25	8	23.95	30	8	27.71	35	8	28.29	40	8	28.33
20	9	19.26	25	9	34.00	30	9	39.35	35	9	40.16	40	9	40.22
20	10	25.22	25	10	44.52	30	10	51.52	35	10	52.59	40	10	52.66
20	11	30.89	25	11	54.52	30	11	63.09	35	11	64.40	40	11	64.49
20	12	35.82	25	12	63.22	30	12	73.16	35	12	74.67	40	12	74.78
20	13	39.77	25	13	70.21	30	13	81.24	35	13	82.92	40	13	83.05
20	14	42.72	25	14	75.41	30	14	87.26	35	14	89.07	40	14	89.20
20	15	44.77	25	15	79.02	30	15	91.44	35	15	93.34	40	15	93.47
20	16	46.10	25	16	81.37	30	16	94.16	35	16	96.11	40	16	96.25
20	17	46.91	25	17	82.81	30	17	95.82	35	17	97.81	40	17	97.95
20	18	47.38	25	18	83.63	30	18	96.78	35	18	98.79	40	18	98.93
20	19	47.64	25	19	84.09	30	19	97.31	35	19	99.32	40	19	99.47
20	20	47.77	25	20	84.32	30	20	97.58	35	20	99.60	40	20	99.74
20	21	47.84	25	21	84.44	30	21	97.71	35	21	99.74	40	21	99.88
20	22	47.87	25	22	84.49	30	22	97.78	35	22	99.80	40	22	99.94
20	23	47.88	25	23	84.52	30	23	97.80	35	23	99.83	40	23	99.97

We would like to estimate the likelihood of the data which follow the normal distribution with a known mean θ and unknown variance σ^2. Thus,

$$f(\delta_i| \theta, \sigma^2) = \frac{1}{\sqrt{2\pi\sigma^2}} \exp\left\{ \frac{-(\delta_i - \theta)^2}{2\sigma^2} \right\} \quad \text{and} \quad \pi(\sigma^2) \equiv 1$$

$$L(\delta_i| \theta, \sigma^2) = \prod_{i=1}^{n} f(\delta_i| \theta, \sigma^2) = \left[2\pi\sigma^2 \right]^{-n/2} \exp\left\{ \frac{-\sum_{i=1}^{n}(\delta_i - \theta)^2}{2\sigma^2} \right\}.$$

As a result, the posterior distribution can be obtained as follows:

$$\pi(\sigma^2| \theta, \delta_i) \propto (\sigma^2)^{\frac{-n}{2}} \exp\left\{ \frac{-\sum_{i=1}^{n}(\delta_i - \theta)^2}{2\sigma^2} \right\}$$

$$\pi(\sigma^2| \theta, \delta_i) \sim \text{Inverse-gamma}\left(\alpha = \frac{n}{2} - 1, \beta = \frac{-\sum_{i=1}^{n}(\delta_i - \theta)^2}{2} \right).$$

Thus, the sample size required for achieving a desired precision can be obtained by following iterative steps:

Step 1: Start with an initial guess for n_0.

Step 2: Generate σ^2 from inverse-gamma $\left(\alpha = \frac{n}{2} - 1, \beta = \frac{-\sum_{i=1}^{n}(\delta_i - \theta)^2}{2} \right).$

Step 3: Calculate the required sample size n with σ^2 (generated from Step 2) by Formula 12.2.

Step 4: If $n \neq n_0$, then let $n_0 = n$ and repeat Steps 1–4. If $n = n_0$, then let $n_b = n$.

The sample size based on the Bayesian approach n_b can be obtained which will converge in probability to n after several iterations.

12.5.4 Remarks

For clinical trials with extremely low incidence rates, the sample size required for achieving a desired power of correctly detecting a small, clinically meaningful calculation if such a difference truly exists is often very large. This huge sample size may not be of practical use. In this section, an alternative approach based on a precision analysis in conjunction with a sensitivity analysis is described. The proposed method reduces the sample size required for achieving a desired precision with certain statistical assurance. As a result, a step-by-step procedure for choosing appropriate sample size is recommended. The proposed procedure for choosing an appropriate sample size is taking the relative improvement into consideration.

For clinical trials with extremely low incidence rate, it will take a large sample to observe a few responses. The time and cost are of great concern to the sponsor of the trial. In practice, it is then of particular interest to stop the trial early if the test treatment will not achieve the study objectives. Along this line, a statistical data safety monitoring procedure based on probability statement is developed to assist the sponsor in making a decision as to whether the trial should stop at the interim. If the observed incidences are within the confidence limits with 95% assurance, then we can check the probabilities for all possible combinations; otherwise, stop the trial.

12.6 Concluding Remarks

As more and more biological/biotechnology-derived proteins are increasingly used as therapeutic agents, the issue of immunogenicity has become a safety concern because these products may induce an unwanted immune response in treated patients. The clinical consequences of such immune reactions to a therapeutic protein could result in either loss of efficacy or severe life-threatening conditions.

Non-clinical studies may contribute to the interpretation of comparability of the immunogenicity potential and of repeat dose toxicity studies. It is essential to adopt an appropriate strategy for the development of adequate screening and confirmatory assays to measure an immune response against a therapeutic protein. Assays should be capable of distinguishing neutralizing from non-neutralizing antibodies, be validated and standardized.

For immunogenicity studies, careful planning of immunogenicity evaluation should include data systematically collected from a sufficient number of patients. The sampling schedule for immunogenicity evaluation should be standardized, adapted for each product on a case-by-case basis and taking a risk-based approach (EMA, 2007). Data on the impact on efficacy and safety should be collected in order to fully understand the clinical consequences of the immune response.

For the clinical evaluation of immunogenicity, a large sample size is expected for achieving a desired power for correctly detecting a relatively small difference at a pre-specified level of significance. As an alternative, a smaller sample size is justifiable based on precision analysis for achieving a certain statistical assurance (inference). With a selected sample size, the statistical procedure for data safety monitoring proposed by Chow and Chiu (2013) is useful for stopping a trial early.

13

CMC Requirements for Biological Products

13.1 Introduction

As indicated in the earlier chapters, there are some fundamental differences between biologics and small-molecule drugs. Small-molecule drugs are prepared by chemical synthesis, which are usually *not* sensitive to process changes, while biological products are made of living cells or organisms, which are very sensitive to process changes. A small change in manufacturing conditions could result in a drastic change in clinical outcomes. In practice, even minor modifications of the manufacturing process can cause variations in important properties of a biological product. Biologics, which possess sophisticated three-dimensional structures and contain mixtures of protein isoforms, are 100-fold or 1000-fold larger than small-molecule drugs. A biological product is a heterogeneous mixture and the current analytical methods cannot characterize these complex molecules sufficiently to confirm structural equivalence with the reference biologics.

Since biological products are manufactured in living systems that are inexact by their nature, they are influenced by the method of the manufacturing system. Along with the manufacturing system, biological products are susceptible to the environmental factors. As a result, the biological products are capable of causing a unique set of pathologies due to their origin during the manufacturing process. Thus, it is important to make sure that biological products are manufactured using a consistent and reproducible process which is in compliance with applicable regulations to ensure the safety, purity, and potency (efficacy) of the biological products.

In the United States, regulatory requirements for biological products are codified in chapter 21, section 600 of the Code of Federal Regulations (21 CFR 600). The CMC requirements for biosimilars in the Europe Union (EU) are those described in the ICH Common Technical Document (CTD) Quality Module 3 with supplemental information demonstrating comparability or similarity in quality attributes to the reference medicine product. At the present time, the United States suggests submission following CTD format for drug substance, which consists of general information, manufacture,

TABLE 13.1

CTD Module 3 Format

Section	Description
3.2.S.1	General information
3.2.S.2	Manufacture
3.2.S.3	Characterization
3.2.S.4	Control
3.2.S.5	Reference standards
3.2.S.6	Container closure system
3.2.S.7	Stability

characterization, control, reference standards, container closure system, and stability (see Table 13.1).

In the next section, CMC requirements for biological products are briefly outlined. Section 13.3 provides brief introduction to product characterization and specification followed by commonly seen errors in biologics license application (BLA) submission. Similarly, Sections 13.4 and 13.5 discuss requirements for manufacturing process validation and quality control/assurance in BLA submission. Section 13.6 reviews CMC requirements for reference standards, container and closure system, and stability. Some concluding remarks are given in the last section of this chapter.

13.2 CMC Development

For manufacturing of biosimilar products, a typical flowchart of manufacturing production is illustrated in Figure 13.1. As it can be seen from Figure 13.1, the development of chemistry, manufacturing, and controls (CMC) for biosimilar products starts with establishment of the expression system (see, e.g., Wolff, 2011). A cell-line is usually selected among bacterial, yeast, and mammalian host strains and then the correct DNA sequence is inserted. Elaborate cell-screening and selection methods are then used to establish a master cell bank (Chen, 2009). Extensive characterization on the master cell bank needs to be carried out to provide microbiological purity or sterility and identity (CBER/FDA, 1993).

As indicated by Chen (2009), bulk protein production involves developing robust and scalable fermentation and purification processes. The goals for fermentation are to increase the expression level, a deficiency, without compromising the correct amino acid sequence and post-translational modification. Achieving high expression requires optimizing culture medium and growth conditions, and efficient extraction and recovery procedures. Correct amino acid sequence and post-translation modification will need to

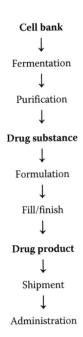

FIGURE 13.1
Typical flowchart of manufacturing production.

be verified. Solubilization and refolding of insoluble proteins are sometimes necessary for proteins which have the tendency to aggregate under the processing condition. Differences in the cell bank and production processes may create impurities that are different from the innovator's product.

Chen (2009) also pointed out that the purification process needs to remove impurities such as host-cell proteins, DNA, medium constituents, viruses, and metabolic by-products as much as possible. It is important for biosimilar manufacturers to accept appropriate yield losses to achieve high purity, because any increase in yield at the expense of purity is unacceptable and can have clinical consequences. The final product is produced by going through formulation, sterile filtration, and fill/finish into the final containers. Selection of formulation components starts from basic buffer species for proper pH control and salt for isotonicity adjustment. Surfactants may be needed to prevent proteins from being absorbed onto the container surface or water–air interface or other hydrophobic surfaces. Stabilizers are required to inhibit aggregation, oxidation, deamidation, and other degradations. The container and closure system can be glass vials, rubber stoppers, and aluminum seals or pre-filled syringes or IV bags. The container and closure integrity needs to be verified by sterility or dye leak test. Biologics are not pure substances. They are heterogeneous mixtures.

In compliance with current good manufacturing practice (cGMP), each batch of a biological products intended for clinical or commercial use needs

TABLE 13.2

Analytical Methods to Characterize Good Drug
Characteristics of Biological Products

Type	Assays
Identity	Western blot, peptide mapping; isoelectric focusing
Strength	Protein concentration by A280
Purity	SDS-PAGE, SEC-HPLC, IEX-HPLC, RP-HPLC
Quality	Appearance, particulates, pH, osmolality
Potency	In vitro or in vivo bioactivity assays
Safety	Endotoxin, sterility, residual DNA, host cell proteins

to be tested for good drug characteristics such as identity, strength, quality, purity, and safety (USP/NF, 2000). These tests are usually done by a panel of assays (given in Table 13.2) to ensure the product meets pre-defined specifications for identity, strength (potency), quality, purity, and safety. Note that the product purity is often measured by multiple assays, which measure different product-related variants (biologically active) or product-related impurities (biologically inactive). It should also be noted that biologics are parenteral drugs and filled into the final containers through the aseptic process so that microbiological control is critical. Thus, it is advisable to set up product specifications for a biosimilar within the variation of the reference biological products for quality assurance/control. Product characterization can be performed on selected batches for primary sequence, high order structures, isoform profiles, heterogeneity, product variants, and impurities and process impurity profiles. Physicochemical characterization tests include IEF, CE, HIC, LCMS, carbohydrate analysis, N- and C-terminal sequencing, amino acid analysis, analytical ultracentrifugation, CD, and DSC (Chirino et al., 2004; Kendrick et al., 2009).

Biologics are highly sensitive to environmental influences during storage, shipment, and handling. Temperature excursion, movement, and exposure to UV light can lead to protein degradation. Product expiry needs to be based on the real-time stability data. Stability program should also include accelerated or stress studies to gain insight of the degradation profiles. In-use stability studies are carried out to verify shipping conditions or handling procedures exert no detrimental effect on the drug product.

13.3 Product Characterization and Specification

13.3.1 General Description

Biosimilar manufacturers usually have no access to the manufacturing process and product specifications of the innovator's products because these are proprietary knowledge. To develop a biosimilar product, a biosimilar manufacturer will need to first identify a marketed biological products to serve as the reference biological products. Then a detailed characterization of the reference biological products can be performed. The information obtained from the characterization of the reference biological products can then be utilized to direct the process development of the biosimilar product and comparative testing to demonstrate similarity between the biosimilar product and the reference biological products. It, however, should be noted that a biosimilar product may be manufactured from a completely new process, which may be based on a different host/vector system with different process steps, facilities, and equipment.

13.3.2 Drug Substance Characterization

Drug substance should be positive for identity and have specified criteria for purity, potency, and microbial contamination. Acceptance criteria for release and stability attributes should be established. Results from release and stability testing should be provided in the IND. Raw data supporting drug substance characterization should be provided in the IND. The following good drug characteristics should be characterized:

Safety—Ensured by the specified limits for bioburden and endotoxin, misc. process-related contaminants, which are usually characterized by the LAL test, the rabbit pyrogen test, and bacterial culture methods.

Purity—Assesses the capability of the purification process to remove process-related impurities (e.g., endogenous viruses, host-cell proteins, DNA, leachables, anti-foam, antibiotics, toxins, solvents, heavy metals), product-related impurities (e.g., aggregates, breakdown products, product variants due to oxidation, deamidation, denaturation, loss of C-term Lys in MAbs), and product substances (product variants that are active). Methods for characterization of purity include, but are not limited to,

1. Reversed-phase HPLC, peptide mapping, MS
2. SDS-PAGE, Western analysis, capillary electrophoresis
3. SEC, AUC, FFF, light scattering
4. Ion exchange chromatography
5. Carbohydrate analysis (capillary electrophoresis, high-pH anion-exchange chromatography, IEF for sialic acid)

Identity—Unique for protein of interest, especially relevant for closely related proteins manufactured in the same facility. Identity is usually characterized by N-terminal sequencing, peptide mapping, or immunoassays (ELISA, Western blotting).

Potency—Required to assess biological activity of the product. The assay should be relevant for protein mechanism of action. For MAb or Fc fusion proteins, a binding assay may be sufficient for early development, but a functional assay relevant for the mechanism of action should be developed. If the mechanism of action is unknown, multiple bioactivities plus elucidating higher-order structure may be required. Potency is usually characterized by animal-based assays, cell-based assays, reporter gene, or biochemical (e.g., enzyme activity).

Strength—Protein content, which can be characterized by RIA, ELISA, UV absorbance, Bradford.

Stability—Drug substance stability should be demonstrated with appropriate stability-indicating assays.

13.3.3 Product Characterization

Similarly, product characterization for the following good drug characteristics such as safety, purity, identity, potency, strength, stability, and container closure should be provided in BLA submission.

Safety—The final drug product for injection should be sterile and within specified limits for endotoxin; immunogenicity should be screened and monitored. Successfully reduced in MAb by replacing murine with human sequences.

Purity and Characterization—Product and process-related impurities and product-related substances should be within specified limits.

Identity—Unique for protein of interest, especially relevant for closely related proteins manufactured in the same facility.

Potency—Assay should be relevant for protein mechanism of action; for MAb or Fc fusion proteins, a binding assay may be sufficient for early development, but a functional assay relevant for the mechanism of action should be developed; if the mechanism of action is unknown, multiple bioactivities plus elucidation of higher-order structure may be required.

Strength—Protein content.

Stability—The drug product should maintain stability for the duration of the clinical trial.

13.3.4 Practical Issues

Commonly seen issues in the process of product characterization include, but are not limited to, (1) establishing specification prior to understanding the product, (2) insufficient knowledge of relationship between protein structure and potential safety/toxicity, (3) lack of the examination of impurity profile, and (4) inadequate process validation/control. Appropriate actions need to be taken in order to correct or resolve these issues for quality assurance/control of the biosimilar product under development.

13.4 Manufacture and Process Validation

13.4.1 Manufacturing Process

A typical manufacturing process for biological product consists of expression vector (plasmid), cell banking system including master cell bank (MCB), working cell bank (WCB), and end of production cells (EOP), drug substance manufacturing and release, and drug product formulation and release (see also Figure 13.2). As an example, consider a manufacturing process for therapeutic biologic protein products. Expression vectors are used for (1) transfer of genes from one organism to another, (2) production of large amounts of protein, (3) description of origin of the construct, (4) plasmid mapping (e.g., restriction sites, integration sites, promoter, copy number) and stability, and (5) sequencing of gene of interest (Markovic, 2007). A WCB is derived from the MCB and is used to initiate a production batch. Table 13.3 provides a list of characterization of cell banks required for CMC. It should be noted that sources of adventitious agents include cell substrate (e.g., endogenous viruses and exogenous microbial contamination, raw materials (e.g., cell culture reagents such as animal and non-animal derived), and environment (e.g., water, air, and humans technicians). As indicated in Figure 13.1, fermentation and purification are two key components of the manufacturing process. The fermentation process and purification process are depicted in Figures 13.2 and 13.3, respectively.

The goal of the manufacturing process is to produce sufficient quantities of quality product in a controlled and reproducible manner. Manufacturing processes are dynamic. Changes can be process-related (e.g., modification of process, increase in scale, or change in location). Changes can be method related (e.g., improvement of analytical method and replacement of one or analytical methods). The manufacturing process should be thoroughly investigated and understood. Quality should be designed into the process, rather than tested into the product via the analytical methods. When evaluating changes, one should focus on (1) that biological products are complex mixtures, that the control starts with the cell banks and on all raw materials, and whether the product is at risk from raw materials, operators, and environment. No change can be assumed to be neutral. Release criteria alone are insufficient to fully evaluate the impact of changes.

13.4.2 Process Validation

As indicated in Chow and Liu (1995), the primary objective of process validation is to provide documented evidence that a manufacturing process does

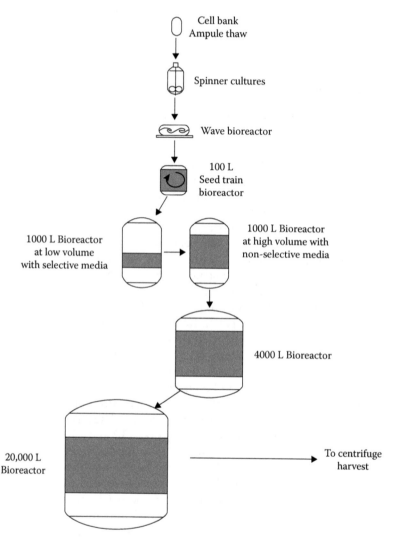

FIGURE 13.2
Fermentation process.

reliably what it purports to do. To accomplish this prospectively, a validation protocol is necessarily developed. A validation protocol should include the characterization of the product, the manufacturing procedure, and sampling plans, acceptance criteria, and testing procedures to be performed at identified critical stages of the manufacturing process. The statistically based sampling plans, testing procedures, and acceptance criteria ensure, with a high degree of confidence, that the manufacturing process does what it purports to do. Since the manufacturing process for a biological product is complex that involves several critical stages, it is important to discuss the following

TABLE 13.3

Characterization of Cell Banks

Test	MCB	WCB	EPC
Viability	×	×	×
Identity	×	×	
Purity	×	×	×
Stability	×		×
Karyology	×	×	
Tumorigenicity	×		×
Sterility	×	×	×
Mycoplasma	×	×	×
Adventitious viruses	×		×
Species-specific	×		
Retrovirus	×		×

Key: MCB, master cell bank; WCB, working cell bank; EOP, end of production cells.

issues with the project scientists to acquire a good understanding of the product and the manufacturing process:

1. Identified critical stages
2. Equipment to be used at each critical stage
3. Possible issues/problems
4. Testing procedures to be performed
5. Sampling plan, testing plan, and acceptance criteria
6. Pertinent information
7. Specification to be used as reference
8. Validation summary

When a problem is observed in a manufacturing process, it is crucial to locate at which stage the problem occurred so that it can be corrected and the manufacturing process can do what it purports to do. In practice, the manufacturing process is usually evaluated by constant monitoring of its critical stages. Therefore, for the validation of a manufacturing process, it is recommended that project scientists be consulted to identify the critical stages of the manufacturing process. At each stage of the manufacturing process, it is also helpful to have knowledge of the equipment to be sued and its components. The equipment may affect the conformance with compendia specifications for product quality. The validation protocol should establish statistically based sampling plans, testing plans, and acceptance criteria. Sampling plans and acceptance criteria are usually chosen such that (1) there is a high probability of meeting the acceptance criteria if the

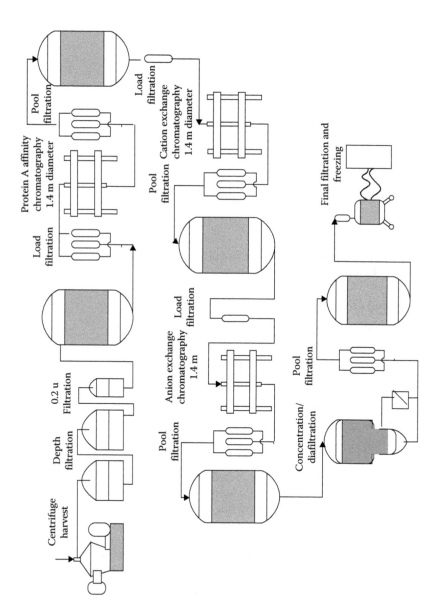

FIGURE 13.3
Purification process.

batch at a given stage is "acceptable" (this probability is 1 – the producer's risk), and (2) there is small probability of meeting the acceptance criteria if the batch at a given stage is "unacceptable" (this probability is the so-called consumer's risk).

13.4.3 Commonly Encountered Issues

Note that commonly seen errors/omissions regarding a manufacturing process include (1) manufacturing and/or testing locations not registered; (2) manufacturing not planned during application review cycle; (3) inadequate raw material control; (4) failure to perform or provide results of process understanding studies and impurity clearance studies; (5) failure to validate commercial process, intermediate hold times, resin and membrane reuse cycles, buffer hold times, reprocessing if included, and shipping of intermediates/drug substance; (6) failure to demonstrate consistency of manufacture (e.g., according to a protocol with pre-specified criteria, using validated test methods, as three successive successful runs); (7) failure to demonstrate comparability between processes during development; and (8) lack of retaining samples to close gaps. Appropriate actions need to be taken in order to correct or resolve these issues for quality control/assurance of the biosimilar product under development.

13.5 Quality Control/Assurance

The manufacture of biological products involves biological processes and materials, such as cultivation of cells or extraction of material from living organisms. These biological processes may display inherent variability, and so the range and nature of by-products are variable. Moreover, the materials used in these cultivation processes provide good substrates for growth of microbial contaminants. Thus, quality control/assurance of biological products usually involves biological analytical techniques which have a greater variability than that of chemical drug products. In-process controls therefore take on a great importance in the manufacture of biological medicinal products.

13.5.1 General Principles

For quality control of biological products, it is suggested that the following general principles should be followed:

In-process controls—In-process controls play an important role in ensuring the consistency of the quality of biological products. Those controls which are crucial for quality (e.g., virus removal), but cannot be carried out on the finished product, should be performed at an appropriate stage of production. Thus, critical stages of the manufacturing process need to be identified and validated accompanied with sampling plan, acceptance criteria, and testing procedure.

Sample retention—It may be necessary to retain samples of intermediate products in sufficient quantities and under appropriate storage conditions to allow the repetition or confirmation of a batch control.

Quality control requirement—Where continuous culture is used, special consideration should be given to the quality control requirements arising from this type of production method.

Statistical process for QC—Continuous monitoring of certain production processes is necessary, for example, fermentation. Such data should form part of the batch record. The statistical process for QC will help in identifying problems or issues early and appropriate actions can be taken to correct the problems or resolve the issues.

13.5.2 Starting Materials

As indicated in WHO (2010), quality and control of the starting material should be documented. Information demonstrating that the starting material meets the quality level appropriate for its intended use should be provided. Thus, the source, origin, and suitability of starting materials should be clearly defined. Where the necessary tests take a long time, it may be permissible to process starting materials before the results of the tests are available. In such cases, release of a finished product is conditional on satisfactory results of these tests.

Note that where sterilization of starting materials is required, it should be carried out where possible by heat. Where necessary, other appropriate methods may also be used for inactivation of biological materials (e.g., irradiation).

13.5.3 Seed Lot and Cell Bank System

For quality and control of the cell bank system of biological medicinal products, it is suggested that the following principles as described in the Guide to Good Manufacturing Practice for Medicinal Products be considered (PIC/S, 2009).

First, in order to prevent the unwanted drift of properties, which might ensue from repeated subcultures or multiple generations, the production of biological medicinal products obtained by microbial culture, cell culture, or propagation in embryos and animals should be based on a system of master and working seed lots and/or cell banks. Second, the number of generations (doublings, passages) between the seed lot or cell bank and the finished product should be consistent with the marketing authorization dossier. Scaling up and post-approval changes of the process should not change this fundamental relationship.

Third, it is strongly recommended that seed lots and cell banks should be adequately characterized and tested for possible contaminants. Their suitability for use should be further demonstrated by the consistency of the characteristics and quality of the successive batches of the product. Seed lots and cell banks should be established, stored, and used in such a way as to minimize the risks of contamination or alteration. A recent incidence of virus contamination is further discussed in the last chapter of this book. It is also important to establish the seed lot and cell bank in a suitably controlled environment in order to protect the seed lot and the cell bank, and, if applicable, the personnel handling it. During the establishment of the seed lot and cell bank, no other living or infectious material (e.g., virus, cell lines, or cell strains) should be handled simultaneously in the same area or by the same person.

Finally, evidence of the stability and recovery of the seeds and banks should be documented. Storage containers should be hermetically sealed, clearly labeled, and kept at an appropriate temperature. An inventory should be meticulously kept. Storage temperature should be recorded continuously for freezers and properly monitored for liquid nitrogen. Any deviation from set limits and any corrective action taken should be recorded. Note that different seed lots or cell banks should be stored in such a way as to avoid confusion or cross-contamination. It is desirable to split the seed lots and cell banks and to store the parts at different locations so as to minimize the risks of total loss.

13.5.4 Operating Principles

From the operating perspective, it is suggested that the growth-promoting properties of culture media should be demonstrated. Addition of materials or cultures to fermenters and other vessels and the taking of samples should be carried out under carefully controlled conditions to ensure that the absence of contamination is maintained. Care should be taken to ensure that vessels are correctly connected when addition or sampling takes place. It should also be noted that centrifugation and blending of products can lead to aerosol formation and containment of such activities. Thus, it is important to prevent transfer of live microorganisms if necessary (PIC/S, 2009).

13.5.5 Premises and Equipment

The assurance of product quality relies on sponsor's commitment and equipment, which involve manufacturing facility, facility design and controls, and robust quality system. Basic considerations for manufacturing facility, facility design and controls, and robust quality system are briefly outlined as follows:

Manufacturing facility—Some basic considerations (commonly seen issues/problems) for manufacturing facility are summarized as follows:

1. Materials of construction are smooth, hard, and cleanable.
2. Edges are coved and seams are sealed.
3. No open floor drains.
4. No clutter.
5. Unidirectional flow of materials, staff, and waste is preferred.
6. Cleaning validation critical for multi-use areas and equipment.
7. Direction of air flow is away from the product.
8. Air returns are low and accessible.
9. Air quality assessed under dynamic conditions.
10. Water is of the highest quality feasible for each step.
11. WFI is introduced as early as feasible in downstream processing.

Facility design and controls—Basic considerations for facility design and controls include the following:

1. Sufficient work space
2. Appropriate equipment
3. Environmental control
4. Validated systems and equipment
5. Validated cleaning procedures using qualified cleaning and sanitizing agents
6. Systems to prevent cross-contamination system to handle waste materials

Robust quality system—Robust quality system should focus on the following:

1. Raw material/inventory control
2. Environmental monitoring programs
3. Maintenance and calibration programs
4. Validation activities including computer systems
5. Staff training requirements
6. Internal audit program
7. Vendor audit program
8. Trending and oversight programs
9. Records review and product release
10. Non-conformance and OOS procedures
11. Change control procedures

13.5.6 Practical Issues

Commonly seen errors in the quality control/assurance of a manufacturing process of biological products include (1) manufacturing/testing locations are not registered; (2) manufacturing is not planned during application review cycle; (3) inadequate raw material control; (4) failure to perform or provide results of impurity clearance studies; (5) failure to validate commercial process, intermediate hold times, resin and membrane reuse cycles, buffer hold times, reprocessing (if included), and shipping of intermediate/drug substance; (6) failure to demonstrate consistency of manufacture according to a protocol with pre-specified criteria; (7) failure to demonstrate comparability between processes during development; and (8) lack of retaining samples to close gaps.

13.6 Reference Standards, Container Closure System, and Stability

In addition to general information regarding manufacturing process/process validation, product characterization/specification, and quality control/assurance, a complete CMC package also requires the inclusion of the establishment of reference standards, the information regarding container closure system, and the evidence of product stability, which are briefly described later.

13.6.1 Reference Standards

Biological medicinal products can be defined by reference to their method of manufacture. Biological medicinal products are usually prepared by the following methods of manufacture:

1. Microbial cultures, excluding those resulting from r-DNA techniques
2. Microbial and cell cultures, including those resulting from recombinant DNA or hybridoma techniques
3. Extraction from biological tissues
4. Propagation of live agents in embryos or animals

Biological medicinal products manufactured by these methods include vaccines, immunosera, antigens, hormones, cytokines, enzymes, and other products of fermentation (including monoclonal antibodies and products derived from r-DNA).

Characterization of reference standard is usually performed using part of the lot used for non-clinical studies. The established reference standard is then used to release the clinical lot. As development progresses, if the lot is too old or there is insufficient amount of the previous lot, a new reference standard may be required to account for change in manufacturing. In this case, a protocol for generating and/or qualifying the new reference standard must be developed to incorporate new methods as new specification evolves. Portion of each reference standard lot must be retained for future use or needs. During the development, reference materials which reflect degradation pathways critical in product quality control are needed as assay development, controls, and validation.

Recently, for the assessment of biosimilarity between a biosimilar (test) product and an innovative (reference) product, a criterion for biosimilarity based on *relative* difference between (T vs. R) and (R vs. R) is recommended. The difference between T and R is compared with the difference between R and R, which is used as a reference standard for comparison. For this purpose, the establishment of the reference standard can be done by either conducting a so-called $R–R$ study or utilizing a three-arm (i.e., T, R, and R) trial (see, e.g., Kang and Chow, 2013). In an $R–R$ study or a three-arm study, it is suggested that the two R's be obtained from either two different batches of the same manufacturing process or two different manufacturing processes (or locations). The establishment of the reference standard will help in addressing the issues of "How similar is considered similar?" and the degree of similarity.

13.6.2 Container Closure System

To fulfill regulatory requirements for license, extractables and leachables studies are often conducted. Extractables are those which migrate from a container closure system and/or other packaging components in a DP vehicle or solvent under exaggerated conditions, while leachables are those which migrate spontaneously from a container closure system and/or other packaging components under normal conditions of use and storage. Extractables are helpful in predicting the potential leachables and in selecting the appropriate container closure system. Leachables are often a subset of extractables, or derived by their chemical modification. Sources of leachables in the product include syringes/prefilled syringes, ampoules, vials, bottles, IV bags, storage bags for product intermediates, closures (screw caps, rubber stoppers), and container liners (e.g., tube liners). Processing equipment usually include stainless steel storage tanks/bioreactors, tubing, gaskets, valves, rings, and filter purification resins.

As indicated by Markovic (2007), leachables could have an impact on safety and product quality. For example, when there is a change from HSA formulation to a polysorbate with unchanged container closure system (prefilled syringes with the uncoated rubber stoppers). The observation of a serious adverse event (PRCA) leads to the hypothesis that leachables acted as adjuvants triggering immunogenicity. For another example, when there is a change from a lyophilized to a liquid formulation (divalent cation leached from the rubber stopper) which might cause activation of metalloprotease (a process-related impurity co-eluted with the API). This could impact product degradation at the N-terminal site (stability study).

Commonly, errors in extractables and leachables studies include absence of data on extractables and leachables from the container closure and absence of assessment of the impact of the extractables/leachables data on product specification and methods (potential to seed microaggregates, potential to alter the immunogenicity profile). In practice, it is suggested that appropriate actions be taken to resolve the issues of extractables and leachables.

13.6.3 Stability

For drug substance and drug product, real-time and accelerated (stress) stability data with several time points under upright and inverted conditions are necessarily collected to establish the expiration dating period of the drug substance and drug product. Stress studies (e.g., UV, exaggerated light, temperature, and pH) are useful to elucidate product degradation pathways and for defining acceptance criteria. Limited time stability studies may be acceptable for short-term stability study. In practice, stability data generated from engineering lots are also acceptable. It should be noted that failure to demonstrate product stability could result in a potential hold issue.

For assessment of stability, the following testing should be performed at a minimum: (1) safety (e.g., bioburden/sterility), (2) purity (including product and process-related impurities and product-related substances), (3) sialic acid (if appropriate), (4) potency, (5) protein content/strength, (6) pH, and (7) appearance leachables (separate study, not part of routine stability testing).

In BLA submission, summary of all stability data includes supporting data from the clinical program; forced degradation data to support choice of stability indicating panel; data assessment to support expiration dating period; stability protocol for commercial lots; data from ICH compliant stability program, with a minimum of 6 months' data under intended storage conditions and conformance lots at commercial scale; and description and validation data for methods used only for assessing stability.

Common errors include insufficient number of lots, insufficient stability data, stability containers not representative of drug substance container closure system, absence of forced degradation data to identify stability indicating assays, and absence of stability protocol. More detailed information regarding requirements, design, and analysis of stability studies are provided in Chapter 15.

13.7 Concluding Remarks

A typical BLA includes (1) form FDA 356h (cover sheet), (2) applicant information, (3) product/manufacturing information, (4) pre-clinical studies, (5) clinical studies, and labeling. Thus, CMC, pre-clinical, and clinical are three critical components in biosimilars development. A full-scale CMC development is required including expression system, culture, purification, formulation, analytics, and packaging. The EU has issued biosimilars guidelines based on comparative testing against the reference biologic drug (the original approved biologic). For approval of biosimilars in the United States, we expect the CMC package will be similar to that in the EU which contains a full quality dossier with a comparability program including detailed product characterization comparison and reduced pre-clinical and clinical requirements.

CMC requirements for biological products have received increasing attention from the regulatory agencies worldwide. The following lists potential CMC hold issues for phase 1 IND:

1. Comparability between preclinical and clinical lots not demonstrated
2. Insufficient characterization of cell banks (e.g., adventitious agents testing, identity)
3. Inadequate product characterization with regards to purity, identity, potency, and safety
4. Lack of final product release testing
5. Lacking or inappropriate specifications for release and stability testing
6. Lacking or inadequate potency assay
7. Data supporting product stability have not been shown for the planned duration of clinical studies
8. Lack or inappropriate immunogenicity assays for high-risk products
9. Lack of evidence for final drug product sterility

Thus, it is suggested that the earlier listed potential CMC issues be resolved before regulatory submission of a BLA for biosimilar product.

14

Test for Comparability in Manufacturing Process

14.1 Introduction

Unlike small-molecular drugs with clearly and well-defined composition and structure, biologic drugs have much more complex ingredients, which are usually biomacromolecules including proteins, nucleic acids (DNA, RNA, antisense oligonucleotides), or living microorganisms like virulence-attenuated viruses and bacteria. Among them, recombinant-protein drugs have been the most common biopharmaceuticals so far. Classes of approved recombinant-protein drugs include hormones, cytokines, clotting factors, monoclonal antibodies, vaccine products, enzymes, and novel conjugates. As indicated earlier, biological products have many fundamental differences from chemical compounds. For example, chemical drugs are usually low-molecular-weight organic compounds (<1000 Da) with simple and definite chemical structures, while biological products have larger sizes and more complex structures. The average molecular weight of biologics ranges from 4,000 Da for nonglycosylated proteins to more than 140,000 Da for monoclonal antibodies (Lanthier et al., 2008). Recombinant-protein drugs fold into three-dimensional structures, which have four distinct levels. Amino acids are polymerized into a linear chain by the formation of an amide linkage between the α-carboxyl group of one amino acid and the α-amino group of the next, which is referred to as the primary structure of proteins. The polypeptide then folds into highly regular local substructures such as an alpha helix and beta strand, forming the secondary structures. The spatial relationship of the secondary structures to one another is referred to as tertiary structure, which is stabilized by nonlocal interactions like the hydrophobic core, salt bridges, hydrogen bonds, disulfide bonds, and posttranslational modifications. Many proteins consist of two or more polypeptide chains, and the manner of these associated protein subunits is called the quaternary structure.

Due to the low molecular weight, it is much easier for chemical compounds to rapidly diffuse across cell membranes and reach intracellular sites of action, compared with biological products. Besides, chemical drugs have generally much higher oral bioavailability, since biologics, usually proteins, will be degraded by proteases in the gastrointestinal tract after oral administration. Thus biologic drugs are usually injected into human bodies and require high purity and safety. Another pharmacokinetic difference is that when chemical drugs enter living organisms, they usually undergo, by the process of drug metabolism, a series of biochemical modifications through specialized enzymatic systems such as the cytochrome P450 superfamily (CYPs). The process usually converts a chemical drug to more water soluble and easily excreted metabolites. It may also contribute to the activity and toxicity of metabolites. But biological products usually do not undergo this kind of drug metabolism since they are generally active biological molecules initially synthesized by human body itself.

Chemical drugs usually have pharmacological functions through binding with targets such as receptors or enzymes and alter activity or function of the targets. For example, small-molecule drug tamoxifen is used as a standard endocrine therapy for steroid hormone receptor-positive breast cancer. It can competitively bind to estrogen receptors on tumors and other tissue targets, producing a nuclear complex that decreases DNA synthesis and inhibits estrogen effects and tumor cell proliferation. The pharmacological mechanisms of biological products are different from those of chemical compounds. Hormones have pharmacological functions through the alleviation of deficiencies. For example, biosynthetic human insulin is used to treat diabetes caused by insulin secretion deficiency, and human growth hormone is used for the treatment of children's growth disorders and adult growth hormone deficiency. Cytokines such as interferon-α can enhance cellular immune responses and have antiviral or antineoplastic effects. Another important class of biological products is monoclonal antibodies. They can specifically inhibit the activity of their targets. For example, bevacizumab is a humanized monoclonal antibody used to treat various cancers by inhibiting vascular endothelial growth factor A and blocking angiogenesis (Los et al., 2007). Accordingly, pharmacological mechanisms are different with biologic medicines and small-molecule chemical drugs.

In the next section, a typical manufacturing process for biological products is briefly outlined. The concept of testing comparability in terms of consistency between raw materials or final products between a biosimilar product and a reference product is introduced in Section 14.3. Statistical tests for comparability in critical quality attributes at various stages between manufacturing processes are studied in Section 14.4. Also included in this section are sampling plans, acceptance criteria, testing procedures, and strategies for statistical quality control (QC)/assurance under various specifications and/or user parameters. Other comparability tests such as pharmacokinetics (PK) comparability test, pharmacodynamics (PD) comparability index, and clinical efficacy comparability study are discussed in Section 14.5. A brief discussion is given in the last section.

14.2 Biologic Manufacturing Process

Unlike small-molecule drugs, which are produced through chemical synthesis procedures, biological products are often recombinant-protein molecules manufactured in living cells. A typical manufacturing process for a biologics from production to drug use is illustrated in Figure 13.1. As it can be seen in Figure 13.1, a typical biological manufacturing process includes several critical stages such as cell bank, fermentation, purification, formulation, and fill/finish. As an example, for manufacturing of a recombinant-protein drug product, the manufacturing processes are highly complex including obtaining an expression of target genes, the optimization and fermentation of gene engineering cells, the clarification and purification of the products, the formulation and testing, aseptic filling and packaging. Each of these procedures contains multiple steps and requires strictly controlled conditions in order to guarantee the efficacy and safety of the biological products, such as the design of bioreactor, pH, OD, PO_2, PCO_2, temperature, concentration, etc. Indeed, since manufacturing details are proprietary, these processes generally cannot be duplicated and differences in any step may result in variations of clinical relevance in important parameters, such as three-dimensional structure of the protein, the quantities of acid–base variants and posttranslational modifications. Thus, in practice, it is hard to produce an identical copy of a biological product.

In practice, since a small change or variation which occurs at any stage of a manufacturing process could result in a drastic change in clinical outcomes (e.g., safety and effectiveness) of the biosimilar product under study, it is suggested that the manufacturing process be validated for QC and assurance. As indicated in the previous chapter, the ultimate goal of manufacturing process validation is to provide documented evidence that a manufacturing process does reliably what it purports to do. Thus, a process validation study is necessarily conducted following a valid validation protocol. A validation protocol should identify critical stages of the manufacturing process. At each identified critical stage, appropriate testing procedures for critical quality attributes should be performed according to the sampling plans and acceptance criteria specified in the validation protocol. Corrected actions can then be taken where a problem is observed.

After regulatory approval of the biosimilar product under development, it is always a great concern to the sponsor that the quality of raw materials, in-process materials, and final products can maintain consistency at post-approval manufacturing process. Thus, it is suggested tests for comparability in raw materials, in-process materials, and final products be performed for QC and assurance of the products manufactured by the process.

14.3 Consistency Index

In this section, we will focus on testing comparability in raw material, in-process (in-use) material, and end product between manufacturing processes. Tse et al. (2006) and Lu et al. (2007) considered testing comparability in terms of a proposed consistency index for traditional Chinese medicine (TCM). The concept of their proposed consistency index can be implemented for developing a valid statistical QC process for quality assurance of the raw materials, in-process materials, and final products of biosimilar products (Chow and Liu, 1995; Tse et al., 2006). In practice, raw materials are often from different resources and the final product may be manufactured in different processes and/or sites (locations). As a result, variabilities from different resources such as process-to-process (or site-to-site or location-to-location), within process (site or location), stage-to-stage are inevitable. Thus, test for comparability (in terms of consistency) in raw materials, in-process materials, and/or final products between manufacturing processes has become an important step in the QC process for the development of biosimilar products.

Tse et al. (2006) proposed a statistical QC method for assessing consistency of raw materials and/or final products between manufacturing processes. The idea is to construct a 95% confidence interval for a proposed consistency index under a prespecified sampling plan. If the constructed 95% confidence lower limit is greater than a prespecified QC lower limit, then we claim that the raw materials or final products of the manufacturing processes are consistent or comparable. To ensure that there is a desired (high) probability for establishing consistency or comparability between manufacturing processes (sites or locations) when truly there is no difference in raw materials or final products between manufacturing processes (sites or locations), an appropriate sampling plan which can draw representative samples at random is necessarily developed.

Let U and W be the characteristics of the biological products under investigation from two different manufacturing processes (sites or locations), where $X = \log U$ and $Y = \log W$ follows normal distributions with means μ_X, μ_Y and variances V_X, V_Y, respectively. Similar to the idea of using $P(X < Y)$ to assess reliability in statistical QC (Church and Harris, 1970; Enis and Geisser, 1971), Tse et al. (2006) proposed the following probability as an index to assess the consistency of raw materials and/or final products from two different manufacturing processes (sites or locations)

$$p = P\left(1 - \delta < \frac{U}{W} < \frac{1}{1 - \delta}\right), \tag{14.1}$$

where $0 < \delta < 1$ and is defined as a limit that allows for consistency. Tse et al. (2006) referred to p as the consistency index. Thus, p tends to 1 as δ tends to 1. For a given δ, if p is close to 1, materials U and W are considered to be identical.

It should be noted that a small δ implies the requirement of high degree of consistency between material U and material W. In practice, it may be difficult to meet this narrow specification for consistency. Under the normality assumption of $X = \log U$ and $Y = \log W$, Equation 14.1 can be rewritten as

$$p = P(\log(1-\delta) < \log U - \log W < -\log(1-\delta))$$

$$= \Phi\left(\frac{-\log(1-\delta)-(\mu_X-\mu_Y)}{\sqrt{V_X+V_Y}}\right) - \Phi\left(\frac{\log(1-\delta)-(\mu_X-\mu_Y)}{\sqrt{V_X+V_Y}}\right),$$

where $\Phi(z_0) = P(Z < z_0)$ with Z being a standard normal random variable. Therefore, the consistency index p is a function of the parameters $\theta = (\mu_X, \mu_Y, V_X, V_Y)$, i.e., $p = h(\theta)$. Suppose that observations $X_i = \log U_i$, $i = 1, \ldots, n_X$ and $Y_i = \log W_i$, $i = 1, \ldots, n_Y$ are collected in an assay study. Then, using the invariance principle, the maximum likelihood estimator (MLE) of p can be obtained as

$$\hat{p} = \Phi\left(\frac{-\log(1-\delta)-(\bar{X}-\bar{Y})}{\sqrt{\hat{V}_X+\hat{V}_Y}}\right) - \Phi\left(\frac{\log(1-\delta)-(\bar{X}-\bar{Y})}{\sqrt{\hat{V}_X+\hat{V}_Y}}\right), \quad (14.2)$$

where $\bar{X} = 1/n_X \sum_{i=1}^{n_X} X_i$, $\bar{Y} = 1/n_Y \sum_{i=1}^{n_Y} Y_i$, $\hat{V}_X = 1/n_X \sum_{i=1}^{n_X}(X_i-\bar{X})^2$, and $\hat{V}_Y = 1/n_Y \sum_{i=1}^{n_Y}(Y_i-\bar{Y})^2$. In other words, $\hat{p} = h(\hat{\theta}) = h(\bar{X},\bar{Y},\hat{V}_X,\hat{V}_Y)$. Furthermore, it can be easily verified that the following asymptotic result holds.

Theorem 14.1

$\hat{p}$ as given in Equation 14.2 is asymptotically normal with mean $E(\hat{p})$ and variance $\text{Var}(\hat{p})$. In other words

$$\frac{\hat{p}-E(\hat{p})}{\sqrt{\text{Var}(\hat{p})}} \to N(0,1), \quad (14.3)$$

where $E(\hat{p}) = p + B(p) + o(1/n)$ and $\text{Var}(\hat{p}) = C(p) + o(1/n)$. The detailed expressions of $B(p)$ and $C(p)$ are given as follows.

Proof
Based on the definitions of $\bar{X}$ and $\hat{V}_X$, it is easy to show that

$$E(\bar{X}) = \mu_X,$$

$$E(\hat{V}_X) = \frac{n_X - 1}{n_X} V_X,$$

$$\mathrm{Var}(\bar{X}) = \frac{V_X}{n_X},$$

and

$$\mathrm{Var}(\hat{V}_X) = \frac{2(n_X - 1)}{n_X^2} V_X^2.$$

Similarly

$$E(\bar{Y}) = \mu_Y,$$

$$E(\hat{V}_Y) = \frac{n_Y - 1}{n_Y} V_Y,$$

$$\mathrm{Var}(\bar{Y}) = \frac{V_Y}{n_Y},$$

and

$$\mathrm{Var}(\hat{V}_Y) = \frac{2(n_Y - 1)}{n_Y^2} V_Y^2.$$

Applying expansion of $\hat{p}$ at p, we have

$$\hat{p} = p + \frac{\partial \hat{p}}{\partial \mu_X}(\bar{X} - \mu_X) + \frac{\partial \hat{p}}{\partial \mu_Y}(\bar{Y} - \mu_Y) + \frac{\partial \hat{p}}{\partial V_X}(\hat{V}_X - V_X) + \frac{\partial \hat{p}}{\partial V_Y}(\hat{V}_Y - V_Y)$$

$$+ \frac{1}{2}\left[\frac{\partial^2 \hat{p}}{\partial \mu_X^2}(\bar{X} - \mu_X)^2 + \frac{\partial^2 \hat{p}}{\partial \mu_Y^2}(\bar{Y} - \mu_Y)^2 + \frac{\partial^2 \hat{p}}{\partial V_X^2}(\hat{V}_X - V_X)^2 + \frac{\partial^2 \hat{p}}{\partial V_Y^2}(\hat{V}_Y - V_Y)^2 \right] + \cdots.$$

The other second-order partial derivatives are not considered because they will lead to expected values of order $O(n^{-2})$ or higher. Taking expectation,

$$E(\hat{p}) = p + \frac{1}{2}\left[\frac{\partial^2 \hat{p}}{\partial \mu_X^2}\frac{V_X}{n_X} + \frac{\partial^2 \hat{p}}{\partial \mu_Y^2}\frac{V_Y}{n_Y} + \frac{\partial^2 \hat{p}}{\partial V_X^2}\left(\frac{2V_X^2}{n_X}\right) + \frac{\partial^2 \hat{p}}{\partial V_Y^2}\left(\frac{2V_Y^2}{n_Y}\right) \right] + O(n^{-2})$$

and

$$\mathrm{Var}(\hat{p}) = \left[\left(\frac{\partial \hat{p}}{\partial \mu_X} \right)^2 \frac{V_X}{n_X} + \left(\frac{\partial \hat{p}}{\partial \mu_Y} \right)^2 \frac{V_Y}{n_Y} + \left(\frac{\partial \hat{p}}{\partial V_X} \right)^2 \left(\frac{2V_X^2}{n_X} \right) + \left(\frac{\partial \hat{p}}{\partial V_Y} \right)^2 \left(\frac{2V_Y^2}{n_Y} \right) \right] + O(n^{-2}).$$

Therefore,

$$B(p) = \frac{1}{2} \left[\frac{\partial^2 \hat{p}}{\partial \mu_X^2} \frac{V_X}{n_X} + \frac{\partial^2 \hat{p}}{\partial \mu_Y^2} \frac{V_Y}{n_Y} + \frac{\partial^2 \hat{p}}{\partial V_X^2} \left(\frac{2V_X^2}{n_X} \right) + \frac{\partial^2 \hat{p}}{\partial V_Y^2} \left(\frac{2V_Y^2}{n_Y} \right) \right] \qquad (14.4)$$

and

$$C(p) = \left[\left(\frac{\partial \hat{p}}{\partial \mu_X} \right)^2 \frac{V_X}{n_X} + \left(\frac{\partial \hat{p}}{\partial \mu_Y} \right)^2 \frac{V_Y}{n_Y} + \left(\frac{\partial \hat{p}}{\partial V_X} \right)^2 \left(\frac{2V_X^2}{n_X} \right) + \left(\frac{\partial \hat{p}}{\partial V_Y} \right)^2 \left(\frac{2V_Y^2}{n_Y} \right) \right]. \qquad (14.5)$$

For the sake of simplicity, denote

$$z_1 = \frac{\log(1-\delta) - (\mu_X - \mu_Y)}{\sqrt{V_X + V_Y}},$$

$$z_2 = \frac{-\log(1-\delta) - (\mu_X - \mu_Y)}{\sqrt{V_X + V_Y}},$$

and

$$\phi(z) = \frac{1}{\sqrt{2\pi}} \exp\left(-\frac{z^2}{2} \right).$$

Then after some algebra, the partial derivatives are given as

$$\frac{\partial \hat{p}}{\partial \mu_X} = -\frac{\partial \hat{p}}{\partial \mu_Y} = \left(\frac{-1}{\sqrt{V_X + V_Y}} \right) [\phi(z_2) - \phi(z_1)],$$

$$\frac{\partial \hat{p}}{\partial V_X} = \frac{\partial \hat{p}}{\partial V_Y} = \left(\frac{-1}{2\sqrt{V_X + V_Y}} \right) [z_2 \phi(z_2) - z_1 \phi(z_1)],$$

$$\frac{\partial^2 \hat{p}}{\partial \mu_X^2} = \frac{\partial^2 \hat{p}}{\partial \mu_Y^2} = \left(\frac{-1}{V_X + V_Y} \right) [z_2 \phi(z_2) - z_1 \phi(z_1)],$$

and

$$\frac{\partial^2 \hat{p}}{\partial V_X^2} = \frac{\partial^2 \hat{p}}{\partial V_Y^2} = \frac{1}{4(V_X + V_Y)^{3/2}} \left[\left(2z_2 - z_2^3\right)\phi(z_2) - \left(2z_1 - z_1^3\right)z_1\phi(z_1) \right].$$

This completes the proof.

Based on the result of Theorem 14.1, an approximate $(1 - \alpha) \times 100\%$ confidence interval for p, i.e., $(LL(\hat{p}), UL(\hat{p}))$, can be obtained. In particular,

$$LL(\hat{p}) = \hat{p} - B(\hat{p}) - z_{\alpha/2}\sqrt{C(\hat{p})} \quad \text{and} \quad UL(\hat{p}) = \hat{p} - B(\hat{p}) + z_{\alpha/2}\sqrt{C(\hat{p})}, \quad (14.6)$$

where z_α is the upper α-percentile of a standard normal distribution.

14.4 Test for Comparability

For a valid statistical QC process, a testing procedure is necessarily performed according to some pre-specified acceptance criteria under an appropriate sampling plan that can draw representative samples at random. In this section, following the idea of Tse et al. (2006), we propose a statistical QC method for assessing consistency of raw materials and/or final products between biosimilar products manufactured by different manufacturing processes (sites or locations). The idea is to construct a 95% confidence interval for a proposed consistency index described earlier under a sampling plan. If the constructed 95% confidence lower limit is greater than a prespecified QC lower limit, then we claim that the raw material or final product has passed the QC and hence can be released for further processing or use. Otherwise, the raw materials and/or final product should be rejected. For a given component (the most active component if possible), the sampling plan is derived to ensure that there is a desired probability for establishing consistency between sites when truly there is no difference in raw materials or final products between sites. In what follows, details regarding the choice of acceptance criteria, sampling plan, and the corresponding testing procedure are briefly outlined.

14.4.1 Acceptance Criteria

In terms of consistency, we propose the following QC criterion. If the probability that the lower limit $LL(\hat{p})$ of the constructed $(1 - \alpha) \times 100\%$ confidence interval of p is greater than or equal to a prespecified QC lower limit, say, QC_L exceeds a prespecified number β (say $\beta = 80\%$), then we claim that U and W are consistent or similar. In other words, U and W are consistent or similar if $P(QC_L \le LL(\hat{p})) \ge \beta$, where β is a prespecified constant.

It should be noted that the selection of β would reflect the degree of consistency or comparability that the sponsor would like to achieve. In practice, it is suggested that β be selected based on the comparison between batches of the reference product manufactured by the same manufacturing process of the reference product.

14.4.2 Sampling Plan

In practice, it is necessary to select a sample size to ensure that there is a high probability or consistency (or comparability), say β, between U and W when in fact U and W are consistent or comparable. It is then suggested that the sample size is chosen such that there is more than 80% chance that the lower confidence limit of p is greater than or equal to the QC lower limit, i.e., β = 0.8. In other words, the sample size is determined such that

$$P\{QC_L \le LL(p)\} \ge \beta. \tag{14.7}$$

Using Equation 14.7, this leads to

$$P\{QC_L \le \hat{p} - B(\hat{p}) - z_{\alpha/2}\sqrt{\mathrm{Var}(\hat{p})}\} \ge \beta.$$

Thus,

$$P\{QC_L + z_{\alpha/2}\sqrt{\mathrm{Var}(\hat{p})} - p \le \hat{p} - p - B(p)\} \ge \beta.$$

This gives

$$P\left\{\frac{QC_L - p}{\sqrt{\mathrm{Var}(\hat{p})}} + z_{\alpha/2} \le \frac{\hat{p} - p - B(p)}{\sqrt{\mathrm{Var}(\hat{p})}}\right\} \ge \beta.$$

Therefore, the sample size required for achieving a probability higher than β can be obtained by solving the following equation:

$$\frac{QC_L - p}{\sqrt{\mathrm{Var}(\hat{p})}} + z_{\alpha/2} \le -z_{1-\beta}. \tag{14.8}$$

Assuming that $n_X = n_Y = n$, the common sample size is given by

$$n \ge \frac{(z_{1-\beta} + z_{\alpha/2})^2}{(p - QC_L)^2}\left\{\left(\frac{\partial \hat{p}}{\partial \mu_X}\right)^2 V_X + \left(\frac{\partial \hat{p}}{\partial \mu_Y}\right)^2 V_Y + \left(\frac{\partial \hat{p}}{\partial V_X}\right)^2 (2V_X^2) + \left(\frac{\partial \hat{p}}{\partial V_Y}\right)^2 (2V_Y^2)\right\}.$$

$$(14.9)$$

The result provided earlier suggests that the required sample size will depend on the choices of α, β, V_X, V_Y, $\mu_X - \mu_Y$, and $p - QC_L$. As it can be seen from the expression in Equation 14.9 that larger sample size is required for smaller α and larger β, i.e., the interval is expected to have high confidence level $(1 - \alpha)$ and high chance that the lower confidence limit is larger than QC_L. Furthermore, if we require QC_L to be close to p, i.e., $p - QC_L$ is small, a relatively large sample size is required. The dependence of the sample size n on the other parameters V_X, V_Y, and $\mu_X - \mu_Y$ is relatively unclear because these parameters are linked to the corresponding partial derivatives. A numerical study is conducted to explore the pattern. Given the large number of parameters involved in Equation 14.9, it is impractical to list the value of n for all the parameters combinations. However, for illustration purpose, we consider only a certain combination of parameters values in an attempt to explore the pattern of dependence of n on the parameters. For the sake of simplicity, define

$$S = \frac{1}{(p-QC_L)^2} \left\{ \left(\frac{\partial \hat{p}}{\partial \mu_X}\right)^2 V_X + \left(\frac{\partial \hat{p}}{\partial \mu_Y}\right)^2 V_Y + \left(\frac{\partial \hat{p}}{\partial V_X}\right)^2 (2V_X^2) + \left(\frac{\partial \hat{p}}{\partial V_Y}\right)^2 (2V_Y^2) \right\}.$$

Then, for given choices of α and β, the required sample size n is equal to $(z_{1-\beta} + z_{\alpha/2})^2 S$. In particular, in our study, $\delta = 0.10, 0.15$, and 0.20; $\mu_X - \mu_Y = 0.5, 1.0$, and 1.5; $p - QC_L = 0.02, 0.05$, and 0.08. V_X is chosen to be 1 and $V_Y = 0.2, 0.5, 1.0, 2.0$, and 5.0. For each combination of these parameters values, the corresponding value of S is listed in Table 14.1. Given the number of parameters involved and the complexity of the mathematical expression of S, it is not easy to detect a general pattern. However, in general, the results suggest that S increases as $\mu_X - \mu_Y$ decreases, and as the variances V_x and V_y differ more from each other. In other words, smaller sample size is required if the difference between the population means is large or the variability of the two sites are of similar magnitude.

As an illustration, if for a study with $\delta = 0.2$, $V_X = 1$, $V_Y = 0.5$, $\mu_X - \mu_Y = 1.0$, and an experiment we expect $p - QC_L$ to be not larger than 0.05, then results in Table 14.1 suggest that $S = 3.024$. Suppose a probability higher than $\beta = 0.8$ at the $\alpha = 0.05$ level of significance is required, the corresponding required sample size is given by

$$n \geq (z_{1-0.8} + z_{0.05/2})^2 S = (0.842 + 1.96)^2 (3.024) = 23.74,$$

i.e., a sample of size at least 24 is required.

14.4.3 Testing Procedure

Hypotheses testing of the consistency index p can also be conducted based on the asymptotic normality of $\hat{p}$. Consider the following hypotheses:

$$H_0: p \leq p_0 \quad \text{versus} \quad H_1: p > p_0.$$

TABLE 14.1

Values of $n/(z_{1-\beta} + z_{\alpha/2})^2$, Where n Is the Required Sample Size

		$\delta = 0.10$			$\delta = 0.15$			$\delta = 0.20$		
		$\Delta = 0.5$	$\Delta = 1.0$	$\Delta = 1.5$	$\Delta = 0.5$	$\Delta = 1.0$	$\Delta = 1.5$	$\Delta = 0.5$	$\Delta = 1.0$	$\Delta = 1.5$
$D = 0.02$	$V_Y = 0.2$	5.693	5.376	4.955	13.403	12.681	11.702	24.861	23.594	21.810
	0.5	4.518	4.289	4.196	10.655	10.134	9.921	19.820	18.901	18.520
	1.0	3.939	3.336	3.237	9.310	7.894	7.662	17.370	14.761	14.333
	2.0	4.231	2.962	2.226	10.020	7.021	5.280	18.756	13.163	9.906
	5.0	5.728	4.159	2.469	13.595	9.876	5.866	25.534	18.558	11.032
$D = 0.05$	0.2	0.911	0.860	0.793	2.144	2.029	1.872	3.978	3.775	3.490
	0.5	0.723	0.686	0.671	1.705	1.622	1.587	3.171	3.024	2.963
	1.0	0.630	0.534	0.518	1.490	1.263	1.226	2.779	2.362	2.293
	2.0	0.677	0.474	0.356	1.603	1.123	0.845	3.001	2.106	1.585
	5.0	0.916	0.666	0.395	2.175	1.580	0.939	4.085	2.969	1.765
$D = 0.08$	0.2	0.356	0.336	0.310	0.838	0.793	0.731	1.554	1.475	1.363
	0.5	0.282	0.268	0.262	0.666	0.633	0.620	1.239	1.181	1.158
	1.0	0.246	0.208	0.202	0.582	0.493	0.479	1.086	0.923	0.896
	2.0	0.264	0.185	0.139	0.626	0.439	0.330	1.172	0.823	0.619
	5.0	0.358	0.260	0.154	0.850	0.617	0.367	1.596	1.160	0.690

Notation: $\Delta = \mu_X - \mu_Y$, $D = p - QC_L$.

We would reject the null hypothesis in favor of the alternative hypothesis of consistency. Under H_0, we have

$$\frac{\hat{p} - p_0 - B(\hat{p})}{\sqrt{\text{Var}(\hat{p})}} \sim N(0,1). \tag{14.10}$$

Thus, we reject the null hypothesis H_0 at the α level of significance if

$$\frac{\hat{p} - p_0 - B(\hat{p})}{\sqrt{\text{Var}(\hat{p})}} > Z_\alpha.$$

This is equivalent to rejecting the null hypothesis H_0 when

$$\hat{p} > p_0 + B(\hat{p}) + Z_\alpha\sqrt{\text{Var}(\hat{p})}.$$

Again, for illustration purposes, Table 14.2 provides critical values of the proposed test for consistency index for various combinations of the parameters. In particular, $\alpha = 0.1$ $p_0 = 0.75, 0.85$, and 0.9, $\delta = 0.10$ and 0.20; $\mu_X - \mu_Y = 0.5, 1.0$, and 1.5. V_X is chosen to be 1 and $V_Y = 0.2, 0.5, 1.0, 2.0$, and 5.0. Note that the critical value is closer to the corresponding p_0 either for larger sample size n, smaller δ, or smaller $\mu_X - \mu_Y$.

14.4.4 Strategy for Statistical Quality Control

In practice, raw materials, in-process materials, and/or final products at different sites are manufactured sequentially in batches or lots. As a result, it is important to perform statistical QC on batches. A typical approach is to randomly select samples from several (consecutive) batches for testing. In this case, observations from the study would be subject to batch-to-batch variability. For the sake of administrative convenience, it is common to have equal number of observations from the batches. Consider the following model:

$$X_{ij} = \mu_X + A_i^X + \varepsilon_{ij}^X, \quad i = 1, \ldots, m_X; j = 1, \ldots, n_X,$$

where
A_i^X accounts for the batch-to-batch variability for the observations collected in site 1 and is normally distributed with mean 0 and variance σ_{b1}^2
m_X is the number of batches collected in the study at site 1
ε_{ij}^X are normal random variables with mean 0 and variance σ_1^2

TABLE 14.2

Critical Values of the Proposed Test for Consistency Index p_0

p_0	δ	V_Y	$\Delta = 0.5$			$\Delta = 1.0$			$\Delta = 1.5$		
			$n = 15$	$n = 30$	$n = 50$	$n = 15$	$n = 30$	$n = 50$	$n = 15$	$n = 30$	$n = 50$
0.75	0.10	0.2	0.7695	0.7640	0.7609	0.7683	0.7632	0.7604	0.7680	0.7629	0.7601
		0.5	0.7673	0.7624	0.7597	0.7665	0.7619	0.7593	0.7665	0.7619	0.7593
		1.0	0.7662	0.7616	0.7590	0.7646	0.7605	0.7582	0.7645	0.7604	0.7581
		2.0	0.7668	0.7620	0.7594	0.7639	0.7600	0.7578	0.7620	0.7586	0.7567
		5.0	0.7697	0.7640	0.7609	0.7667	0.7619	0.7593	0.7628	0.7592	0.7572
	0.20	0.2	0.7907	0.7791	0.7727	0.7884	0.7777	0.7717	0.7878	0.7771	0.7712
		0.5	0.7863	0.7760	0.7703	0.7846	0.7749	0.7695	0.7847	0.7749	0.7695
		1.0	0.7839	0.7743	0.7689	0.7807	0.7721	0.7673	0.7805	0.7719	0.7671
		2.0	0.7853	0.7753	0.7697	0.7793	0.7710	0.7664	0.7754	0.7682	0.7642
		5.0	0.7915	0.7797	0.7731	0.7853	0.7752	0.7697	0.7771	0.7694	0.7651
0.85	0.10	0.2	0.8695	0.8640	0.8609	0.8683	0.8632	0.8604	0.8680	0.8629	0.8601
		0.5	0.8673	0.8624	0.8597	0.8665	0.8619	0.8593	0.8665	0.8619	0.8593
		1.0	0.8662	0.8616	0.8590	0.8646	0.8605	0.8582	0.8645	0.8604	0.8581
		2.0	0.8668	0.8620	0.8594	0.8639	0.8600	0.8578	0.8620	0.8586	0.8567
		5.0	0.8697	0.8640	0.8609	0.8667	0.8619	0.8593	0.8628	0.8592	0.8572
	0.20	0.2	0.8907	0.8791	0.8727	0.8884	0.8777	0.8717	0.8878	0.8771	0.8712
		0.5	0.8863	0.8760	0.8703	0.8846	0.8749	0.8695	0.8847	0.8749	0.8695
		1.0	0.8839	0.8743	0.8689	0.8807	0.8721	0.8673	0.8805	0.8719	0.8671
		2.0	0.8853	0.8753	0.8697	0.8793	0.8710	0.8664	0.8754	0.8682	0.8642
		5.0	0.8915	0.8797	0.8731	0.8853	0.8752	0.8697	0.8771	0.8694	0.8651
0.90	0.10	0.2	0.9195	0.9140	0.9109	0.9183	0.9132	0.9104	0.9180	0.9129	0.9101
		0.5	0.9173	0.9124	0.9097	0.9165	0.9119	0.9093	0.9165	0.9119	0.9093
		1.0	0.9162	0.9116	0.9090	0.9146	0.9105	0.9082	0.9145	0.9104	0.9081
		2.0	0.9168	0.9120	0.9094	0.9139	0.9100	0.9078	0.9120	0.9086	0.9067
		5.0	0.9197	0.9140	0.9109	0.9167	0.9119	0.9093	0.9128	0.9092	0.9072
	0.20	0.2	0.9407	0.9291	0.9227	0.9384	0.9277	0.9217	0.9378	0.9271	0.9212
		0.5	0.9363	0.9260	0.9203	0.9346	0.9249	0.9195	0.9347	0.9249	0.9195
		1.0	0.9339	0.9243	0.9189	0.9307	0.9221	0.9173	0.9305	0.9219	0.9171
		2.0	0.9353	0.9253	0.9197	0.9293	0.9210	0.9164	0.9254	0.9182	0.9142
		5.0	0.9415	0.9297	0.9231	0.9353	0.9252	0.9197	0.9271	0.9194	0.9151

Notation: $\Delta = \mu_X - \mu_Y$.

Similarly,

$$Y_{ij} = \mu_Y + A_i^Y + \varepsilon_{ij}^Y, \quad i = 1, \ldots, m_Y; \quad j = 1, \ldots, n_Y,$$

where
A_i^Y accounts for the batch-to-batch variability for the observations collected in site 2 and is normally distributed with mean 0 and variance σ_{b2}^2
m_Y is the number of batches collected in the study at site 2
ε_{ij}^Y are normal random variables with mean 0 and variance σ_2^2

Therefore, the total variability of the most active component at the two sites is given by Var $X = V_X = \sigma_{b1}^2 + \sigma_1^2$ and Var $Y = V_Y = \sigma_{b2}^2 + \sigma_2^2$, respectively.

Furthermore, let $\bar{X}_{i.} = 1/n_X \sum_{j=1}^{n_X} X_{ij}$ and $\bar{X} = 1/m_X \sum_{i=1}^{m_X} \bar{X}_{i.}$. Then, the observed sums of squares are $SSA_1 = n_X \sum_{i=1}^{m_X} (\bar{X}_{i.} - \bar{X})^2$, $SSE_1 = \sum_{i=1}^{m_X} \sum_{j=1}^{n_X} (X_{ij} - \bar{X}_{i.})^2$, and $SST_1 = SSA_1 + SSE_1$. Following the results in Chow and Tse (1991), the MLEs of σ_{b1}^2 and σ_1^2 are

$$\hat{\sigma}_{b1}^2 = \begin{cases} \dfrac{1}{n_X}\left(\dfrac{1}{m_X} SSA_1 - \dfrac{1}{m_X(n_X - 1)} SSE_1 \right) & \text{if } \dfrac{1}{m_X} SSA_1 \geq \dfrac{1}{m_X(n_X - 1)} SSE_1 \\[6pt] 0 & \dfrac{1}{m_X} SSA_1 < \dfrac{1}{m_X(n_X - 1)} SSE_1 \end{cases}$$

(14.11)

and

$$\hat{\sigma}_1^2 = \begin{cases} \dfrac{1}{m_X(n_X - 1)} SSE_1 & \text{if } \dfrac{1}{m_X} SSA_1 \geq \dfrac{1}{m_X(n_X - 1)} SSE_1 \\[6pt] \dfrac{1}{n_X m_X} SST_1 & \dfrac{1}{m_X} SSA_1 < \dfrac{1}{m_X(n_X - 1)} SSE_1 \end{cases} \qquad (14.12)$$

Furthermore, the MLE of the total variability V_X is given by $\hat{V}_X = (1/n_X m_X) SST_1$. The MLEs of σ_{b2}^2, σ_2^2, and V_Y, denoted by $\hat{\sigma}_{b2}^2$, $\hat{\sigma}_2^2$, and $\hat{V}_Y$, respectively, can be obtained in a similar way using observations Y_{ij}. Comparison of the estimates $\hat{\sigma}_{b2}^2$ and $\hat{\sigma}_{b1}^2$ would give an idea of the magnitude of the batch-to-batch variability at the two sites.

14.5 Other Comparability Tests

In addition to comparability tests for in vivo and in vitro critical quality attributes that may be encountered in a manufacturing process, there are several important comparability tests during the development of biosimilar products.

These comparability tests include, but are not limited to, PK comparability test, PD comparability test, and clinical efficacy comparability study, which are briefly described later.

14.5.1 PK Comparability Test

The PK comparability test is nothing but test for equivalence in drug absorption profile between a test product and a reference product in terms of AUC (area under the blood or plasma concentration–time curve) and C_{max} (maximum concentration). As discussed extensively in the first few chapters of this book, the PK comparability test includes the assessment of average bioequivalence, population bioequivalence, and individual bioequivalence (IBE). For average bioequivalence, two drug products are considered comparable if the 90% confidence interval of the geometric mean ratio (GMR) is within (80%, 125%). For highly variable drug products, the assessment of average bioequivalence may be done using the scaled average bioequivalence (SABE) criterion.

For assessment of population bioequivalence, PBE criterion, PBE can be claimed if the following null hypothesis in

$$H_0 : \lambda \geq 0 \quad \text{versus} \quad H_a : \lambda < 0$$

is rejected at the 5% level of significance and the observed GMR is within the limits of 80% and 125%, where

$$\lambda = \delta^2 + \sigma_{TT}^2 - \sigma_{TR}^2 - \theta_{PBE} \max(\sigma_{TR}^2, \sigma_0^2)$$

and θ_{PBE} is a constant specified in the 2003 FDA draft guidance. Note that PBE can be claimed if the one-sided 95% upper confidence bound for λ is less than a prespecified bioequivalence limit.

For assessment of IBE, IBE can be claimed if the null hypothesis

$$H_0 : \gamma \geq 0 \quad \text{versus} \quad H_a : \gamma < 0$$

is rejected at the 5% level of significance and the observed GMR is within the limits of 80% and 125%, where

$$\gamma = \delta^2 + \sigma_D^2 + \sigma_{WT}^2 - \sigma_{WR}^2 - \theta_{IBE} \max(\sigma_{WR}^2, \sigma_{W0}^2)$$

and θ_{IBE} is a constant specified in the 2003 FDA draft guidance. Note that IBE can be claimed if the one-sided 95% upper confidence bound for γ is less than a prespecified bioequivalence limit.

14.5.2 PD Comparability Index

The following PD comparability index is often considered to compare PD responses between a test product (T) and a reference product (R)

$$f_{PD} = 2 \times \frac{\min\left(E_{max}^R - E_{min}^R, E_{max}^T - E_{min}^T\right)}{max\left(E_{max}^R - E_{min}^R, E_{max}^T - E_{min}^T\right) + \sqrt{1/T \sum_{j=1}^{T} w_j \left(y_j^R - y_j^T\right)^2}} - 1,$$

where

   T is the number of time points

   w_j is the optional weight factor

   E_{max} and E_{min} are from the PK/PD model (e.g., E_{max} model) or PD profile

This index is then transformed to scale within (0, 1). Thus, comparability is claimed if the lower 95% confidence interval limit of the defined index for T/R is greater than the lower limit of index value for R/R or ≥0.54, which is corresponding to 30% profile changes, provided that the point estimate of the index for T/R is greater than 0.8

14.5.3 Clinical Efficacy Comparability Study

Comparability in clinical efficacy is referred to as that the biosimilar is no better and no worse than the innovator. In practice, a couple of questions have been raised. First, is there a need to show biosimilar is better than the placebo? Second, should an equivalence trial or a non-inferiority trial be conducted? To address the questions described earlier, the recent FDA guidance on non-inferiority trials is helpful.

In practice, the selection of equivalence limit (for equivalence trial) or non-inferiority margin (for non-inferiority trial) is the key to the success of clinical efficacy comparability study. A typical approach is to obtain information such as variability of the reference product from the comparison of a reference product to itself, which we will refer to as an R–R study. In an R–R study, the reference products could come from different lots (batches), manufactured at different times, and/or different times on shelf.

Once the acceptance criteria (i.e., the equivalence limit for equivalence trial or non-inferiority margin for non-inferiority trial) have been determined, Liao and Heyse (2011) considered T and R are comparable if (1) T and R are comparable in distribution for the clinical endpoint, if the 95% confidence interval of T–R is within an R–R plausibility interval (PI) and the point estimate of T/R is within (0.8, 1.25), and (2) T is clinically effective, if $B_{TP} > 0$ and

$$B_{TR} + (1-\lambda)B_{PR} > 0,$$

where
   λ is the assay effect
   B represents treatment effect

Note that condition (1) guarantees that T and R are comparable in distribution for the clinical endpoint, while condition (2) assures that T is clinically effective as compared to the placebo.

14.6 Concluding Remarks

In this chapter, we focus on statistical QC for testing comparability (consistency) in raw material and/or end product of a biosimilar product obtained from different manufacturing processes or sites. The idea is to construct a 95% confidence interval for a proposed consistency index under a sampling plan. If the constructed 95% confidence lower limit is greater than a prespecified QC lower limit, then we claim that the two manufacturing processes are comparable (or consistent in producing similar biological products). Sampling plan is derived to ensure that there is a desired high probability for establishment of consistency between manufacturing processes or sites when truly there is no difference in raw materials and/or end products between manufacturing processes or sites.

When there are more than one test for comparability (e.g., there are more than one quality attribute) between manufacturing processes, the method proposed by Tse et al. (2006) can be modified and extended to test the following consistency index:

$$p = P\left(1-\delta_k < \frac{U_k}{W_k} < \frac{1}{1-\delta_k}; \quad k=1,2,\ldots,K\right),$$

where $0 < \delta_k < 1$ and is the limit that allows for consistency for the kth quality attribute of U_k and W_k from the two manufacturing processes or sites. Thus, we have

$$p = P\left(1-\delta_k < \frac{U_k}{W_k} < \frac{1}{1-\delta_k}; \quad k=1,2,\ldots,K\right)$$

$$= \prod_{k=1}^{K} P\left(1-\delta_k < \frac{U_k}{W_k} < \frac{1}{1-\delta_k}\right)$$

$$= \prod_{k=1}^{K} p_k,$$

where p_k can be estimated using Equation 14.2, based on the observations obtained from the kth quality attribute. In particular,

$$\hat{p} = \prod_{k=1}^{K} \Phi\left(\frac{-\log(1-\delta_k)-(\bar{X}_k-\bar{Y}_k)}{\sqrt{\hat{V}_{k,X}+\hat{V}_{k,Y}}}\right) - \Phi\left(\frac{\log(1-\delta_k)-(\bar{X}_k-\bar{Y}_k)}{\sqrt{\hat{V}_{k,X}+\hat{V}_{k,Y}}}\right),$$

where $\bar{X}_k$, $\bar{Y}_k$, $\hat{V}_{k,X}$, $\hat{V}_{k,Y}$ are the sample means and sample variances based on the kth quality attribute of the biological products from the two manufacturing processes or sites, respectively. Statistical properties of $\hat{p}$, however, needs further research.

In its recent draft guidances on the assessment of biosimilarity of biosimilar products, the FDA proposed the concept of totality-of-the-evidence for assessment of biosimilarity. The totality-of-the-evidence is, in effect, global biosimilarity across different domains (e.g., critical quality attributes at various stages in a manufacturing process). The FDA seems to suggest that similarity (comparability) in critical quality attributes should be demonstrated across different stages of the manufacturing process. The degree of similarity or comparability in different stages, however, may have different degrees of impact on the clinical outcomes (i.e., safety and effectiveness). As a result, it is suggested that different criteria for similarity (comparability) in critical quality attribute at different stages of the manufacturing process should be considered for providing the totality-of-the-evidence for global similarity. In addition, since a small change or variation at any stage of the manufacturing process could have an impact on the safety and effectiveness of the biosimilar product under development, the manufacturing process must be validated. At each critical stage of the manufacturing process, *sampling plan, acceptance criteria,* and *testing procedure* must be described in detail in the protocol for process validation. Tests for comparability in critical quality attributes between raw materials, in-process (in-use) materials, and end products of manufacturing processes should be conducted based on some prespecified *criteria for comparability.*

15

Stability Analysis of Biosimilar Products

15.1 Introduction

Schellekens (2005) pointed out that small-molecule drug products tend to follow Arrhenius behavior (i.e., thermally dependent molecular motion) and thus have predictable stability based on acceleration studies. In contrast, the activity and biological function of proteins are highly dependent on their unique spatial conformation, which is the reason why biologics are much less stable than small-molecule compounds. First, proteins may shift between several related structures, in conformational changes, usually induced by the binding of a substrate molecule to an enzyme's active site, or the physical region of the protein that participates in chemical catalysis. Second, many environmental factors such as temperature, pH, pressure, concentrated in organic salt or organic solvent will cause proteins lose their tertiary and secondary structure in a process called denaturation. Third, enzymolysis and hydrolysis will lead to protein degradation and the loss of their functions. Accordingly, slight variations in the manufacturing process may affect protein stability and efficacy of the biopharmaceuticals. Thus, stability profiles of the biosimilar product and the reference biological products need to be studied by placing the product under stressed conditions. The rate of degradation and degradation profiles (oxidation, deamidation, aggregation, and other degradation reactions) should be compared. If unknown degradation species are detected, they need to be studied to determine if they affect safety and efficacy. If differences in product purities and stability profiles are present between the biosimilar product and the reference biological products, these differences need to be justified using scientific knowledge or pre-clinical or clinical data.

Since biosimilars are often very sensitive to environmental factors, their assessment requires advanced analytical capabilities integrated stability programs in compliance with current good manufacturing practices (cGMP) in order to evaluate their quality and change with time while being stored under various conditions of temperature and humidity. Stability study requirements are described in ICH guidelines Q1A (R2) "Stability Testing of New Drug Substances and Products" and Q5C "Quality of Biotechnological

Products—Stability Testing of Biotechnologicals/Biological Products." During early development, accelerated stability studies can help to provide key data and information on the effect of short-term exposure to environmental conditions. Short-term stability studies are typically performed over a 6 month period. Long-term stability studies (12 months and longer) allow evaluation of the quality of the drug both during and beyond its projected shelf-life.

Stability studies are conducted not only to provide evidence on how the quality of a drug substance or drug product varies with time under the influence of a variety of environmental factors such as temperature, humidity, and light but also to establish a retest period for the drug substance or a shelf-life for the drug product and recommended storage conditions (Chow, 2007). For a newly developed biosimilar product, accelerated testing is required for 6 months, and long-term testing is required for the length of shelf-life. Thus the cost of the stability studies can be substantial. This leads quite naturally to statistically designed stability studies, which are called *matrix* designs, or studies where a selected subset of the total number of possible samples for all factor combinations is tested at a specified time point.

In the next section, ICH stability guideline Q5C for biotechnology products is briefly described. Section 15.3 provides the definition and determination of expiration dating period (or shelf-life) of a biosimilar product following both the FDA and the ICH stability guidelines (FDA, 1987; ICH, 1993, 2003). Sections 15.4 and 15.5 focus on the design and analysis of stability studies, respectively. Section 15.6 provides brief concluding remarks of this chapter.

15.2 Regulatory Stability Guidelines on Biologicals

15.2.1 ICH/EMA Guidelines on Stability

Between 1993 and 2003, the ICH published a number of guidelines on stability for drug substances and drug products. These guidelines are listed in Table 15.1. As can be seen from Table 15.1, ICH Q1A R2 is a revision of the

TABLE 15.1

ICH Guidelines on Stability

Q1A—Stability testing for new drug substances and products (R2-2003)
Q1B—Stability testing of new drug substances and products (1996)
Q1C—Stability testing for new dosage forms (1996)
Q1D—Bracketing and matrixing designs for stability testing for new drugs substance and products (2002)
Q1E—Evaluation of stability data (2003)
Q5C—Stability testing of biotechnological/biological products (1995)

TABLE 15.2

EU EMA Stability Guidelines on Biologicals

CPMP/QWP/609/96	Declaration of storage condition
CPMP/QWP/2934/99	In-use stability testing
CPMP/QWP/159/96	Maximum shelf-life for sterile products after first opening or following reconstitution

parent guideline published in 1993, which defines the stability data package for registration of a new molecular entity as a drug substance/drug product. ICH Q1B makes recommendations on photostability testing, while ICH Q1C gives some recommendations on new dosage forms for authorized medicinal products. ICH Q1D provides specific principles for the bracketing and matrixing designs for stability studies. ICH Q1E suggests how to establish shelf-life or retest period based on the performed stability studies. The ICH Q5C is the main reference for biological medicinal substances and products. However, the principles defined in ICH Q1 guidelines are also applicable.

Table 15.2 lists guidances on stability by EU EMA. As can be seen from Table 15.2, CPMP/QWP/609/96 provides a declaration of storage conditions. CPMP/QWP/2934/99 focuses on in-use stability testing, while CPMP/QWP/159/96 discusses maximum shelf-life for sterile products after first opening or following reconstitution. It should be noted that although regulatory requirements for stability testing for biologics from EU EMA are slightly different from those of ICH, they are similar enough for the harmonization of regulatory requirements for stability testing of biosimilars. Thus, in this chapter, we shall focus on the ICH Q5C stability guideline for biological products.

15.2.2 ICH Q5C Stability Guideline

15.2.2.1 Scope

The ICH Q5C stability guideline was published as an annex to the Tripartite ICH *Guideline for Stability of New Drug Substance and Products*. ICH Q5C intends to give guidance to applicants regarding the type of stability studies to be provided in support of marketing authorization applications for biological medicinal products. The ICH Q5C applies to well-characterized proteins and polypeptides, their derivatives, and products of which they are components, and which are isolated from tissues, body fluids, cell cultures, or produced using rDNA technology. Table 15.3 lists medicinal products covered by ICH Q5C.

15.2.2.2 Batch Selection

As indicated by the ICH Q5C guideline, stability evaluation should be done on active substances (bulk material), intermediates, and medicinal products

TABLE 15.3

Coverage of ICH Q5C Stability Guideline

Cover	Does Not Cover
Cytokines (IFN, IL, CSF, TNF)	Antibiotics
EPO	Allergenic extracts
Plasminogen activators	Heparins
Blood products	Vitamins
Growth hormones	Whole blood
Insulins	Cellular/blood components
Monoclonal antibodies	products
Vaccines	

(final container products). For stability data of drug substances, the ICH Q5C requires at least three batches representative of the manufacturing scale of production to be tested. Representative data are referred to as representative of (1) the quality of batches used in pre-clinical and clinical studies, (2) the manufacturing process and storage conditions, and (3) containers/closures. If the shelf-life to be claimed is longer than 6 months, a minimum of 6 months stability data at the time of submission should be submitted. On the other hand, if the shelf-life to be claimed is less than 6 months, the minimum amount of stability data in the initial submission should be determined on a case-by-case basis. Data from pilot-plant-scale batches of an active substance produced at a reduced scale of fermentation and purification may be provided at the time the dossier is submitted to the regulatory agencies with a commitment to place the first three manufacturing scale batches into a long-term stability program after approval.

In practice, stability data for intermediates may be critical to the production of a finished product. Thus, hold time and storage steps should be identified. The ICH Q5C suggests that the manufacturer should generate in-house data and process limits that assure their stability within the bounds of the developed process. Along this line, appropriate validation and/or stability studies should be performed.

For stability data of the final drug product, similarly, the ICH Q5C guideline requires at least three batches representative of the manufacturing scale of the production being tested. Drug product batches should be derived from different batches of the drug substance. If the shelf-life to be claimed is longer than 6 months, a minimum of 6 months of stability data at the time of submission should be submitted. On the other hand, if the shelf-life to be claimed is less than 6 months, the minimum amount of stability data in the initial submission should be determined on a case-by-case basis. Shelf-life should be derived from representative real-time/real-conditions data. Data can be provided during the review and evaluation process. Here, representative data are referred to as representative of (1) the quality of batches used in pre-clinical and clinical studies, (2) manufacturing process and storage conditions, and (3) the use of final containers/closures.

15.2.2.3 Study Design

Regarding study design and sample selection criteria, the ICH Q5C guideline recommends that a bracketing design or a matrixing design be used (see, e.g., Chow, 1992; Helboe, 1992; Carstenson et al., 1992; Nordbrock, 1989, 1991, 1994a,b,c; Fairweather et al., 1994; DeWoody and Raghavarao, 1997; Pong and Raghavarao, 2000; Chow, 2007). Samples can then be selected for the stability program on the basis of a matrixing system and/or by bracketing. A bracketing design is a design that only samples on the extremes of certain design factors which are tested at all time points. Stability at the intermediate levels is considered being represented by the stability of the extremes. Bracketing is generally not applicable for drug substances. Bracketing can be applied to studies with multiple strength of identical or closely related formulation. In this case, only samples on the extremes of certain design factors (e.g., strength, container size, fill) are tested at all time points. A bracketing design can also be applied to studies with the same container closure system with either the fill volume and/or the container size change.

A matrixing design is a statistical design of a stability study that allows different fractions of samples to be tested at different sampling time points (see, e.g., Nordbrock, 1992; Chow, 2007). Each subset of samples represents the stability of all samples at a given time point. Differences in the samples should be identified as covering different batches, different strengths, and different sizes of the same container closure system. A matrixing design should be balanced such that each combination of a factor is tested to the same extent over the duration of the studies. It should be noted that all samples should be tested at the last time point before the submission of application. For the purpose of illustration, the following examples exhibit matrixing in a long-term stability study for one storage condition: (1) one-half reduction eliminates one in every two time points (Table 15.4) and (2) one-third design eliminates one in every three time points (Table 15.5).

15.2.2.4 Storage Conditions

The ICH Q5C guideline also defines storage conditions such as humidity, temperature, accelerated/stress conditions, light, container/closure, and stability after reconstitution of the freeze-dried product. The ICH Q5C indicates that products are generally distributed in containers protecting against humidity. If it is demonstrated that containers (storage conditions) provide sufficient protection against high and low humidity, relative humidities can be omitted. If humidity protecting containers are not used, appropriate data should be provided. While most biologics need precisely defined storage temperatures, real-time/real-temperature studies are confined to the proposed

TABLE 15.4

Example of Matrixing Design—One-Half
Reduction

Strength	Time Point (Months)							
	0	3	6	9	12	18	24	36
S1								
Batch 1	T	T		T	T		T	T
Batch 2	T	T		T	T	T		T
Batch 3	T		T		T	T		T
S2								
Batch 1	T		T		T		T	T
Batch 2	T	T		T	T	T		T
Batch 3	T		T		T		T	T

Key: T = Sample tested.

TABLE 15.5

Example of Matrixing Design—One-Third
Reduction

Strength	Time Point (Months)							
	0	3	6	9	12	18	24	36
S1								
Batch 1	T	T		T	T		T	T
Batch 2	T	T	T		T	T		T
Batch 3	T		T	T	T	T	T	T
S2								
Batch 1	T		T	T	T	T	T	T
Batch 2	T	T		T	T		T	T
Batch 3	T	T	T		T			T

Key: T = Sample tested.

storage temperature. Requirements for light should be evaluated on a case-by-case basis. For accelerated and stress conditions, shelf-life is established based on real-time/real-temperature data. In practice, accelerated studies can not only be supportive to established shelf-life but also provide information on post-development changes, the validation of stability indicating tests. Accelerated testing conditions are normally one step higher than real storage conditions, which will help in elucidating the degradation profile. Stress testing can not only determine the best product stability indicators but also reveal patterns of degradation. They are representative of accidental exposures to other conditions. The ICH Q5C guideline indicates that accelerated and stress conditions should be carefully selected on a case-by-case basis. ICH Q1A recommends accelerated conditions (Table 15.6) related to long-term studies (ICH Q1A addresses climatic zones I and II).

TABLE 15.6

Accelerated Testing Conditions

Long Term	Accelerated	Stress
≤−20° ± 5°C	+5°C ± 3°C and/or +25°C ± 2°C/60%RH	Temperature, pH, light, oxidation, shaking, freeze/thaw, etc.
+5°C ± 3°C	+25°C ± 2°C/60%RH	
+25°C ± 2°C/60%RH or +35°C ± 2°C/65%RH	+40°C ± 2°C/75%RH	

TABLE 15.7

Recommended Testing Intervals

Stability Demonstration			
Long Term	Accelerated (6 Months)	Storage Statement	Additional Statement[a]
+25°C ± 2°C/60%RH or +30°C ± 2°C/65%RH	+40 ± 2°C/75%RH	No special storage conditioned	Do not refrigerate or freeze
+25°C ± 2°C/60%RH or +30°C ± 2°C/65%RH	—	Do not store above +30°C or +25°C	Do not refrigerate or freeze
+5°C ± 3°C	—	Store at +2°C to +8°C	Do not freeze
<0°C	—	Store at −XX°C	—

[a] Where relevant.

15.2.2.5 Testing Frequency

Shelf-lives for biological products usually vary. ICH stability guidelines are based on shelf-lives of 6 months to 5 years for most biological products. The recommended testing intervals for long-term studies in pre-licensing are given in Table 15.7.

15.2.2.6 General Principles

The ICH stability guideline suggests the following general principles for the evaluation of stability of biosimilar products. These general principles indicate that the applicant should

1. Develop data to support the claimed shelf-life.
2. Consider any external conditions affecting potency, purity, and quality.
3. The primary data to support the requested shelf-life should be based on long-term, real-time, real-condition stability studies. The design of the long-term stability program is critical.
4. Retest periods are not appropriate for biotech/biological.

15.3 Stability Indicating Profile and Expiration Dating Period

15.3.1 Stability Indicating Assay

In practice, there is no single assay indicating stability. The stability indicating assay should be product-specific and allow the detection of any changes in purity, identity, and potency. The analytical methods must be validated at the time of submission. Stability studies for biologics and biosimilars can require a diverse range of protein analysis techniques conducted in accordance with GLP or cGMP requirements such as

1. 1-D and 2-D SDS–PAGE
2. Western blot
3. Isoelectric focusing
4. Amino acid analysis
5. Capillary electrophoresis (CE)
6. Peptide fingerprinting
7. Peptide mapping and sequencing by LC–MS/MS
8. Total protein quantification
9. Glycan characterization
10. Immunochemistry techniques
11. cGMP cell-based bioassays

Note that alternative analytical techniques may also be required to investigate post-translational modifications such as

1. Di-sulfide bridge mapping by MALDI–MS
2. Carbohydrate analysis
3. Higher-order structure characterization by CD, NMR, FTIR
4. Protein aggregation state analysis by dynamic light scattering

15.3.2 Expiration Dating Period

As indicated in the 1987 FDA stability guideline and the 1993 ICH stability guideline, the expiration dating period of a drug product can be determined as the time at which the average drug characteristic remains within an approved specification (e.g., USP/NF) after manufacture (FDA, 1987; ICH, 1993; Chow, 2007). FDA suggests that an expiration dating period of a drug product be determined as the time point at which the 95% lower confidence bound of the mean drug characteristic intersects the approved lower specification of the drug product. The use of the one-sided 95% lower confidence bound of the mean degradation of the drug product is to assure that the drug product will remain within the approved specification for the identity, strength, quality, and purity prior to the expiration date.

FDA's approach for determination of the expiration dating period of a given batch of a drug product is briefly described in the following. For a given batch, let y_j be the assay result at a time x_j, $j = 1, 2, ..., n$. The following simple linear model is usually assumed:

$$y_j = \alpha + \beta x_j + e_j, \quad j = 1, ..., n,$$

where α and β are unknown parameters, x_j's are deterministic time points (storage times) selected in the stability study, and e_j's are measurement errors independently and identically distributed as a normal (Gaussian) random variable with mean 0 and variance σ^2. According to the method suggested by the FDA, for a fixed time point, the 95% lower confidence bound for $\alpha + \beta x$ is given by

$$L(x) = \hat{\alpha} + \hat{\beta} x - \hat{\sigma} t_{n-2} \sqrt{\frac{1}{n} + \frac{(x - \bar{x})^2}{S_{xx}}}$$

where
t_{n-2} is the 95th percentile of the t-distribution with $n-2$ degrees of freedom
$\bar{x}$ is the average of x_j's

$$\hat{\sigma}^2 = \frac{1}{n-2} \left(\frac{S_{yy} - S_{xy}^2}{S_{xx}} \right)$$

in which

$$S_{yy} = \sum_{j=1}^{n} (y_j - \bar{y})^2 \quad S_{xx} = \sum_{j=1}^{n} (x_j - \bar{x})^2 \quad S_{xy} = \sum_{j=1}^{n} (x_j - \bar{x})(y_j - \bar{y})$$

and $\bar{y}$ is the average of y_j's

In practice, if $L(x)$ is larger than the lower product specification, we claim that the product meets the product specification up to the time x.

15.4 Stability Designs

Since stability data are analyzed using a linear regression, the selection of observations that will give the minimum variance for the slope is made by taking one-half at the beginning of the study and one-half at the end.

The beginning of the stability study is usually called $t = 0$. Stability studies are typically done at several different times. In practice, there is no unique best design. Thus, the choice of design must use the fact that analyses will be done after additional data are collected. Nordbrock (1992; 2003) introduced several designs that are commonly considered in stability studies. These designs are briefly described later.

15.4.1 Basic Matrix 2/3 on Time Design

A complete long-term study for one strength of a dosage form in one package has three batches, with all three tested every 3 months in the first year, every 6 months in the second year, and annually thereafter. Thus if a 36 month shelf-life is desired and the complete study is used, each of the three batches is tested at 0, 3, 6, 9, 12, 18, 24, and 36 months. The basic matrix 2/3 on time design has only two of the three batches tested at intermediate time points (other than at times of 0 and 36), as presented in Table 15.8. If an analysis is to be done after 18 months (e.g., for a registration application), the basic matrix 2/3 on time design can be modified by testing all batches at 18 months.

15.4.2 Matrix 2/3 on Time Design with Multiple Packages

The first extension of the basic design is when one strength is packaged into three packages (i.e., when each batch is packaged into each of three packages). The basic matrix 2/3 on time design is applied to each package in a balanced fashion, as presented in Tables 15.9 and 15.10. *Balance* is defined as each batch is tested twice at each intermediate time point, and each package

TABLE 15.8

Basic Matrix 2/3 on Time Design

Batch			Test Times					
A	0	3		9	12			24	36
B	0	3	6		12	18		36
C	0		6	9		18	24	36

TABLE 15.9

Matrix 2/3 on Time Design with Multiple Packages

Batch	Pkg 1	Pkg 2	Pkg 3
A	T1	T2	T3
B	T2	T3	T1
C	T3	T1	T2

Note: Pkg 1 = Package 1, etc.

TABLE 15.10

Test Code Definitions

Code	Test Times after Time 0					
T1	3		9	12		24	36
T2	3	6		12	18		36
T3		6	9		18	24	36

Note: Batches are tested at time 0.

is tested twice at each intermediate time point. If an analysis will be done after 18 months (e.g., for a registration application), this design can be modified by testing all batch-by-package combinations at 18 months.

15.4.3 Matrix 2/3 on Time Design with Multiple Packages and Multiple Strengths

When three strengths (say, 10, 20, and 30) are manufactured using different weights of the same formulation, giving nine sub-batches, we further assume that there are three packages for each strength. In this case, the basic matrix 2/3 on time design can be applied to each of the nine sub-batches in a balanced fashion (see Table 15.11). In this design, each sub-batch is tested twice at each intermediate time point, each package is tested twice at each intermediate time point for each batch, each batch is tested six times at each intermediate time point, and each package is tested six times at each intermediate time point. If an analysis will be done after 18 months (e.g., for a registration application), this design can be modified by testing all batch-by-strength-by-package combinations at 18 months.

TABLE 15.11

Matrix 2/3 on Time Design with Multiple Packages and Multiple Strengths

Batch	Strength	Pkg 1	Pkg 2	Pkg 3
A	10	T1	T2	T3
A	20	T2	T3	T1
A	30	T3	T1	T2
B	10	T2	T3	T1
B	20	T3	T1	T2
B	30	T1	T2	T3
C	10	T3	T1	T2
C	20	T1	T2	T3
C	30	T2	T3	T1

Note: Pkg 1 = Package 1, etc.

TABLE 15.12

Basic Matrix 1/3 on Time Design

Batch	Test Times						
A	0	3		12			36
B	0		6		18		36
C	0			9		24	36

15.4.4 Matrix 1/3 on Time Design

A further reduction in the amount of testing is accomplished by reducing the testing in each of the preceding designs from 2/3 to 1/3. For example, the basic 1/3 on time design has one of the three batches tested at each intermediate time point, as presented in Table 15.12. If an analysis will be done after 18 months (e.g., for a registration application), the basic matrix 1/3 on time design can be modified by testing all batches at 18 months.

15.4.5 Matrix on Batch × Strength × Package Combinations

If there are multiple strengths and multiple packages, one could also choose to test only a portion of the batch-by-strength-by-package combinations. An example of when this might be appropriate is when there are three batches, each made into two strengths, giving six sub-batches. Although three packages will be used, the batch size is small and only two packages can be manufactured in each strength sub-batch. A matrix design on batch × strength × package combinations is presented in Table 15.13, with two packages selected for each of the six sub-batches, and where time is also matrixed by the factor 1/2. This design is approximately balanced because two packages are tested per sub-batch, one or two strengths are tested for each selected package by batch, four sub-batches are tested for each package, etc. Similar statements for the balance on time can be made.

TABLE 15.13

Matrix 1/2 on Time and Matrix on Batch × Strength × Package

Batch	Strength	Pkg 1	Pkg 2	Pkg 3
A	10	T1	T2	—
A	20	T2	—	T1
B	10	T2	—	T1
B	20	—	T1	T2
C	10	—	T1	T2
C	20	T1	T2	—

15.4.6 Uniform Matrix Design

Another approach to design is the uniform matrix design, for which the same time protocol is used for all combinations of the other design factors (Murphy, 1996). The strategy is to delete certain times (e.g., 3, 6, 9, and 18 month time points); therefore, testing is done only at 12, 24, and 36 months. This design has the advantages of simplifying the data entry of the study design and eliminating time points that add little to reducing the variability of the slope of the regression line. The disadvantage is that if there are major problems with the stability, there is no early warning because early testing is not done. Further, it may not be possible to determine if the linear model is appropriate (e.g., it may not be possible to determine whether there is an immediate decrease followed by very little decrease). However, the major disadvantage is that this design is probably not acceptable to some regulatory agencies.

15.4.7 Comparison of Designs

Nordbrock (1992, 2003) compared designs based on the power approach. This approach computes the probability that a statistical test will be significant when there is a specified alternative slope configuration. Power can be computed easily in SAS. The strategy is to compute power for several designs and then to choose the design that has acceptable power and the smallest sample size (or cost). Acceptable power is not well defined at this stage. Other methods of comparing designs are given in Ju and Chow (1995) and Pong and Raghavarao (2000), where the criterion is the precision for estimating shelf-life.

When evaluating designs, it is also important to answer the question "What is the probability of being able to defend the desired shelf-life with the study?" (see, e.g., Nordbrock, 2003). In other words (assuming that the parameter is expected to decrease over time), what is the probability that the 95% one-sided lower confidence bound for the slope will be acceptable for specified values of the slope(s) for particular subsets of data, which may include, for example, only one strength and/or only one package? It is important to know at the design stage what the statistical penalty (with respect to shelf-life) might be if differences among packages and/or strengths are found. Similarly, Nordbrock (2009) compared matrix designs to full designs using the probability of achieving the desired shelf-life.

15.4.8 Factors Acceptable to Matrix

In the foregoing, examples have been used to present possible matrix designs. In this section, a summary of when it is acceptable to matrix is given based on a document prepared by the PhRMA Stability Working

Group (Nordbrock and Valvani, 1995), on FDA presentations (Chen, 1996; Lin, 1997) and on ICH Q1D.

1. It is acceptable to matrix at all stages of development for a drug product and also for a drug substance. It is acceptable for new drug application (NDA) studies, investigational new drug application (IND) studies, supplements, and marketed product studies.

2. It is acceptable to matrix for all types of products, such as solids, semisolids, liquids, and aerosols.

3. It is acceptable to matrix after bracketing.

4. It is acceptable to matrix when there are multiple sources of raw materials (e.g., drug products).

5. It is acceptable to matrix if there are multiple sites of drug product manufacture.

6. It is acceptable to matrix when identical formulations are manufactured into several strengths.

7. It is acceptable to matrix if formulations are closely related (e.g., difference in colorant or flavoring).

8. Matrixing is applicable to the orientation of container during storage.

9. Matrixing may be acceptable in certain cases when closely related formulations are used for different strengths (e.g., if an inactive is replaced by an active).

10. Matrix across container and closure systems may be applicable if justified.

11. It is acceptable to matrix within a package composition type, e.g., of different sizes if the fill (i.e., head space) is the same, or if of the same size but different fills (head space). It may be acceptable to matrix if the container size and fill size change, if there is an adequate explanation. It is not acceptable to matrix across package composition types (e.g., blisters and HDPE).

12. It is not acceptable to matrix across storage conditions. However, it is acceptable to do a separate matrix design for each storage condition.

13. It is not acceptable to matrix across parameters, such as dissolution and potency. However, it is acceptable to do a separate design for each parameter.

14. Matrixing is applicable regardless of the method precision; however, it should be remembered that when using a matrix design, the resulting shelf-life is generally shorter than when a complete design is used. Also, when the method precision is larger, the difference between a complete design and a matrixed design will be larger (i.e., a larger penalty to the sponsor, resulting in a shorter shelf-life for the matrix design than the complete design).

15. Matrixing is applicable regardless of the stability of the product. However, comments similar to those in the preceding point apply, and it should be remembered that if a product has a poor stability profile (e.g., a shelf-life of 1 year), matrixing will usually result in an even shorter shelf-life.

16. The latest guideline should be consulted for applicability.

15.4.9 General Rules

Several general rules should be followed when designing studies:

1. Matrix designs should be approximately balanced (i.e., for all one-way, two-way combinations of batch, package, and strength that are ever tested, approximately the same number of tests should be done cumulatively to every time point).

2. When every batch-by-strength-by-package combination is not tested, every strength-by-package combination that is ever tested should be tested in at least two batches (i.e., for every package-by-strength combination that is ever tested, there should be at least two batches tested).

3. Unless there are manufacturing restrictions such as in the foregoing example, it is probably acceptable to matrix on batch × strength × package combinations only when there are more than three strengths or more than three packages.

15.5 Statistical Analysis

Although there may be instances when a linear regression is not appropriate, the rest of this discussion assumes that a straight-line linear regression of the parameter of interest on time is relevant. Further, it is assumed that the parameter of interest is expected to decrease over time. For long-term data with a single package and a single strength, the ICH Q1E Guidance (ICH Q1E, 2004) specifies that the 95% one-sided lower confidence bound for the mean regression line must be above the lower specification at all times prior to the shelf-life. When there are multiple strengths and/or multiple packages, according to ICH Q1E, there are three possible approaches for analysis. The first approach is to analyze each package-by-strength combination separately—in other words, to do multiple analyses. The second approach is to model all data with one analysis, with separate intercepts and separate slopes for each batch by strength by package, without testing for poolability, so there is no reduced model. The third approach is to model all data with one analysis and test for poolability and then select the appropriate reduced model.

15.5.1 Separate Analysis Approach

In the first approach, multiple analyses are conducted, with a separate analysis of each package-by-strength-by-batch. A shelf-life is calculated for each of the separate analyses, and the product shelf-life is the minimum of all the package-by-strength-by-batch shelf-lives.

15.5.2 One Analysis Approach without Testing Poolability

In the second approach, one analysis is done which includes all data. A shelf-life is estimated using individual intercepts, individual slopes, and the pooled mean square error from the entire data set. Shelf-life for each batch-by-package-by-strength is taken as the time the batch-by-package-by-strength remains within acceptable limits, i.e., the time that the 95% one-sided lower confidence bound for the mean regression line remains above specification.

If there are multiple batches but only one package and one strength, the SAS model is $Y = B + A + B \times A$, where B is a class term for batch and A is the covariate for age. The 95% one-sided lower confidence bound for the mean regression line is calculated for each batch. The shelf-life of each batch is such that the confidence bound is within the specification at all times prior to the shelf-life. The shelf-life of the product is the minimum of the batch shelf-lives.

If there are multiple batches and multiple packages but only one strength, and if the initials for a particular batch are applicable to all packages, then the SAS model is $Y = B + A + B \times A + P \times A + B \times P \times A$, where B is a class term for batch, P is a class term for package, and A is the covariate for age. This model has separate slopes for each batch-by-package, separate intercepts for each batch, and a common intercept for all packages from the same batch. For example, if initials are tested using a bulk product (before the product is packaged), and all packages are entered into the study at the same time, then this model is typically appropriate. The 95% one-sided lower confidence bound for the mean regression line is calculated for each batch by package. The shelf-life of each batch-by-package is such that the confidence bound is within the specification at all times prior to the shelf-life. The shelf-life of the product is the minimum of all batch-by-package shelf-lives.

15.5.3 One Analysis Testing Poolability

When using the model-building (poolability test) approach, it is very important that the full model reflect the manufacturing process. In this section, it is assumed that there are multiple strengths and multiple packages and that a batch is manufactured into multiple strengths by using different weights of the same exact formulation. It is assumed that a granulation batch is split into sub-batches, where each sub-batch is manufactured into a different-strength product using different weights of the granulation, and it is assumed that every strength is manufactured from every granulation batch. It is further assumed that the time 0 samples are collected from each tablet sub-batch, and every tablet sub-batch is packaged into all packages.

The full model includes slope terms for all two-way interactions of package, strength, and batch, and it includes intercept terms that reflect the manufacturing process. The manufacturing process dictates that each tablet sub-batch must have a separate intercept in the full model, but there is no need to allow packages in each tablet sub-batch to have separate intercepts. (Process validation provides evidence that the entire tablet sub-batch is uniform.)

Thus in the example, the full SAS model is

$$Y = B + S + B(S) + A + B \times A + P \times A + S \times A + B \times P \times A + B \times S \times A$$
$$+ P \times S \times A,$$

with B as a class term for granulation batch, P as a class term for package, S as a class term for strength, and A as a covariate for time. The model building begins by testing the slope two-way interactions to determine if any can be deleted, using a significance level of 0.25 when the batch is part of the term and 0.05 otherwise. Then the main-effect slope terms are tested, using the 0.25 (batch) or 0.05 (not batch) level. Terms that are not significant are deleted, except that any main-effect slope included in a non-deleted two-way slope term cannot be deleted.

After deleting slope terms, the intercept terms are tested (using the same criterion for significance as was used for slopes) and insignificant terms are deleted. Using the final model, the 95% one-sided lower confidence bound for the mean regression line(s) is (are) found, and a shelf-life is assigned for each package-by-strength combination such that the 95% one-sided lower confidence bound(s) is (are) within specification at all times prior to the shelf-life. Slightly different algorithms for deleting terms from the full model have been proposed (Fairweather et al., 1995; Tsong et al., 2008).

Note that SAS programs for analysis of stability data developed by FDA statisticians are given in Chow (2007).

15.6 Concluding Remarks

Biological substances are complex molecules which include primary structure (e.g., the amino acid sequence of polypeptide chain), secondary structure (e.g., α-helix, β-sheet—stabilized by hydrogen bonds), tertiary structure (e.g., the three-dimensional structure of a single molecule folded into a compact globule, stabilized by non-specific hydrophobic interactions and specific interactions such as salt bridges, H-bonds, and –S–S-bonds), and quaternary structure (e.g., assembly of several polypeptide chains: no-covalent interactions, –S–S-bonds). Thus, biological products are particularly sensitive to environmental factors such as temperature, oxidation, light, and ionic content. In practice, stringent conditions for storage are usually necessary. As a result, the evaluation of stability may necessitate complex analytical methodologies. Physicochemical tests alone are insufficient to characterize the product sufficiently to permit prediction of the biological activity. In practice, the most commonly employed analytical tests include tests for deamidation (e.g., hydrolysis of asparagine and glutamine side chain amides), oxidation (e.g., of methionine, histidine, cysteine, tyrosine, and tryptophane residues), denaturation (e.g., loss of three-dimensional structure), aggregation (e.g., association of monomers or native multimers, covalent or non-covalent), and glycoproteins (e.g., most common instability of glycosylation hydrolysis of sialic acid residues).

As indicated earlier, during the early development of biosimilar products, accelerated stability studies can help provide key data and information on the effect of short-term exposure to environmental conditions. Short-term stability studies are typically performed over a 6 month period. Long-term stability studies (12 months and longer) allow evaluation of the quality of the drug both during and beyond its projected shelf-life. Matrix designs described in this chapter are generally applicable to many situations and can result in significant savings, with the 1/3 matrix on time readily acceptable for stable products. There are two basic approaches when analyzing data from a matrix design. There are several methods used to evaluate and to compare potential designs.

For the estimation of expiration dating period (or shelf-life) of a drug, the FDA stability guideline requires that at least three batches, and preferably more, be tested in a stability analysis to account for batch-to-batch variation so that a single shelf-life is applicable to all future batches manufactured under similar circumstances. Under the assumption that the drug characteristic decreases linearly over time, the FDA stability guideline indicates that if there is no documented evidence for batch-to-batch variation (i.e., all the batches have the same shelf-life), the single shelf-life can be determined, based on the ordinary least-squares method, as the time point at which the 95% lower confidence bound for the degradation curve of the drug characteristic intersects the approved lower specification limit. Along this line, a typical approach is to perform a stability analysis by combining the three batches as *fixed batches*. This method is referred to as stability analysis with fixed batches. However, as indicated in the 1987 FDA stability guideline, the batches used in long-term stability studies for the establishment of a drug shelf-life should constitute a random sample from the population of future population batches. In addition, the guideline requires that all estimated expiration dating periods be applicable to all future batches. In this case, a stability analysis with fixed batches may not be appropriate. Alternatively, it is suggested that statistical methods based on a random-effects model be considered (see, e.g., Chow and Shao, 1991; Shao and Chow, 1994; Shao and Chen, 1997). This approach is referred to as stability analysis with random batches.

It should be noted that some drug products must be stored at specific temperatures, such as −20°C (frozen temperature), 5°C (refrigerator temperature), and 25°C (room temperature) in order to maintain stability until use. In this case, a typical shelf-life statement usually consists of multiple phases with different storage temperatures. For example, a commonly adopted shelf-life statement could be 24 months at −20°C followed by 2 weeks at 5°C. As a result, the drug shelf-life is determined based on a two-phase stability study. However, no discussion of the statistical methods for the estimation of two-phase shelf-life is available in either the FDA stability guidance or the ICH stability guidelines. Shao and Chow (2001) proposed a method for a two-phase stability study using a two-phase linear regression based on the statistical principle described in both the FDA and the ICH stability guidelines (see also Chow, 2007).

16

Assessing Biosimilarity
Using Biomarker Data

16.1 Introduction

As indicated in Chow and Liu (2008), the assessment of bioequivalence for small-molecule drug products is performed under the *Fundamental Bioequivalence Assumption*. This Assumption considers pharmacokinetic responses such as AUC and C_{max} as surrogate endpoints for clinical endpoints for the evaluation of the safety and efficacy of the drug products under study. Following a similar idea, statistical methods for the assessment of biosimilarity between a biosimilar product and an innovator product can be derived under a *Fundamental Biosimilarity Assumption* and a probability-based criterion for biosimilarity using biomarker data by assuming that the biomarker is predictive of the clinical outcome of the biological products (Chow et al., 2010).

For the assessment of bioequivalence or similarity between drug products, several criteria have been proposed in the literature. For example, criteria for the assessment of average bioequivalence (ABE) based on average of bioavailability, population bioequivalence (PBE) based on total variability of bioavailability, and individual bioequivalence (IBE) based on inter- and intra-subject variabilities and the variability due to subject-by-product interaction have been proposed in the FDA guidances (see, e.g., FDA, 2001, 2003). Among these criteria for the assessment of bioequivalence, a common ground is that the comparison is moment-based, i.e., the comparison is based on the moments of the two populations. Alternatively, probability-based criteria, which are based on the comparison of the probabilities, have also been proposed to evaluate equivalence/similarity. For example, Schall and Luus (1993) proposed a probability-based measure for the expected discrepancy in pharmacokinetic (PK) responses between drug products, which is based on the probability that the absolute difference of PK responses between drug products is smaller than a pre-specified positive constant. Tse et al. (2006) proposed a probability-based index for traditional Chinese medicine to assess the *consistency* between raw materials from different resources and/or between final products by different manufacturing processes. The consistency index is defined by the probability that the ratio of characteristics of the products from different resources is within a pre-specified interval. Thus, following these ideas, the similarity of two drugs can be assessed by measures which are either moment-based or probability-based.

For some drug products, the FDA indicates that an in vitro dissolution test may serve as a surrogate for an in vivo bioequivalence test by comparing the corresponding dissolution profiles. Two drug products are considered to have similar drug absorption profiles if their dissolution profiles (measurement of drug release) are similar. These drug products include (1) pre-1962 classified "AA" drug products; (2) lower strength products; (3) scale-up and post-approval changes; (4) products demonstrating in vitro and in vivo correlation (Chow and Shao, 2002). Along this line, two drug products may be considered to have similar drug absorption profiles if their genomic profiles are similar, provided that there is a relationship between PK and genomic data and/or an appropriate adjustment is made to account for their difference. Thus, Chow et al. (2004) proposed to use genomic prediction as a surrogate for the PK response in assessing bioequivalence. The objective of this chapter is to derive statistical methods for the assessment of average biosimilarity using biomarker(s) data according to both the moment-based criterion and the probability-based criterion under a parallel-group design, assuming that the biomarker(s) is/are predictive of clinical outcomes for the evaluation of safety and efficacy of the follow-on biologics.

In the next section, moment-based and probability-based criteria for the assessment of biosimilarity currently available in regulatory guidelines/guidances or the literature are briefly reviewed. Following a similar idea of Chow et al. (2004), statistical methods for the assessment of biosimilarity using biomarker data are derived under both moment-based and probability-based criteria in Section 16.3. In Section 16.4, a numerical study was conducted to evaluate the performance of the derived methods under both the moment-based and probability-based criteria. Brief concluding remarks are given in the last section.

16.2 Assessment of Biosimilarity

16.2.1 Moment- and Probability-Based Criteria

In this section, we shall focus on both moment-based and probability-based criteria to assess biosimilarity between biological products. In particular, the following criteria are considered. Let Y_T and Y_R be the same study endpoints of interest for the test product T and reference product R, respectively. In particular, $E(Y_i) = \mu_i$, $i = T, R$.

16.2.1.1 *Moment-Based Criterion*

The two biological products are concluded to be biosimilar if the 90% confidence interval for μ_T/μ_R falls within the similarity limit of $(1 - \Delta, 1/1 - \Delta)$, where $0 < \Delta < 1$ is a pre-specified constant.

16.2.1.2 *Probability-Based Criterion*

The two biological products are biosimilar if the 90% confidence lower bound of p is larger than p_0, where $0 < p_0 < 1$ is a similarity limit and

$$p = P\left\{1 - \delta < \frac{Y_T}{Y_R} < \frac{1}{1 - \delta}\right\}, \tag{16.1}$$

with $0 < \delta < 1$ as a pre-specified constant.

16.2.2 Assessing Biosimilarity Using Genomic Data

As indicated earlier, Chow et al. (2004) proposed to use the genomic prediction x as a surrogate for the PK response in assessing bioequivalence. Their idea is briefly outlined in the following. Let x be a genomic prediction of a PK response under consideration. Typically, x is a function of genomic data such as genetic markers, DNA sequence, mRNA transcription profiling, linkage and physical maps, gene location, and quantitative trait loci (QTL) mapping. In this chapter, the genomic prediction x is used as a surrogate for the PK response in assessing biosimilarity. More specifically, if we can claim biosimilarity between two drug products using x in place of the PK response but the same statistical test designed for PK data, can we claim biosimilarity between the two drug products without a bioavailability/bioequivalence study? The answer is affirmative if x is a perfect prediction of the PK response. In practice, however, genomic prediction is usually not perfect, because of the existence of variability, model misspecification, and/or missing important genomic variables. The idea of Chow et al. (2004) is to evaluate the impact of the differences between the distribution of the genomic prediction and PK response on the assessment of bioequivalence/biosimilarity. For ABE, a tolerance limit for this difference was derived so that if the difference is within the tolerance limit, then ABE can be assessed by using the genomic prediction.

Consider the usual model under a standard 2×2 crossover design as described in Chinchilli and Estinhart (1996):

$$y_{ijk} = \mu_i + \gamma_{ij} + S_{ijk} + e_{ijk},$$

where

μ_i is the ith treatment effect ($i = T, R$)

γ_{ij} is the fixed effect of treatment i in the sequence j with constraint $\sum_j \gamma_{ik} = 0$ for each i

(S_{Tjk}, S_{Rjk}) are the random effects of the kth subject in the jth sequence that are independent and identically distributed bivariate normal random vectors with mean 0 and $\text{Var}(S_{ijk}) = \sigma_{Bi}^2$, $i = T, R$, and $\text{Cov}(S_{Tjk}, S_{Rjk}) = \rho\sigma_{BT}\sigma_{BR}$

e_{ijk} are independent normal random errors with mean 0 and $\text{Var}(e_{ijk}) = \sigma_{Wi}^2$, $i = T, R$

(S_{Tjk}, S_{Rjk}) and e_{ijk} are assumed independent

Let x be the genomic prediction of y. One of the concerns is how to test ABE by using x_{ijk}, the genomic prediction of y_{ijk}. Chow et al. (2004) assume that x_{ijk} values follow the same model of y_{ijk} but with all parameters changed. In particular, treatment effects μ are changed to v values and variance components σ^2's are changed to τ^2 values. Chow et al. (2004) then defined

$$\epsilon = (\mu_T - \mu_R) - (v_T - v_R).$$

Note that $\epsilon = 0$ if the genomic predictions are unbiased. Because of possible model misspecification and/or missing important genomic variables, however, ϵ may not be 0. Let $\bar{y}$ or $\bar{x}$ be the average of y-values or x-values with a dot in the subscript indicating over which index is being averaged. Also, let

$$\hat{\delta}_y = \bar{y}_{T..} - \bar{y}_{R..}$$

and

$$s_y^2 = \frac{1}{n_1 + n_2 - 2} \sum_{j,k} (y_{Tjk} - y_{Rjk} - \bar{y}_{Tj\cdot} + \bar{y}_{Rj\cdot})^2.$$

Then, $\hat{\delta}_y$ is normally distributed with mean $\delta = \mu_T - \mu_R$ and $(n_1 + n_2 - 2)s_y^2/\sigma^2$ is chi-square distributed with $n_1 + n_2 - 2$ degrees of freedom, where

$$\sigma = \sigma_{BT}^2 + \sigma_{BR}^2 - 2\rho\sigma_{BT}\sigma_{BR} + \sigma_{WT}^2 + \sigma_{WR}^2$$

$\hat{\delta}_y$ and s_y^2 are independent.

According to the 2003 FDA guidance on bioequivalence, ABE can be claimed if the 90% confidence interval for δ, denoted by $(\hat{\delta}_{y-}, \hat{\delta}_{y+})$, falls within $(-\eta, \eta)$, where

$$\hat{\delta}_{y\pm} = \hat{\delta}_y \pm t_{0.95, n_1 + n_2 - 2} \frac{s_y}{2} \sqrt{\frac{1}{n_1} + \frac{1}{n_2}}$$

$t_{a,m}$ denotes the ath quantile of the central t-distribution with m degrees of freedom.

Now, let $\widehat{\leq \delta}_{x\pm}$ be the same as $\hat{\delta}_{y\pm}$ but calculated with y-data replaced by x-values. If $(\hat{\delta}_{x-}, \hat{\delta}_{x+})$ is within $(-\eta, \eta)$, it is of interest to know whether we can claim ABE. Statistically speaking, if the genomic prediction x is the perfect prediction of y, then we can claim ABE. However, there is a difference between the distributions of y and x. If ϵ is known, then a 90% confidence interval for $\delta = \mu_T - \mu_R$ is $(\hat{\delta}_{x-} + \epsilon, \hat{\delta}_{x+} + \epsilon)$. Consequently, ABE can be claimed if

$$-\eta < \hat{\delta}_{x-} + \epsilon \quad \text{and} \quad \hat{\delta}_{x+} + \epsilon < \eta.$$

The parameter ϵ is typically unknown. If $\epsilon_- \leq \epsilon \leq \epsilon_+$ and the bounds $\epsilon_\pm$ are known, then ABE can be claimed if

$$-\eta < \hat{\delta}_{x-} + \epsilon_- \quad \text{and} \quad \hat{\delta}_{x+} + \epsilon_+ < \eta.$$

The tolerance limits for ε to claim ABE are then given by

$$\hat{\epsilon}_- = -\eta - \hat{\delta}_{x-} \quad \text{and} \quad \hat{\epsilon}_+ = \eta - \hat{\delta}_{x+}.$$

For PBE and IBE, Chow et al. (2004) considered a sensitivity analysis of prediction bias and variation difference within some pre-determined limits. Note that in their study, Chow et al. (2004) assumed that a well-established relationship between PK data and genomic data could be identified and in particular the relationship is assumed to be linear. However, in many cases, this assumption may not be true. Thus, it may be misleading assuming a linear relationship when in fact the relationship is essentially nonlinear. Lu et al. (2009) study the impact of misspecification (or the departure from the linearity) on ABE assessment in terms of controlling type I error and requiring the sample size to achieve a desired power.

16.3 Statistical Test for Biosimilarity Using Biomarker Data

16.3.1 General Idea

For the assessment of biosimilarity, the primary study endpoint may be costly or time-consuming to observe. In such cases, it is desirable to find a surrogate response which is relatively easy or less expensive to observe. Following the ideas of Chow et al. (2004, 2010) proposed a valid statistical test for testing biosimilarity using data collected from surrogate or biomarker endpoints, assuming that there is a well-established relationship between the surrogate endpoint or biomarker and the primary study endpoint. Denote by y the primary study endpoint and by x the surrogate endpoint or biomarker. For simplicity, the following first-order model is considered:

$$\log y_i = \beta_0 + \beta_1 x_i + \varepsilon_i, \tag{16.2}$$

where
β_0 and β_1 are known coefficients
x_i is normally distributed with mean μ_{Xi} and variance σ_{Xi}^2
ε_i are random normal errors with mean 0 and variance σ_{Yi}^2, $i = T, R$
x_i and ε_i are independent

It is easy to show that $\log(y_i)$ is normally distributed with mean $\beta_0 + \beta_1 \mu_{Xi}$ and variance $\beta_1^2 \sigma_{Xi}^2 + \sigma_{Yi}^2$. Since y_i is log-normally distributed

$$E(y_i) = \mu_i = \exp\left\{ \beta_0 + \beta_1 \mu_{Xi} + 0.5(\beta_1^2 \sigma_{Xi}^2 + \sigma_{Yi}^2) \right\}. \tag{16.3}$$

Suppose that the surrogate endpoint or biomarker x is observed from a two-group parallel design. Let x_{ij} be the observation from the jth subject in the ith group, $i = T, R$ and $j = 1, 2, \ldots, n_i$. Let $\hat{y}_{ij} = \exp\{\beta_0 + \beta_1 x_{ij}\}$ be the "predicted" value of the corresponding primary study endpoint. Denote by v_i the expected value of $\hat{y}_{ij}$. Then, based on the aforementioned assumptions,

$$v_i = E(\hat{y}_{ij}) = \exp\left\{ \beta_0 + \beta_1 \mu_{Xi} + 0.5\beta_1^2 \sigma_{Xi}^2 \right\}. \tag{16.4}$$

16.3.2 Moment-Based Criterion for Assessing Biosimilarity

In this section, the confidence interval for the ratio of the means μ_T and μ_R, or equivalently, for $\log \mu_T - \log \mu_R$ is derived under the moment-based criterion. Furthermore, the power of the proposed test for biosimilarity is derived to facilitate the determination of the required sample size to achieve a desired level of power.

16.3.2.1 Confidence Interval Estimation

Similar to the assessment of bioequivalence between two drug products, say, treatment (T) versus reference (R), the following hypotheses are considered to assess biosimilarity between two biological products:

$$H_0 : \frac{\mu_T}{\mu_R} \leq 1 - \Delta \quad \text{or} \quad \frac{\mu_T}{\mu_R} \geq \frac{1}{1-\Delta} \quad \text{versus} \quad H_1 : 1 - \Delta < \frac{\mu_T}{\mu_R} < \frac{1}{1-\Delta},$$

where $0 < \Delta < 1$ is a pre-specified constant; or equivalently

$$H_0 : \left|\log \mu_T - \log \mu_R\right| \geq \delta \quad \text{versus} \quad H_1 : \left|\log \mu_T - \log \mu_R\right| < \delta, \quad (16.5)$$

where δ is a positive constant. From Equations 16.4 and 16.5,

$$\log \mu_T - \log \mu_R = \log v_T - \log v_R + 0.5\sigma_{Wd}^2 = \beta_1 \mu_{Xd} + 0.5\left(\beta_1^2 \sigma_{Xd}^2 + \sigma_{Wd}^2\right), \quad (16.6)$$

where

$$\mu_{Xd} = \mu_{XT} - \mu_{XR}, \quad \sigma_{Wd}^2 = \sigma_{WT}^2 - \sigma_{WR}^2, \quad \text{and} \quad \sigma_{Xd}^2 = \sigma_{XT}^2 - \sigma_{XR}^2.$$

Let

$$\hat{\mu}_{Xi} = \frac{1}{n_i} \sum_{j=1}^{n_i} x_{ij}$$

and

$$\hat{\sigma}_{Xi}^2 = \frac{1}{n_i - 1} \sum_{j=1}^{n_i} (x_{ij} - \hat{\mu}_{Xi})^2, \quad i = T, R.$$

Further, let z_α, $t_{\alpha,n}$ and $\chi_{\alpha,n}^2$ be the αth-quantile of the standard normal distribution, the student t-distribution with n degrees of freedom, and the chi-squared distribution with n degrees of freedom, respectively. Note that it is in general not easy to construct an exact confidence interval for $\log \mu_T - \log \mu_R$, which is a linear combination of parameters involving variance components. However, for this type of parameters, the modified large-sample method (MLS) can be used to give an approximate confidence interval, which has better finite sample performance than many other approximation methods including the normal approximation method. Details can be found in Howe (1974), Graybill and Wang (1980),

Ting et al. (1990), Hyslop et al. (2000). Thus, using the MLS method, a $(1 - 2\alpha) \times 100\%$ confidence interval of $\log v_T - \log v_R$ is given as $(\hat{\eta}_l, \hat{\eta}_u)$, where

$$\hat{\eta}_l = \hat{d}_x - \sqrt{\beta_1^2 \sum_{i=T,R} \frac{\hat{\sigma}_{Xi}^2 t_{1-\alpha,n_i}^2}{n_i} + \frac{1}{4}\beta_1^4 \left[\hat{\sigma}_{XT}^4 \left(\frac{n_T - 1}{\chi_{1-\alpha,n_T-1}^2} - 1 \right)^2 + \hat{\sigma}_{XR}^4 \left(\frac{n_R - 1}{\chi_{\alpha,n_R-1}^2} - 1 \right)^2 \right]},$$

and

$$\hat{\eta}_u = \hat{d}_x + \sqrt{\beta_1^2 \sum_{i=T,R} \frac{\hat{\sigma}_{Xi}^2 t_{1-\alpha,n_i}^2}{n_i} + \frac{1}{4}\beta_1^4 \left[\hat{\sigma}_{XT}^4 \left(\frac{n_T - 1}{\chi_{\alpha,n_T-1}^2} - 1 \right)^2 + \hat{\sigma}_{XR}^4 \left(\frac{n_R - 1}{\chi_{1-\alpha,n_R-1}^2} - 1 \right)^2 \right]},$$

with

$$\hat{d}_x = \log \hat{v}_T - \log \hat{v}_R = \beta_1(\hat{\mu}_{XT} - \hat{\mu}_{XR}) + \frac{1}{2}\beta_1^2 \left(\hat{\sigma}_{XT}^2 - \hat{\sigma}_{XR}^2 \right).$$

The idea of Schuirmann's two one-sided tests can be used to test the hypotheses defined in Equation 16.5 (Schuirmann, 1987). In particular, the null hypothesis H_0 is decomposed into the following two one-sided hypotheses:

$$H_{01} : \log \mu_T - \log \mu_R > \delta \quad \text{and} \quad H_{02} : \log \mu_T - \log \mu_R < -\delta.$$

Equivalently, both H_{01} and H_{02} are rejected at an α-level of significance if the $(1 - 2\alpha)$ confidence interval of $\log \mu_T - \log \mu_R$ falls within $(-\delta, \delta)$.

If σ_{Wd}^2 is known, then a $(1-2\alpha) \times 100\%$ confidence interval for $\log \mu_T - \log \mu_R$ is $(\hat{\eta}_l + 0.5\sigma_{Wd}^2, \hat{\eta}_u + 0.5\sigma_{Wd}^2)$. Consequently, the two biological products are claimed to be biosimilar according to the moment-based criterion if

$$\hat{\eta}_l + 0.5\sigma_{Wd}^2 > -\delta \quad \text{and} \quad \hat{\eta}_u + 0.5\sigma_{Wd}^2 < \delta. \tag{16.7}$$

If σ_{Wd}^2 is unknown, suppose that $\sigma_{Wd-}^2 \leq \sigma_{Wd}^2 \leq \sigma_{Wd+}^2$ with σ_{Wd-}^2 and σ_{Wd+}^2 as the known limits. Then the two biological products are claimed to be biosimilar according to the moment-based criterion if

$$\hat{\eta}_l + 0.5\sigma_{Wd-}^2 > -\delta \quad \text{and} \quad \hat{\eta}_u + 0.5\sigma_{Wd+}^2 < \delta. \tag{16.8}$$

16.3.2.2 Type I Error Rate and Power

Note that $(\hat{\eta}_l, \hat{\eta}_u)$ is a $(1-2\alpha) \times 100\%$ confidence interval for $\log v_T - \log v_R$. If the null hypothesis $H_0 : |\log \mu_T - \log \mu_R| \geq \delta$ is true, the type I error rate of the test for biosimilarity should be controlled at the nominal level α if the rule in

Equation 16.7 is adopted when σ_{Wd}^2 is known. But, if only the bounds for σ_{Wd}^2 are known, the type I error rate depends on the bounds for σ_{Wd}^2. In particular, the type I error rate is smaller for larger bounds. Thus, in general, the rule given in Equation 16.8 is conservative which would lead to a smaller type I error rate than the nominal level α.

Suppose that the primary study endpoint y is observed and biosimilarity is assessed using the y data. Let y_{ij} be the observation of y from the jth subject in the ith treatment group, $j = 1, \ldots, n_i; i = T, R$. Let $z_{ij} = \log(y_{ij})$, $\bar{z}_i = 1/n_i \sum_{j=1}^{n_i} z_{ij}$ and $S_{Z_i}^2 = 1/(n_i - 1) \sum_{j=1}^{n_i} (z_{ij} - \bar{z}_i)^2$. Then a $(1 - 2\alpha) \times 100\%$ confidence interval based on the MLS method is given as $\left(\hat{\eta}_{y-}, \hat{\eta}_{y+}\right)$, where

$$\hat{\eta}_{y-} = \hat{d}_y - \sqrt{\sum_{i=T,R} \frac{S_{Z_i}^2 t_{1-\alpha,n_i}^2}{n_i} + \frac{1}{4} S_{ZT}^4 \left(\frac{n_T - 1}{\chi_{1-\alpha,n_T-1}^2} - 1\right)^2 + \frac{1}{4} S_{ZR}^4 \left(\frac{n_R - 1}{\chi_{\alpha,n_R-1}^2} - 1\right)^2},$$

and

$$\hat{\eta}_u = \hat{d}_y + \sqrt{\sum_{i=T,R} \frac{S_{Z_i}^2 t_{1-\alpha,n_i}^2}{n_i} + \frac{1}{4} S_{ZT}^4 \left(\frac{n_T - 1}{\chi_{\alpha,n_T-1}^2} - 1\right)^2 + \frac{1}{4} S_{ZR}^4 \left(\frac{n_R - 1}{\chi_{1-\alpha,n_R-1}^2} - 1\right)^2},$$

with $\hat{d}_y = \log \hat{\mu}_{Ty} - \log \hat{\mu}_{Ry} = \bar{z}_T - \bar{z}_R + 0.5(S_{ZT}^2 - S_{ZR}^2)$. Then, the power of claiming the two biological products are biosimilar using the y-data can be approximated by

$$\Phi\left(\frac{\delta - (\log \mu_T - \log \mu_R)}{\sqrt{V_Y}} - z_{1-\alpha}\right) - \Phi\left(\frac{-\delta - (\log \mu_T - \log \mu_R)}{\sqrt{V_Y}} + z_{1-\alpha}\right), \quad (16.9)$$

where $V_Y = \sum_{i=T,R} \left[n_i^{-1}(\beta_1^2 \sigma_{Xi}^2 + \sigma_{Wi}^2) + 0.5(n_i - 1)^{-1}(\beta_1^2 \sigma_{Xi}^2 + \sigma_{Wi}^2)^2 \right]$ and $\Phi(\cdot)$ is the cumulative distribution function of the standard normal distribution. The required sample size using the y-data can be obtained by taking the minimum of n_T and n_R such that the probability given in Equation 16.9 is larger than the desired level. On the other hand, if only the x-data are observed and the rule given in Equation 16.8 is adopted, the power of the test for biosimilarity is approximately equal to

$$\Phi\left(\frac{\delta - 0.5(\sigma_{Wd+}^2 - \sigma_{Wd}^2) - d}{\sqrt{V_X}} - z_{1-\alpha}\right) - \Phi\left(\frac{-\delta + 0.5(\sigma_{Wd}^2 - \sigma_{Wd-}^2) - d}{\sqrt{V_X}} + z_{1-\alpha}\right),$$

$$(16.10)$$

where $d = \log \mu_T - \log \mu_R$ and $V_X = \sum_{i=T,R} \left[n_i^{-1}\beta_1^2 \sigma_{Xi}^2 + 0.5(n_i - 1)^{-1}\beta_1^4 \sigma_{Xi}^4 \right]$. Note that the power based on the x-data given in Equation 16.10 is decreasing in

V_X, $\sigma^2_{Wd+} - \sigma^2_{Wd}$ and $\sigma^2_{Wd} - \sigma^2_{Wd-}$. Thus, the power is smaller for larger bounds of σ^2_{Wd}. However, the power of the test based on the x-data is not necessarily smaller than the power of the test based on the y-data since $V_X < V_Y$. Similarly, the required sample size to achieve a desired power level is obtained as the minimum of n_T and n_R such that the probability given in Equation 16.10 is larger than the target level.

16.3.3 Probability-Based Criterion for Assessing Biosimilarity

To test whether two biological products are biosimilar based on the PB criterion, the following hypotheses are considered:

$$H_0 : p \leq p_0 \quad \text{versus} \quad H_1 : p > p_0, \tag{16.11}$$

where
 p is defined in Equation 16.1
 p_0 is the similarity limit

16.3.3.1 Estimation

Based on the assumptions for Model 16.2, $\log Y_T - \log Y_R$ follows a normal distribution $N(\beta_1 \mu_{Xd}, \sigma^2_{LT} + \sigma^2_{LR})$, where $\sigma^2_{Li} = \beta^2_1 \sigma^2_{Xi} + \sigma^2_{Wi}$, $i = T, R$. Then, the probability is equal to

$$p = \Phi\left(\frac{-\log(1-\delta) - \beta_1 \mu_{Xd}}{\sqrt{\sigma^2_{LT} + \sigma^2_{LR}}} - z_{1-\alpha} \right) - \Phi\left(\frac{\log(1-\delta) - \beta_1 \mu_{Xd}}{\sqrt{\sigma^2_{LT} + \sigma^2_{LR}}} + z_{1-\alpha} \right). \tag{16.12}$$

If σ^2_{WT} and σ^2_{WR} are known, then based on the x-data, p can be estimated by

$$\hat{p}_1 = \Phi\left(\frac{-\log(1-\delta) - \beta_1 \hat{\mu}_{Xd}}{\sqrt{\beta^2_1(\hat{\sigma}^2_{XT} + \hat{\sigma}^2_{XR}) + \sigma^2_{WT} + \sigma^2_{WR}}} - z_{1-\alpha} \right)$$

$$- \Phi\left(\frac{\log(1-\delta) - \beta_1 \hat{\mu}_{Xd}}{\sqrt{\beta^2_1(\hat{\sigma}^2_{XT} + \hat{\sigma}^2_{XR}) + \sigma^2_{WT} + \sigma^2_{WR}}} + z_{1-\alpha} \right), \tag{16.13}$$

where $\hat{\mu}_{Xd} = \beta_1(\hat{\mu}_{XT} - \hat{\mu}_{XR})$. However, in general, σ^2_{WT} and σ^2_{WR} are unknown. In this case, we assume $\sigma^2_{WT} + \sigma^2_{WR} \leq \sigma^2_{W+}$, where σ^2_{W+} is known. Then, p can be estimated by

$$\hat{p}_2 = \Phi\left(\frac{-\log(1-\delta) - \beta_1 \hat{\mu}_{Xd}}{\sqrt{\beta^2_1(\hat{\sigma}^2_{XT} + \hat{\sigma}^2_{XR}) + \sigma^2_{W+}}} - z_{1-\alpha} \right) - \Phi\left(\frac{\log(1-\delta) - \beta_1 \hat{\mu}_{Xd}}{\sqrt{\beta^2_1(\hat{\sigma}^2_{XT} + \hat{\sigma}^2_{XR}) + \sigma^2_{W+}}} + z_{1-\alpha} \right).$$

$$\tag{16.14}$$

On the other hand, based on the y-data, p can be estimated by

$$\hat{p} = \Phi\left(\frac{-\log(1-\delta)-(\bar{z}_T-\bar{z}_R)}{\sqrt{S_{ZT}^2+S_{ZR}^2}} - z_{1-\alpha}\right) - \Phi\left(\frac{\log(1-\delta)-(\bar{z}_T-\bar{z}_R)}{\sqrt{S_{ZT}^2+S_{ZR}^2}} + z_{1-\alpha}\right),$$

$$(16.15)$$

where $\bar{z}_T-\bar{z}_R$, S_{ZT}^2 and S_{ZR}^2, given in Section 3.2.2, are the unbiased estimators of $\beta_1\mu_{Xd}$, σ_{LT}^2 and σ_{LR}^2 based on the y-data, respectively.

16.3.3.2 Power and Sample Size

The distribution of $\hat{p}$ is needed in order to assess the power and for the required sample to achieve a target power level. Following the similar idea of Tse et al. (2006), it can be verified that

$$\frac{\hat{p}-p-B(\hat{\theta})}{\sqrt{C(\hat{\theta})}} \xrightarrow{d} N(0,1),$$

where $B(\hat{\theta})$, $C(\hat{\theta})$ and $\hat{\theta}=(\bar{z}_T-\bar{z}_R, S_{ZT}^2, S_{ZR}^2)$ are the estimators of $B(\theta)$, $C(\theta)$, and $\theta=(\beta_1\mu_{Xd},\sigma_{LT}^2,\sigma_{LR}^2)$, respectively. The derivations of $B(\theta)$, $C(\theta)$, $B_2(\psi)$, and $C_2(\psi)$ are outlined as follows.

Taking Taylor expansion of $\hat{p}$ at p, we obtain

$$\hat{p} = p + \frac{\partial p}{\partial \mu_{Xd}}\left(\beta_1^{-1}(\bar{z}_T-\bar{z}_R)-\mu_{Xd}\right) + \frac{\partial p}{\partial\sigma_{LT}^2}\left(S_{ZT}^2-\sigma_{LT}^2\right) + \frac{\partial p}{\partial\sigma_{LR}^2}\left(S_{ZR}^2-\sigma_{LR}^2\right)$$

$$+\frac{1}{2}\left[\frac{\partial^2 p}{\partial\mu_{Xd}^2}\left(\beta_1^{-1}(\bar{z}_T-\bar{z}_R)-\mu_{Xd}\right)^2 + \frac{\partial^2 p}{\partial(\sigma_{LT}^2)^2}\left(S_{ZT}^2-\sigma_{LT}^2\right)^2\right.$$

$$\left.+\frac{\partial^2 p}{\partial(\sigma_{LR}^2)^2}\left(S_{ZR}^2-\sigma_{LR}^2\right)^2\right]+\cdots.$$

The other terms of the second order partial derivatives are not considered because they will lead to expected values of order $O(n^{-2})$ or higher. Note that $\bar{z}_T-\bar{z}_R$ follows $N(\beta_1\mu_{Xd}, n_T^{-1}\sigma_{LT}^2+n_R^{-1}\sigma_{LR}^2)$ and that $(n_i-1)S_{Zi}^2/\sigma_{Li}^2$ is chi-square distributed with n_i-1 degrees of freedom. In addition, $\partial p/\partial\sigma_{LT}^2 = \partial p/\partial\sigma_{LR}^2$ and $\partial^2 p/\partial(\sigma_{LT}^2)^2 = \partial^2 p/\partial(\sigma_{LR}^2)^2$. Consequently, $E(\hat{p})=p+B(\theta)+O(n^{-2})$ and $Var(\hat{p})=C(\theta)+O(n^{-2})$, where

$$B(\theta) = \frac{1}{2}\left[\frac{\partial^2 p}{\partial\mu_{Xd}^2}\beta_1^{-2}\left(\frac{\sigma_{LT}^2}{n_T}+\frac{\sigma_{LR}^2}{n_R}\right)+\frac{2\partial^2 p}{\partial(\sigma_{LT}^2)^2}\left(\frac{\sigma_{LT}^4}{n_T-1}+\frac{\sigma_{LR}^4}{n_R-1}\right)\right],$$

and

$$C(\theta) = \left[\left(\frac{\partial p}{\partial \mu_{Xd}} \right)^2 \beta_1^{-2} \left(\frac{\sigma_{LT}^2}{n_T} + \frac{\sigma_{LR}^2}{n_R} \right) + 2 \left(\frac{\partial p}{\partial \sigma_{LT}^2} \right)^2 \left(\frac{\sigma_{LT}^4}{n_T - 1} + \frac{\sigma_{LR}^4}{n_R - 1} \right) \right].$$

The partial derivatives are given as

$$\frac{\partial p}{\partial \mu_{Xd}} = \left(\frac{-\beta_1}{\sqrt{\beta_1^2(\sigma_{XT}^2 + \sigma_{XR}^2) + \sigma_{WT}^2 + \sigma_{WR}^2}} \right) [\phi(z_2) - \phi(z_1)], \qquad (16.16)$$

$$\frac{\partial p}{\partial \sigma_{LT}^2} = \left(\frac{-1}{2 \left[\beta_1^2(\sigma_{XT}^2 + \sigma_{XR}^2) + \sigma_{WT}^2 + \sigma_{WR}^2 \right]} \right) [z_2\phi(z_2) - z_1\phi(z_1)], \qquad (16.17)$$

$$\frac{\partial^2 p}{\partial \mu_{Xd}^2} = \left(\frac{-\beta_1^2}{\beta_1^2(\sigma_{XT}^2 + \sigma_{XR}^2) + \sigma_{WT}^2 + \sigma_{WR}^2} \right) [z_2\phi(z_2) - z_1\phi(z_1)], \qquad (16.18)$$

$$\frac{\partial^2 p}{\partial (\sigma_{LT}^2)^2} = \frac{1}{4 \left[\beta_1^2(\sigma_{XT}^2 + \sigma_{XR}^2) + \sigma_{WT}^2 + \sigma_{WR}^2 \right]^2} \left[(3z_2 - z_2^3)\phi(z_2) - (3z_1 - z_1^3)z_1\phi(z_1) \right],$$

$$(16.19)$$

where

$$z_1 = \frac{\log(1-\delta) - \beta_1\mu_{Xd}}{\sqrt{\sigma_{LT}^2 + \sigma_{LR}^2}}, \quad z_2 = \frac{-\log(1-\delta) - \beta_1\mu_{Xd}}{\sqrt{\sigma_{LT}^2 + \sigma_{LR}^2}}, \quad \text{and}$$

$$\phi(z) = \frac{1}{\sqrt{2\pi}} \exp(-0.5z^2).$$

Following similar ideas, we obtain the following results for $\hat{p}_2$:

$$E(\hat{p}_2) = p_2 + B_2(\psi) + O(n^{-2}),$$

and

$$\text{var}(\hat{p}_2) = C_2(\psi) + O(n^{-2}),$$

where

$$B_2(\psi) = \frac{1}{2} \left[\frac{\partial^2 p_2}{\partial \mu_{Xd}^2} \left(\frac{\sigma_{XT}^2}{n_T} + \frac{\sigma_{XR}^2}{n_R} \right) + \frac{2\partial^2 p_2}{\partial (\sigma_{LT}^2)^2} \beta_1^4 \left(\frac{\sigma_{XT}^4}{n_T - 1} + \frac{\sigma_{XR}^4}{n_R - 1} \right) \right]$$

and

$$C_2(\psi) = \left[\left(\frac{\partial p_2}{\partial \mu_{Xd}} \right)^2 \left(\frac{\sigma_{XT}^2}{n_T} + \frac{\sigma_{XR}^2}{n_R} \right) + 2 \left(\frac{\partial p_2}{\partial \sigma_{LT}^2} \right)^2 \beta_1^4 \left(\frac{\sigma_{XT}^4}{n_T - 1} + \frac{\sigma_{XR}^4}{n_R - 1} \right) \right],$$

with $\partial p_2/\partial \mu_{Xd}$, $\partial p_2/\partial \sigma_{LT}^2$, $\partial^2 p_2/\partial \mu_{Xd}^2$, and $\partial^2 p_2/\partial(\sigma_{LT}^2)^2$ being the same as $\partial p/\partial \mu_{Xd}$, $\partial p/\partial \sigma_{LT}^2$, $\partial^2 p/\partial \mu_{Xd}^2$, and $\partial^2 p/\partial(\sigma_{LT}^2)^2$ in Equations 16.6 through 16.19, respectively, but with $\sigma_{WT}^2 + \sigma_{WR}^2$ being replaced by σ_{W+}^2 (including those in z_1 and z_2). Consequently, an approximate $(1-\alpha) \times 100\%$ lower confidence bound for p is given by

$$\hat{p}_L = \hat{p} - B(\hat{\theta}) - z_{1-\alpha}\sqrt{C(\hat{\theta})}. \tag{16.20}$$

The null hypothesis H_0 defined in Equation 16.11 is rejected at an α level of significance if $\hat{p}_L > p_0$. Thus, the power of the test based on the PB criterion can be approximated by

$$1 - \Phi\left(\frac{p_0 - p}{\sqrt{C(\theta)}} + z_{1-\alpha} \right).$$

Let $n = n_T = n_R$. Based on the expression of $C(\theta)$, the required sample size to achieve a power level of $(1-\beta)$ is given as

$$n = \frac{(z_{1-\alpha} + z_{1-\beta})^2}{(p - p_0)^2} \left[\left(\frac{\partial p}{\partial \mu_{Xd}} \right)^2 \beta_1^{-2} \left(\sigma_{LT}^2 + \sigma_{LR}^2 \right) + 2 \left(\frac{\partial p}{\partial \sigma_{LT}^2} \right)^2 \left(\sigma_{LT}^4 + \sigma_{LR}^4 \right) \right]. \tag{16.21}$$

Based on the asymptotic normality of $\hat{p}_2$, an approximate $(1-\alpha) \times 100\%$ lower confidence bound for p_2 is given as

$$\hat{p}_{2L} = \hat{p}_2 - B_2(\hat{\psi}) - z_{1-\alpha}\sqrt{C_2(\hat{\psi})},$$

where $\hat{p}_2$ is obtained by replacing $\sigma_{WT}^2 + \sigma_{WR}^2$ with σ_{W+}^2 in Equation 16.13, $B_2(\hat{\psi})$, $C_2(\hat{\psi})$, and $\hat{\psi} = (\hat{\mu}_{Xd}, \hat{\sigma}_{XT}^2, \hat{\sigma}_{XR}^2)$ are the estimators of $B_2(\psi)$, $C_2(\psi)$, and $\psi = (\mu_{Xd}, \sigma_{XT}^2, \sigma_{XR}^2)$, respectively. The detailed expressions of $B_2(\psi)$ and $C_2(\psi)$ are given in the Appendix. Using the x-data, the null hypothesis defined in Equation 16.11 is rejected at the α level of significance if $\hat{p}_{2L} > p_0$. Thus, the power of the test based on the PB criterion can be approximated by

$$1 - \Phi\left(\frac{p_0 - p_2}{\sqrt{C_2(\psi)}} + z_{1-\alpha} \right).$$

Let $n = n_T = n_R$. Using the expression of $C_2(\theta)$ given earlier, based on the x-data, the required sample size to achieve a power level $(1 - \beta)$ is given as

$$n = \frac{(z_{1-\alpha} + z_{1-\beta})^2}{(p_2 - p_0)^2}\left[\left(\frac{\partial p_2}{\partial \mu_{Xd}}\right)^2\left(\sigma_{XT}^2 + \sigma_{XR}^2\right) + 2\left(\frac{\partial p_2}{\partial \sigma_{XT}^2}\right)^2\left(\sigma_{XT}^4 + \sigma_{XR}^4\right)\right]. \qquad (16.22)$$

16.4 Numerical Study

For the MB criterion, a numerical study gets some insights into the effect of the random error and the bounds for its variance on the required sample size. Without loss of generality, assume $\beta_1 = 1$ and for simplicity let $n = n_T = n_R$. Note that sample size calculations for both criteria do not include β_0. In all the numerical studies conducted, $\alpha = 0.05$ and $1 - \beta = 0.80$. Let $1 - \Delta = 0.80$, i.e., $\delta = 0.223$, which is the limit for assessing ABE suggested by FDA (2003). For the chosen values of μ_{Xd}, σ_{Xi}^2, and σ_{Wi}^2 ($\sigma_{WR}^2 = 0.04$), the required sample size n for the primary study endpoint y is presented in Table 16.1. The sample size is determined as the minimum n such that the power in Equation 16.9 is larger than 0.80. Suppose that the rule given in Equation 16.8 is adopted. Then, for simplicity, assume $\sigma_{Wd+}^2 = -\sigma_{Wd-}^2$. Several values of σ_{Wd+}^2 are selected such that $\sigma_{Wd+}^2 \geq \sigma_{XT}^2 - \sigma_{XR}^2$ for all the chosen values of σ_{XT}^2 and σ_{XR}^2 in Table 16.1. Table 16.2 shows the required sample sizes for surrogate study endpoint x, which is determined as the minimum n such that the power in Equation 16.10 is larger than 0.80. From the results presented in Table 16.1, for given values of μ_{Xd}, σ_{Xd}^2,

TABLE 16.1

Sample Sizes for the Study Endpoint y (Moment Based)

		$\sigma_{XT}^2 = 0.10$			$\sigma_{XT}^2 = 0.20$			$\sigma_{XT}^2 = 0.30$			$\sigma_{XT}^2 = 0.40$		
	σ_{XR}^2	0.05	0.10	0.15	0.15	0.20	0.25	0.25	0.30	0.35	0.35	0.40	0.45
$\mu_{Xd} = 0.00$	$\sigma_{WT}^2 = 0.02$	40	50	65	81	91	111	125	135	161	172	183	214
	$\sigma_{WT}^2 = 0.04$	46	53	66	88	94	110	133	139	158	183	186	209
	$\sigma_{WT}^2 = 0.06$	52	57	68	97	99	111	145	144	158	198	193	207
$\mu_{Xd} = 0.04$	$\sigma_{WT}^2 = 0.02$	51	53	59	102	96	101	158	144	146	219	195	194
	$\sigma_{WT}^2 = 0.04$	62	60	64	120	107	107	183	158	153	251	212	202
	$\sigma_{WT}^2 = 0.06$	77	70	70	143	121	115	215	176	163	293	236	214
$\mu_{Xd} = 0.08$	$\sigma_{WT}^2 = 0.02$	85	75	70	172	137	119	267	205	172	369	278	229
	$\sigma_{WT}^2 = 0.04$	110	92	81	213	164	135	326	242	194	447	326	257
	$\sigma_{WT}^2 = 0.06$	143	114	96	268	198	157	403	289	223	548	387	294

TABLE 16.2

Sample Sizes for the Study Endpoint x (Moment Based)

		$\sigma^2_{XT} = 0.10$			$\sigma^2_{XT} = 0.20$			$\sigma^2_{XT} = 0.30$			$\sigma^2_{XT} = 0.40$		
	σ^2_{XR}	0.05	0.10	0.15	0.15	0.20	0.25	0.25	0.30	0.35	0.35	0.40	0.45
$\mu_{Xd} = 0.00$	$\sigma^2_{Wd+} = 0.02$	33	41	55	77	85	101	126	132	152	179	183	207
	$\sigma^2_{Wd+} = 0.04$	36	45	60	86	93	112	140	145	168	198	201	229
	$\sigma^2_{Wd+} = 0.06$	40	50	67	95	103	125	155	160	187	220	222	255
$\mu_{Xd} = 0.04$	$\sigma^2_{Wd+} = 0.02$	46	47	53	109	97	98	179	152	147	254	211	200
	$\sigma^2_{Wd+} = 0.04$	52	53	58	126	109	108	205	170	162	291	235	220
	$\sigma^2_{Wd+} = 0.06$	61	59	64	146	122	119	238	191	179	338	265	244
$\mu_{Xd} = 0.08$	$\sigma^2_{Wd+} = 0.02$	84	75	68	204	155	127	333	243	191	474	337	260
	$\sigma^2_{Wd+} = 0.04$	102	87	77	247	181	144	405	283	217	575	394	295
	$\sigma^2_{Wd+} = 0.06$	126	103	89	306	215	165	501	336	249	713	466	338

and σ^2_{Wd}, the sample size is increasing in σ^2_{Wi} and σ^2_{Xi}, $i = T, R$. This pattern can be verified based on the power function given in Equation 16.9. On the other hand, the results in Table 16.2 suggest that the sample size is increasing in σ^2_{Wd+}. In other words, $n_X - n_Y$ is increasing in σ^2_{Wd+} for given values of the other parameters in Equation 16.9, where n_x and n_y are the sample sizes for the test based on the x-data and y-data, respectively. However, for the same value of μ_{Xd}, σ^2_{Xi}, and β_1, n_X may be larger or smaller than n_Y. This pattern is consistent with the conclusion drawn at the end of Section 16.3. Similar to the results shown in Table 16.1, the sample size is increasing in σ^2_{Xi} for given values of μ_{Xd}, σ^2_{Xd}, and σ^2_{Wd+}.

The performance of the test under the model defined in Equation 16.2 based only on the x-data is investigated by simulation. Using the sample sizes given in Table 16.2, the empirical power of the test according to the rule given in Equation 16.8 is obtained by a simulation study with 50,000 iterations. The results given in Table 16.3 suggest that the test shows very good performance when the two biological products are biosimilar. It should be noted that if the power in Equation 16.10 is approximated by

$$2\Phi\left(\frac{\delta - 0.5\sigma^2_{Wd+} - |\log v_T - \log v_R|}{\sqrt{V_X}} - z_{1-\alpha}\right) - 1,$$

when $\sigma^2_{Wd+} = -\sigma^2_{Wd-}$, then the sample size, in general, is seriously overestimated. For the combinations of parameter values given in Table 16.2, simulation results show that most of empirical powers are larger than 0.88, which are much larger than the nominal value 0.80. Furthermore, it is worth noting that when the null hypothesis that $|\log \mu_T - \log \mu_R| = \delta$ is true, simulation results

TABLE 16.3

Power (%) of the Test Using x with Sample Sizes from Table 16.2

	σ^2_{XR}	$\sigma^2_{XT} = 0.10$			$\sigma^2_{XT} = 0.20$			$\sigma^2_{XT} = 0.30$			$\sigma^2_{XT} = 0.40$		
		0.05	0.10	0.15	0.15	0.20	0.25	0.25	0.30	0.35	0.35	0.40	0.45
$\mu_{Xd} = 0.00$	$\sigma^2_{Wd+} = 0.02$	80.00	79.31	79.98	79.37	80.00	79.35	79.33	80.06	79.53	79.58	80.11	79.73
	$\sigma^2_{Wd+} = 0.04$	79.49	79.25	79.22	79.65	79.72	79.64	79.72	79.97	79.58	79.62	79.64	80.01
	$\sigma^2_{Wd+} = 0.06$	79.75	79.95	79.50	79.37	80.34	79.75	79.41	79.87	79.51	79.44	79.48	80.08
$\mu_{Xd} = 0.04$	$\sigma^2_{Wd+} = 0.02$	79.34	79.81	80.24	79.94	79.79	79.97	79.53	79.62	79.50	79.78	79.80	79.76
	$\sigma^2_{Wd+} = 0.04$	79.08	80.25	79.92	79.71	80.09	80.07	79.40	79.82	79.41	79.74	79.79	79.59
	$\sigma^2_{Wd+} = 0.06$	79.57	79.60	79.80	79.28	79.72	79.84	79.78	79.73	79.61	79.67	79.55	79.80
$\mu_{Xd} = 0.08$	$\sigma^2_{Wd+} = 0.02$	79.26	79.91	79.95	79.73	80.18	80.09	79.81	79.92	80.12	79.88	79.99	79.92
	$\sigma^2_{Wd+} = 0.04$	79.38	79.66	80.14	79.82	79.84	80.16	79.52	79.75	80.24	79.83	79.90	79.61
	$\sigma^2_{Wd+} = 0.06$	79.39	79.82	80.52	79.96	80.23	80.14	79.44	79.70	80.04	79.81	79.98	79.90

(not shown here) with a sample size of 50 and 100 suggest that the type I error rate is controlled at the nominal level and is decreasing in σ^2_{Wd+} and σ^2_{Xi}.

For the PB criterion, a similar procedure is used to investigate the effect of the random error ε_i in Equation 16.2 and the bound for its variance. The biosimilar limit p_0 is set to be 0.60. Let $\delta = 0.40$ and $\sigma^2_{WR} = 0.02$. The corresponding sample sizes for selected values of other parameters are presented in Table 16.4 and Table 16.5 for the test based only on y-data and x-data, respectively.

TABLE 16.4

Sample Sizes for the Study Endpoint y (Probability Based)

		$\sigma^2_{XT} = 0.06$			$\sigma^2_{XT} = 0.08$			$\sigma^2_{XT} = 0.10$			$\sigma^2_{XT} = 0.12$		
	σ^2_{XR}	0.14	0.16	0.18	0.14	0.16	0.18	0.10	0.12	0.14	0.10	0.12	0.14
$\mu_{Xd} = 0.00$	$\sigma^2_{WT} = 0.01$	33	50	81	46	73	127	29	43	68	42	66	112
	$\sigma^2_{WT} = 0.02$	38	60	100	55	91	167	35	53	86	53	84	151
	$\sigma^2_{WT} = 0.03$	46	73	127	68	117	230	42	66	112	67	111	212
$\mu_{Xd} = 0.04$	$\sigma^2_{WT} = 0.01$	34	53	85	48	77	134	30	45	71	44	69	118
	$\sigma^2_{WT} = 0.02$	40	63	105	58	96	177	36	55	91	55	89	160
	$\sigma^2_{WT} = 0.03$	48	77	134	71	124	246	44	69	118	70	117	227
$\mu_{Xd} = 0.08$	$\sigma^2_{WT} = 0.01$	39	60	98	54	89	158	34	52	83	51	81	141
	$\sigma^2_{WT} = 0.02$	45	72	122	67	112	214	41	64	107	64	105	195
	$\sigma^2_{WT} = 0.03$	54	89	158	83	147	306	51	81	141	82	140	284

TABLE 16.5

Sample Sizes for the Study Endpoint x (Probability Based)

		$\sigma^2_{XT} = 0.06$			$\sigma^2_{XT} = 0.08$			$\sigma^2_{XT} = 0.10$			$\sigma^2_{XT} = 0.12$		
	σ^2_{XR}	0.14	0.16	0.18	0.14	0.16	0.18	0.10	0.12	0.14	0.10	0.12	0.14
$\mu_{Xd} = 0.00$	$\sigma^2_{W+} = 0.05$	32	53	95	47	84	171	27	44	78	44	76	150
	$\sigma^2_{W+} = 0.06$	36	63	120	56	107	240	31	53	99	53	96	211
	$\sigma^2_{W+} = 0.07$	42	77	159	69	141	369	36	64	131	64	127	323
$\mu_{Xd} = 0.04$	$\sigma^2_{W+} = 0.05$	33	56	100	50	89	184	29	47	83	47	81	162
	$\sigma^2_{W+} = 0.06$	38	66	128	59	114	261	33	56	106	56	103	230
	$\sigma^2_{W+} = 0.07$	44	82	170	73	152	408	38	69	141	69	137	359
$\mu_{Xd} = 0.08$	$\sigma^2_{W+} = 0.05$	38	65	120	58	107	230	34	55	100	55	98	204
	$\sigma^2_{W+} = 0.06$	44	78	155	71	140	340	39	67	130	67	127	302
	$\sigma^2_{W+} = 0.07$	52	98	213	88	192	567	46	83	178	83	174	503

The results in Table 16.4 suggest that the required sample size is increasing in μ_{Xd}, σ^2_{Wi}, and σ^2_{Xi}. The pattern shown in Table 16.4 is different from that exhibited in Table 16.1. The results in Table 16.5 indicate that the sample size is increasing in μ_{Xd}, σ^2_{W+}, and σ^2_{Xi}. However, these patterns do not hold for μ_{Xd} and σ^2_{Xi} in Table 16.2. Note that the MB criterion is proposed for the ratio of means of Y_T and Y_R which depends on σ^2_{Xd} and σ^2_{Wd} (or σ^2_{Wd+}), but not on σ^2_{Xi} and σ^2_{Wi}. On the other hand, the PB criterion is set for the ratio of Y_T and Y_R. Thus, σ^2_{Xi} and σ^2_{Wi} play a role in the index p defined in the PB criterion. Consequently, the PB criterion requires small values of σ^2_{Xi} and σ^2_{Wi} to ensure that $p > p_0$.

Consider the case that only x-data are observed and the rule of the test is that two biological products are claimed to be biosimilar if $\hat{p}_{2L} > p_0$. Based on the sample sizes given in Table 16.5, the empirical power of the test is obtained by a simulation study with 50,000 iterations. The results given in Table 16.6 suggest that the test shows good performance when the two biological products are biosimilar. Furthermore, the power of the test is much closer to the nominal value. For example, the powers in the third column are larger than those in the first column to about 2% in each block corresponding to a value of σ^2_{XT} in Table 16.6. Additional simulations show that when the required sample size is smaller than 30, the corresponding power is in general smaller than 0.75. This may be due to the inaccuracy of the normal approximation of $\hat{p}_2$ and/or the approximation of the bias and variance of $\hat{p}_2$ when the sample size is not sufficiently large. When the null hypothesis $H_0 : p = p_0$ is true, the simulation results given in Table 16.7 based on 50,000 iterations with a sample size of 100 show that the resulting type I error rate is inflated but to a tolerable extent.

16.5 Concluding Remarks

Chow et al. (2010) compared the moment-based criterion with the probability-based criterion for the assessment of biosimilarity using biomarker data under a parallel-group design. The results indicate that the probability-based criterion is not only a much more stringent criterion but also is sensitive to any small change in variability. This justifies the use of the probability-based criterion for the assessment of biosimilarity if a certain level of precision and reliability of biosimilarity is desired.

As indicated earlier, biosimilars are fundamentally different from generic chemical drugs. Important differences include the size and complexity of the active substance and the nature of the manufacturing process. Unlike classical generics, biosimilars are not identical to their originator products and therefore should not be brought to market using the same procedure applied to generics. This is partly a reflection of the complexities of manufacturing

TABLE 16.6

Power (%) for the Test Using x with Sample Sizes from Table 16.5

	σ^2_{XR}	$\sigma^2_{XT} = 0.06$			$\sigma^2_{XT} = 0.08$			$\sigma^2_{XT} = 0.10$			$\sigma^2_{XT} = 0.12$		
		0.14	0.16	0.18	0.14	0.16	0.18	0.10	0.12	0.14	0.10	0.12	0.14
$\mu_{Xd} = 0.00$	$\sigma^2_{W+} = 0.05$	76.31	77.40	78.15	76.68	77.87	79.36	74.72	76.46	78.15	76.63	78.17	79.05
	$\sigma^2_{W+} = 0.06$	76.19	77.56	78.68	76.97	78.45	78.92	74.75	77.58	78.22	77.02	78.26	79.13
	$\sigma^2_{W+} = 0.07$	76.21	77.61	78.90	77.93	78.97	79.20	75.19	77.20	78.83	77.22	78.43	79.31
$\mu_{Xd} = 0.04$	$\sigma^2_{W+} = 0.05$	75.93	77.77	78.18	77.20	78.13	79.02	75.82	77.35	78.07	77.51	78.35	79.23
	$\sigma^2_{W+} = 0.06$	76.43	77.70	78.56	77.15	78.50	79.15	75.83	77.28	78.20	77.49	78.43	79.35
	$\sigma^2_{W+} = 0.07$	76.20	78.09	78.37	77.66	78.86	79.21	75.75	77.43	78.78	77.81	78.67	79.51
$\mu_{Xd} = 0.08$	$\sigma^2_{W+} = 0.05$	76.58	77.84	78.68	76.93	78.36	79.02	76.48	77.21	78.40	77.42	78.43	79.26
	$\sigma^2_{W+} = 0.06$	76.37	77.97	78.48	77.80	78.50	79.45	76.21	78.03	78.42	77.53	78.99	79.55
	$\sigma^2_{W+} = 0.07$	77.08	78.07	78.99	78.05	79.13	79.76	76.73	77.54	78.67	77.26	78.78	79.32

TABLE 16.7

Type I Error Rate (%) for Testing Biosimilarity Based on x

		$\sigma^2_{XT} = 0.06$			$\sigma^2_{XT} = 0.08$			$\sigma^2_{XT} = 0.10$			$\sigma^2_{XT} = 0.12$		
	σ^2_{XR}	0.14	0.16	0.18	0.14	0.16	0.18	0.10	0.12	0.14	0.10	0.12	0.14
$\mu_{Xd} = 0.00$	$\sigma^2_{W+} = 0.05$	6.102	5.930	6.044	5.754	5.714	5.700	5.648	5.398	5.670	5.590	5.534	5.362
	$\sigma^2_{W+} = 0.06$	5.964	5.822	5.986	5.804	5.730	5.926	5.530	5.542	5.696	5.548	5.474	5.494
	$\sigma^2_{W+} = 0.07$	5.882	5.960	6.058	5.658	5.750	5.786	5.604	5.512	5.496	5.562	5.336	5.354
$\mu_{Xd} = 0.04$	$\sigma^2_{W+} = 0.05$	5.846	5.852	5.856	5.824	5.794	5.506	5.520	5.616	5.662	5.672	5.364	5.418
	$\sigma^2_{W+} = 0.06$	5.818	5.914	5.874	5.776	5.592	5.928	5.626	5.898	5.502	5.624	5.488	5.420
	$\sigma^2_{W+} = 0.07$	5.916	5.996	6.058	5.728	5.826	5.674	5.666	5.392	5.746	5.544	5.544	5.294
$\mu_{Xd} = 0.08$	$\sigma^2_{W+} = 0.05$	6.010	5.900	5.962	5.646	5.730	5.704	5.750	5.656	5.644	5.690	5.576	5.438
	$\sigma^2_{W+} = 0.06$	5.922	6.022	6.146	5.834	5.808	5.910	5.756	5.666	5.584	5.614	5.482	5.562
	$\sigma^2_{W+} = 0.07$	5.914	6.202	5.808	5.812	5.888	5.888	5.802	5.808	5.692	5.648	5.556	5.378

and safety and efficacy controls of biosimilars when compared to their small-molecule generic counterparts (see, e.g., Chirino and Mire-Sluis, 2004; Schellekens, 2004; Crommelin et al., 2005; Roger, 2006; Roger and Mikhail, 2007). As biological products are usually recombinant protein molecules manufactured in living cells, manufacturing processes for biological products are highly complex and require hundreds of specific isolation and purification steps. In practice, it is impossible to produce an identical copy of a biological products, as changes to the structure of the molecule can occur with changes in the production process. Since a protein can be modified (e.g., a side chain may be added, the structure may have changed due to protein misfolding, and so on) during the process, different manufacturing processes may invariably lead to structural differences in the final product, which may result in differences in efficacy and may have a negative impact on patient immune responses. As a result, the development of follow-on biologics or biosimilars is very sensitive to small variations during the manufacturing process. Thus, current regulation for the assessment of bioequivalence may not be appropriate (or may be too loose to be applied) for the assessment of biosimilarity of follow-on biologics. Even though the probability-based criterion is more stringent than the moment-based criterion, it is strongly recommended that biosimilarity in variability (perhaps, in addition to average biosimilarity) between a follow-on biologic and the innovator biological products be assessed.

In this chapter, we considered assessing biosimilarity between biological products using biomarker data based on both a moment-based criterion and a probability-based criterion under the *Fundamental Biosimilarity Assumption.* Statistical methods for the assessment of biosimilarity in the average of biomarker responses between follow-on biologics are derived under a parallel-group design based on both MB and PB criteria. Even though a similar idea can be applied to derive statistical methods for the assessment of biosimilarity in the variability of biomarkers between biosimilar products if the similarity between variabilities is of primary concern, further research is needed in this area.

17

Current Issues in Biosimilar Studies

17.1 Introduction

Like bioequivalence assessment for the generic approval of small-molecule drug products, the process for assessing the biosimilarity of biosimilar products includes endpoint selection, criteria for biosimilarity, study design, statistical methods for data analysis, and regulatory submission, review, and approval. As indicated in the previous chapters, biosimilar products are made of living cells or organisms with mixed, complicated structures which are difficult, if not impossible, to characterize fully. Thus, standard methods for the assessment of bioequivalence for small-molecule drug products cannot be appropriately and directly applied to assess biosimilarity. Besides, biosimilar products are known to be sensitive to environmental factors such as light and temperature as a small change or variation at any critical stage of the manufacturing process could result in a drastic change in clinical outcomes.

Following the passage of the BPCI Act, in order to obtain input on specific issues and challenges associated with the implementation of the BPCI Act, the FDA conducted a 2 day public hearing on the *Approval Pathway for Biosimilar and Interchangeability Biological Products* on November 2–3, 2010, at the FDA in Silver Spring, Maryland. At the public hearing, several scientific factors and/or practical issues were discussed. These scientific factors and/or issues that related to statistics include (1) How similar is considered to be (highly) similar? (2) What endpoints should be used for the assessment of biosimilars? (Or, is a clinical trial always required?) (3) What criteria for assessing biosimilars should be adopted? (Or, is the one-size-fits-all criterion for PK parameters appropriate?) (4) Is a crossover design appropriate for assessing biosimilars? (5) Should tests for comparability in a manufacturing process in terms of critical quality attributes be conducted? and (6) Are there any differences in regulatory requirements for CMC (chemistry, manufacturing, and control)? In addition, the issues regarding the interpretation and assessment of drug interchangeability of biosimilar products were also discussed. Some of these scientific factors and/or issues were also discussed at the subsequent public meeting for user fees held on December 16, 2011, at the FDA in Silver Spring, Maryland. On February 9, 2012, the FDA circulated three draft guidances for comments. One of the three draft guidances is related to scientific considerations for the assessment of biosimilar products. In this guidance, the FDA introduces the concept of stepwise approach and the totality-of-the-evidence for the assessment of biosimilarity. However, the issue of drug interchangeability was not mentioned (see, FDA, 2012a,b,c). To obtain public comments and input on the FDA's draft guidances, a public hearing was held on May 11, 2012, at the FDA in Silver Spring (see, e.g., Chow et al., 2013).

In this chapter, comments on these scientific factors and some current issues related to the assessment of biosimilarity and drug interchangeability will be described in the next two sections followed by a section of concluding remarks.

17.2 Scientific Factors

In this section we shall focus on the scientific factors of endpoint selection, one-size-fits-all criterion, the degree of similarity (i.e., how similar is considered highly similar?), study design, and test for comparability in critical quality attributes at various stages of manufacturing process.

17.2.1 Endpoint Selection

Endpoint selection is related to the following questions:

1. Is a pharmacokinetic/pharmacodynamic (PK/PD) or bioavailability/ bioequivalence (BA/BE) study sufficient for the assessment of biosimilarity?
2. Is a clinical trial always required for the assessment of biosimilarity?
3. How many studies are required in order to achieve totality-of-the- evidence to support biosimilarity as called for in the FDA draft guidance?

In addition, the following questions are commonly asked:

1. What if we pass some of the studies but fail to pass the remaining studies?
2. Which of these studies utilizing different study endpoints is telling the truth?
3. Can these study endpoints translate one another?

In what follows, an attempt will be made to address or at least to comment on these questions. First, endpoint selection depends upon the specific biosimilar studies conducted. For example, AUC (area under the blood or plasma concentration time curve) and C_{max} (maximum concentration) are the study endpoints for pharmacokinetic and/or bioavailability/bioequivalence studies, while in clinical investigations, outcomes such as response rate (efficacy) and the incidence rate of adverse events (safety) should be considered. Second, to address the question whether a clinical trial should always be conducted, we may revisit the definition of biosimilarity as described in the BPCI Act. A biological product that is demonstrated to be highly similar to an FDA-licensed biological product may rely on certain existing scientific knowledge about *safety*, *purity* (quality), and *potency* (efficacy) of the reference product. Thus, if one would like to show that the safety and efficacy of a biosimilar product are highly similar to those of the reference product, then a clinical trial must be conducted. In some cases, clinical trials for the assessment of biosimilarity may be waived if there exists substantial evidence that surrogate endpoints or biomarkers are predictive of the clinical outcomes. On the other hand, clinical trials are required for the assessment of drug interchangeability in order to show that the safety and efficacy between a biosimilar product and a reference product are similar in *any given patient* of the patient population under study as described in the BPCI Act. Similarly, if it is required by the regulatory agencies to demonstrate that a biosimilar product is highly similar in purity (quality) to that of the reference product, then some in vitro studies for assessment of biological activities are required.

Third, how many studies are required in order to support biosimilarity between a biosimilar product and a reference product? Ideally, the sponsor should conduct as many studies as possible to demonstrate that the test product is highly similar with the reference product in terms of important good drug characteristics such as *identity*, *purity*, *strength*, *safety*, *quality*, and *stability* as described in the USP/NF (2000) if significant differences in these characteristics have an impact on the clinical outcomes of the biosimilar product under investigation. For example, if it is known that a small change in a specific critical quality attribute at a specific stage of the manufacturing process would have an impact on the clinical outcomes, then a comparability study is necessary to conduct in order to show that there is no clinically meaningful difference between the test product and the reference product in terms of the quality attributes at the specific stage of the manufacturing process of the biosimilar product. According to the FDA guidance, it is suggested that how many studies are required for the assessment of biosimilarity depends upon whether these studies are sufficient to achieve the totality-of-the-evidence for the assessment of biosimilarity. Thus, consultation and/or communication with members of the Biosimilar Review Committee (BRC) at the FDA is strongly recommended prior to the conduct of these biosimilar studies.

Regarding the question that "Which of these study endpoints is telling the truth?" since the development/manufacturing of a biosimilar product is a very complex process, it cannot be fully described by a *single* or *multiple* endpoints in a *single study* or some study endpoints from some other biosimilar studies alone. That is why the FDA requires that the totality-of-the-evidence (including important quality attributes across all functional areas or domains of the manufacturing process) be achieved for an overall evaluation of the biosimilar product under investigation. Finally, *calibration* studies need to be conducted in order to address the issue of translations among study endpoints which may be related to one another in certain ways.

17.2.2 One-Size-Fits-All Criterion

The one-size-fits-all criterion for bioequivalence assessment of small-molecule drug products has been in practice since the 1970s across all therapeutic areas. The one-size-fits-all criterion, which was developed based on the assessment of average of bioavailability (measurement of drug absorption), has been criticized by many researchers and/or scientists from the academia and the pharmaceutical industry (see, e.g., Chow and Liu, 2008). It is suggested that a more flexible criterion be considered (1) by adjusting for the intra-subject variability and/or therapeutic index (window) or (2) by adopting asymmetric boundaries (depending upon efficacy and safety therapeutic index). Along this line, the FDA published guidances for the assessment of individual bioequivalence (IBE) and population bioequivalence (PBE), which attempted to adjust the one-size-fits-all criterion by taking into consideration the intra-subject and inter-subject variabilities and the variability due to subject by product interaction.

If we were to adopt the one-size-fits-all criterion for all required biosimilar studies, chances would be that we would pass some of the studies but fail other studies. In this case, it is suggested that flexible criteria for the assessment of biosimilarity be considered for certain biosimilar studies because differences observed in some studies may be insensitive to the clinical outcomes. For those studies which are less sensitive to clinical outcomes, it may be more appropriate to use a wider biosimilarity limit.

Regarding the use of a more flexible criterion for bioequivalence assessment of small-molecule drug products, most recently, the FDA recommends the use of the scaled average bioequivalence (SABE) criterion for highly variable drug products (Haidar et al., 2008). The SABE criterion for highly variable drug products is a flexible criterion adjusting for the variability of the reference product. EMA suggested a closely related approach (EMA, 2010c). Whether the SABE criterion can be applied to assessing biosimilar products has recently attracted much attention since biosimilar products usually have relatively large variability.

17.2.3 How Similar Is Similar?

As indicated in the BPCI Act, a biosimilar product is defined as one that is *highly similar* to the reference product. However, no definition regarding highly similar was given, mentioned, or discussed in both the BPCI Act and the FDA draft guidances. This has raised the following questions. First: How similar is considered to be highly similar? What is the criterion for similarity? How to define the degree of similarity for highly similar?

Current criteria for the assessment of bioequivalence in terms of PK responses such as AUC and C_{max} are useful for determining whether a biosimilar product is similar to a reference product. However, they do not provide additional information regarding the *degree* of similarity. As indicated in Chapters 4 and 5, we may consider a relative distance between "T and R," denoted by $d(T, R)$ and "R and itself," defined as $d(R, R)$, i.e.,

$$rd = \frac{d(T, R)}{d(R, R)}$$

We may claim that T is highly similar to R if rd is close to 1. For example, rd could be within (90%, 110%), the limits used in the assessment of in vitro bioequivalence testing for locally acting drug products. Alternatively, we may consider assessing the average biosimilarity first and then comparing biosimilarity in variability. If we pass average biosimilarity, we may consider the two products to be similar. If we also pass biosimilarity in variability, we may claim that they are highly similar. These criteria for assessing similarity and high similarity have been proposed in the literature. In the recent draft guidances of the FDA, however, there is no definition of highly similar and little or no discussion regarding the degree of similarity was provided.

In practice, it is also of concern to the sponsor that "what if a biosimilar product turns out to be superior to the reference product?" A simple answer to the concern is that the test product under investigation is not similar. As indicated in Chapter 7, the concept of testing for non-inferiority consists of the concept of testing for equivalence and the concept of testing for superiority. Thus, it is suggested that a non-inferiority test be performed. We may test for non-superiority once the non-inferiority has been established without paying any statistical penalty due to the nature of closed testing procedure.

17.2.4 Study Design

Unlike small-molecule drug products for which a crossover design is the design of choice for bioequivalence assessment, parallel design is often considered for the assessment of biosimilar products due to the fact that most biosimilar products have relatively long half-lives. Although a parallel design can be employed to assess similarity between drug products, it suffers from the following drawbacks. First, we are unable to compare the test product and the reference product within each individual subject. In addition, we are unable to estimate within-subject (intra-subject) variability. In practice, it is recognized that (1) biosimilar products are generally very sensitive to environmental factors such as light and temperature, (2) a small change (variation) at any critical stage of the manufacturing process could cause a drastic change in clinical outcomes. To overcome this problem, the three-arm design proposed by Kang and Chow (2013) is useful. In practice, if a two-arm parallel group design is used, one may consider to randomly split the reference arm into two groups a large number of times in order to obtain some insight information regarding the comparison of the reference product with itself.

Alternatively, it is suggested that a Balaam's design, which is a combination of a parallel design and a crossover design, be considered. Let T and R denote the test product and the reference product, respectively. The Balaam's design can be expressed as:

Balaam's design— (TT, RR, TR, RT), which is a 4×2 (four-sequence, two-period) crossover design. Note that the first two sequences constitute a repeated parallel design. Under Balaam's design, we are able to estimate both within-subject and between-subject variabilities for both the test product and the reference product. Alternatively, one may consider a 2×2 crossover design, i.e., (TR, RT), but repeat the second period. In other words, the following design is commonly considered as an alternative design to the Balaam's design:

The 2 × 3 crossover design— (TRR, RTT).

In addition, the following 2 × 3 crossover designs are useful designs for the assessment of biosimilarity:

The 2 × 3 dual design— (TRT, RTR)
The 2 × 3 extra-reference design— (TRR, RTR)

Zhang et al. (2013) compared relative advantages and limitations of the previously described study designs for the assessment of biosimilarity and suggested that the 2×3 extra-reference design (TRR, RTR) be used for achieving the desired power with an adequate control of the overall type I error rate.

For the assessment of drug interchangeability in terms of alternating and switching, the BPCI Act indicated that for a biological product that is administered more than once to an individual, the risk in terms of safety or diminished efficacy of alternating or switching between the use of the biological product and the reference product is not greater than the risk of using the reference product without such alternation or switch. An appropriate study design should allow the assessment of T–T, T–R, R–T, and R–R for switching and the assessment of R–T–R and T–R–T for alternating. For this purpose, the study designs for switching, alternating, and switching/alternating as described in Chapter 11 may be useful.

17.2.5 Test for Comparability in Critical Quality Attributes

As clearly stated in the BPCI Act, a biosimilar product is defined as a product that is *highly similar* to the reference product notwithstanding minor differences in clinically inactive components, and there are no clinically meaningful differences in terms of safety, purity, and potency. Based on this definition, we would interpret that a biological medicine is biosimilar to a reference biological medicine if it is highly similar to the reference in safety, purity, and potency. In other words, a biological product that is demonstrated to be highly similar to an FDA-licensed biological product may rely on certain existing scientific knowledge about safety, purity, and potency of the reference product. High similarity in purity is viewed as high similarity in critical quality attributes at critical stages of the manufacturing process including raw materials, in-process (or in-use) materials, and end-product. Thus, tests for comparability in critical quality attributes play an important role for achieving the totality-of-the-evidence for the assessment of biosimilarity.

Tests for the comparability in critical quality attributes involve (1) the establishment of product specifications at each critical stage of the manufacturing process and release targets for the end-product; (2) in-process or in-use materials quality assurance and quality control; and (3) test for stability. Since a small change and/or variation at each critical stage of the manufacturing process could result in a drastic change in clinical outcomes (e.g., safety and/or efficacy), it is suggested that much tighter acceptance criteria or release targets should be used for controlling variabilities associated with each critical stage of the manufacturing process and, consequently, improving the quality of the product.

As indicated earlier, the manufacturing process for a biological product is very complex and involves the characterization of mixed structures. As a result, protocols should be developed for comparability studies which include sampling plans, acceptance criteria, and testing procedures in order to obtain representative samples (data) for an accurate and unbiased assessment of the comparability between (1) different batches of the same manufacturing process, (2) different manufacturing processes (locations), (3) and a test product and a reference product. Under an approved protocol of a comparability study, statistical methods can be derived based on the sampling plan and acceptance criteria employed (see, e.g., Chow and Liu, 1995). Although general principles for testing comparability of biological products have been described, specific guidances for sampling plans and/or acceptance criteria for specific quality attributes at critical stages of a specific manufacturing process are still not available.

17.3 Current Issues

For the assessment of biosimilarity and drug interchangeability, there are many practical issues in addition to the scientific factors outlined in the previous section. These practical issues are briefly described later. For each practical issue, valid statistical methods are necessarily developed under a valid study design.

17.3.1 Reference Standards

In practice, important information regarding the reference product is generally not available. Thus, it is important to conduct an R–R study (i.e., a study comparing the reference product to itself). Note that for an R–R study, the reference product could come from two different manufacturing processes (locations) or different batches from the same manufacturing process in order to obtain important information regarding the reference product. The R–R study will provide not only the information regarding the variability associated with the reference product but also establish baseline (i.e., similarity between R and R) for a comparison (i.e., comparison between T vs. R and R vs. R).

For this purpose, prospectively, one may consider a three-arm parallel design (i.e., one arm with test product and two arms with the reference product) proposed by Kang and Chow (2013). For a post-study approach for a two-arm study, one could randomly split the reference arm into two groups, say R_1 and R_2 of equal sample size, a large number of times. One can then establish a standard (or specification) for the reference product. Based on the established standards, the determination of the degree of similarity for *highly similar* is possible.

17.3.2 Criteria for Biosimilarity

Current thinking regarding the criteria for biosimilarity is based on the concept of bioequivalence in average bioavailability or of individual/PBE which takes variabilities (both inter-subject and intra-subject variabilities) into consideration. Due to the complexity, heterogeneity, and complication mechanisms of biological drug products, difference in variability between biosimilar and innovator biological products in PK, PD, and clinical responses will be much larger than the difference observed between the conventional generic and the innovator chemical drug product. Therefore, biosimilarity in average alone may not be sufficient to establish biosimilarity. On the other hand, because of masking effect, the aggregate metrics for population and IBE fail to address the closeness of the distributions of the responses between the biosimilar and the innovator biological products (Liu, 1998; Carrasco and Jover, 2003). Disaggregate metrics can address the masking effect suffered by the aggregate metrics and find the sources of in-equivalence. However, determination of individual equivalence margins with different interpretations is not an easy task. In addition, because of the involved multiparameters, any procedure will tend to be conservative if it is based on a disaggregate metric for the evaluation of equivalence between follow-on and innovator biological products, especially in small samples. Furthermore, all current methods derived from the probability-based, moment-based, aggregate, or disaggregate criteria are based on the normality assumption, which is either extremely difficult to verify or simply not true. To resolve the previously mentioned dilemmas regarding the evaluation of equivalence (similarity), Chow and Liu (2010) proposed the following concept of stochastic equivalence or stochastic non-inferiority:

Let $F(x)$ and $G(y)$ be the cumulative distribution functions of the responses for biosimilar and innovator biological products, respectively. Assuming that a large response value indicates better efficacy, the follow-on and innovator biological products are said to be stochastically equivalent (two-sided) if the absolute difference between $F(x)$ and $G(x)$ is within some prespecific margins for all x. In other words, metric $\theta = \sup|F(x) - G(x)|$, and the hypothesis for equivalence becomes

$$H_0 : \sup|F(x) - G(x)| \geq \eta, \quad \text{for some } x$$

vs. (17.1)

$$H_1 : \sup|F(x) - G(x)| < \eta, \quad \text{for all } x.$$

Similarly, the biosimilar product is said to be stochastically non-inferior to the innovator counterpart if the difference between $F(x)$ and $G(x)$ is larger than $-\eta$. The corresponding hypothesis is given as

$$H_0 : \sup|F(x) - G(x)| \leq -\eta, \quad \text{for some } x$$

versus (17.2)

$$H_1 : \sup|F(x) - G(x)| > -\eta, \quad \text{for all } x,$$

However, the hypotheses in Equations 17.1 and 17.2 can be used only for the evaluation of equivalence with respect to one study endpoint such as AUC or some primary efficacy endpoint. They cannot be utilized to assess whether the equivalence in a product characteristic such as AUC can be extrapolated to equivalence in a primary efficacy endpoint. Both well-defined product characteristics and primary efficacy endpoint are measured for each patient. Therefore, group means of a well-defined product characteristic can be computed for each dose level for the biosimilar and the innovator's product, respectively. Using the group means of the well-defined characteristic as the independent variable, a simple linear regression equation can be fit to the primary efficacy endpoint (dependent variable) for the biosimilar and innovator's biological products, respectively. It follows that the concept of the relative potency in the parallel-line bioassay can then be employed to investigate the ability to extrapolate the equivalence in product characteristic to the equivalence in efficacy (Finney, 1979). In other words, if the relative potency between the biosimilar and the innovator's biological products is within some predefined margins, then it can be concluded that equivalence in the product characteristic can be extrapolated to equivalence in efficacy.

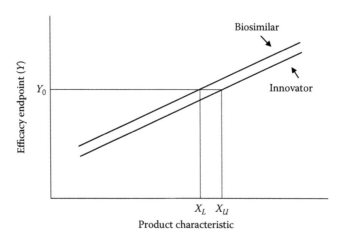

FIGURE 17.1
Parallel-line assays to evaluation of extrapolation ability.

Figure 17.1 provides a graphical depiction of the application of the parallel-line assay to the evaluation of the extrapolation ability of equivalence in product characteristic to equivalence in efficacy. Let ρ be the relative potency of the biosimilar product to the innovator's biological product. The hypothesis of extrapolation ability is as follows:

$$H_0: \rho \leq \rho_L \quad \text{or} \quad \rho \leq \rho_U \quad \text{versus} \quad H_a: \rho_L < \rho < \rho_U, \tag{17.3}$$

where $0 < \rho_L < 1 < \rho_U$.

Even though the methods based on Kolmogorov–Smirnov type of statistics have been extensively investigated (Serfling, 1980), relatively little literature exists on the statistical tests for stochastic equivalence or non-inferiority. One method is to employ the naïve asymptotic confidence band for $\theta = \sup|F(x) - G(x)|$ or $\theta = \sup[F(x) - G(x)]$ as the test statistics for Hypotheses 17.1 and 17.2. If the $(1-2\alpha) \times 100\%$ confidence band is totally contained within the band formed by the equivalence margins $(-\eta, \eta)$, then equivalence between the biosimilar and the originator's biological products can be concluded at the α significance level. Similarly, if the $(1-\alpha) \times 100\%$ lower confidence band is above the lower band formed by the lower margin $-\eta$, then non-inferiority of the biosimilar product to the innovator's biological product can be established at the α significance level. Derivation of the test statistics for Hypotheses 17.1 and 17.2 at the boundary margins of the null hypothesis and the corresponding distribution and confidence interval require further research. However, permutation and bootstrap techniques can also be used to find the distribution of the test statistics and the corresponding confidence intervals empirically.

17.3.3 Criteria for Interchangeability

As pointed out by Chow (2013), there is clear distinction between biosimilarity and interchangeability of biosimilar products according to the definitions given in the BPCI Act. The assessment of biosimilarity focuses on the comparison between T (test product) and R (reference product). However, interchangeability is referred to the comparison (relative risk) between a number of Ts and R. In the recent FDA draft guidances on biosimilar products, drug interchangeability and criteria for assessing interchangeability were not mentioned. Based on past experience with small-molecule drug products, it is recognized that drug interchangeability (in terms of the concepts of drug prescribability and drug switchability) is related to the variability due to subject-by-drug interaction. However, it is not clear whether criterion for interchangeability should be based on the variability due to subject-by-drug interaction or the variability due to subject-by-drug interaction adjusted for intra-subject variability of the reference drug. Unlike small-molecule drug products, the BPCI Act gives a clear definition of drug interchangeability in terms of the concepts of switching and alternating (see Chapter 11).

Current issues regarding drug interchangeability of biosimilar products include (1) the definition and interpretation of the interchangeability in terms of switching and alternating as described in the BPCI Act, (2) criteria for interchangeability, and (3) appropriate study designs and development of valid statistical methods for data analysis. As the BPCI Act states, the interchangeability is expected to produce the *same* clinical result in *any given patient*, which can be interpreted as that the same clinical result can be expected in *every single patient*. In reality, conceivably, lawsuits may be filed if adverse effects are recorded in a patient after switching from one product to another. Chow (2013) interpreted the interchangeability as producing the *same* clinical result in *any given patient* with certain assurance. If this interpretation is acceptable to the FDA, then criteria for interchangeability based on either variability or CV can be developed.

17.3.4 Criteria for Comparability

The concept of testing for comparability involves (1) the validation of a manufacturing process and (2) the testing for comparability between manufacturing processes.

The primary objective of process validation is to provide documented evidence that a manufacturing process does reliably what it purports to do. To accomplish this prospectively, a validation protocol is usually developed. A validation protocol should include: (1) critical stages of the manufacturing process, (2) equipment to be used at each critical stage, (3) possible problems, (4) tests to be performed, (5) sampling plans, (6) testing plans, (7) acceptance criteria, (8) pertinent information, (9) test or specification to be used as reference, and (10) validation summary. When a problem is observed in the manufacturing process, it is crucial to locate at which stage the problem occurred so that it can be corrected and the manufacturing process can do what it purports to do.

For testing comparability between manufacturing processes of a biosimilar product and a reference product, critical quality attributes at critical stages of the manufacturing processes need to be identified. Since small changes or variations can occur at any of the critical stages of the manufacturing processes, these could result in drastic changes in clinical outcome. Therefore, it is suggested that sources of variations and the possible causes of variations be identified, eliminated, and/or control for quality assurance/control during the process of manufacturing. In practice, sources of variations can be classified into the categories of (1) expected and controllable, (2) expected but not controllable, (3) unexpected but controllable, and (4) unexpected and uncontrollable. For those critical quality attributes that are expected and/or controllable, statistical processes with tighter criteria for quality assurance/control are necessarily developed. Once the process is out of control (i.e., out of in-house QA/QC specifications), appropriate actions must be taken to reduce or control the variability in order to improve the quality. The impact of the variability on clinical outcomes should be examined whenever possible.

17.3.5 Determination of Non-Inferiority Margin

As indicated in Chapter 7, testing for non-inferiority consists of testing for equivalence and testing for superiority (both statistical superiority and clinical superiority). As a result, non-inferiority is considered a one-sided equivalence. Thus, the non-inferiority margin is the same as the equivalence limit. In clinical research, the determination of equivalence limit or non-inferiority margin is critical and yet extremely controversial.

After a series of internal discussions, a draft guidance on non-inferiority clinical trials is currently being distributed by the FDA for comments (FDA, 2010). Basically, this draft guidance consists of four parts, which are (1) a general discussion of regulatory, study design, scientific, and statistical issues associated with the use of non-inferiority studies when these are used to establish the effectiveness of a new drug, (2) details of some of the issues such as the quantitative analytical and statistical approaches used to determine the non-inferiority margin for use in non-inferiority studies, (3) Q&A of some commonly asked questions, and (4) five examples of successful and unsuccessful efforts for determining non-inferiority margins and the conduct of non-inferiority studies.

In principle, the 2010 FDA draft guidance is very similar to the ICH E10 guideline. However, the 2010 FDA draft guidance provides more details regarding study design and statistical issues. For example, the 2010 FDA draft guidance defines two non-inferiority margins, namely M_1 and M_2, where M_1 is defined as the entire effect of the active control assumed to be present in the non-inferiority study, and M_2 is referred to as the largest clinically acceptable difference (degree of inferiority) of the test drug compared to the active control. As indicated in the 2010 FDA draft guidance, M_1 is based on (1) the treatment effect estimated from the historical experience with the active control drug, (2) the assessment of the likelihood that the current effect of the active control is similar to the past effect (the constancy assumption), and (3) the assessment of the quality of the non-inferiority trial, particularly looking for defects that could reduce a difference between the active control and the new drug. On the other hand, M_2 is a clinical judgment which is never to be larger than M_1, even if for active control drugs with small effects, a clinical judgment might argue that a larger difference is not clinically important. Ruling out a difference between the active control and the test drug that is larger than M_1 is a critical finding that supports the conclusion of effectiveness.

As indicated in the draft guidance, there are essentially two different approaches to analysis of the non-inferiority study: one is the fixed margin method (or the two confidence interval method) and the other one is the synthesis method. In the fixed margin method, the margin M_1 is based on estimates of the effect of the active comparator in previously conducted studies, making any needed adjustment for changes in trial circumstances. The non-inferiority margin is then prespecified and it is usually chosen as a margin smaller than M_1 (i.e., M_2). The synthesis method combines (or synthesizes) the estimate of treatment effect relative to the control from the non-inferiority trial with the estimate of the control effect from a meta-analysis of historical trials. This method treats both sources of data as if they came from the same randomized trial to project what the placebo effect would have been had the placebo been present in the non-inferiority trial.

17.3.6 Bridging Bioequivalence Studies

Generic drugs are very crucial for the health and welfare of the people of developing countries. For example, in some countries, generic drugs in fact account for more than 70% of total prescriptions. To ensure efficacy, safety, and quality of the generic drugs, approval of generic drugs is a very important task for the regulatory authorities in developing countries. However, the generic drugs in these countries are either from foreign countries or from local generic sponsors of their own countries. Consequently, the approval of generic copies is a very complicated and challenging issue that the regulatory authorities of the developing countries have to face.

In this subsection we describe one of the situations often encountered for the approval of generic drugs in developing countries. In what follows, a new region is denoted as a generic name for the developing countries. Suppose that for some reasons such as the price of the innovative drug or the market size of the new region, the innovative drug product of the original region was not marketed in the new region. After the patent of the innovative drug product expired in the original region, a generic copy manufactured in the original region was approved by the regulatory authority of the original region. However, because of its affordability, this generic copy of the original region was introduced and approved by the regulatory authority for marketing in the new region. Another generic copy of the innovative drug manufactured by a local sponsor is seeking for marketing approval in the new region. However, equivalence between two generic copies does not imply bioequivalence between the local generic copy and the innovative drug (Chow and Liu, 1997; Fleming, 2000). To ensure the equivalent efficacy and safety of the local generic copy, therefore, the regulatory authority in the new region may still require the evidence of average bioequivalence between the local generic copy and the innovative drug despite the fact that the latter is not available in the new region.

Because the generic copy from the original region has been approved by both the original and the new regions, following the bridging concept suggested in the ICH E5 Guideline on *Ethnic Factors in the Acceptability of Foreign Clinical Data* (ICH, 1998), one could utilize the data provided by the bioequivalence study conducted in the original region to evaluate average bioequivalence between the local generic copy of the new region and the innovative drug of the original region. This problem is referred to as the *bridging bioequivalence problem* and the innovative drug of the original region is called the original reference formulation. Suppose that a local bioequivalence study is conducted to compare the local generic copy to the generic copy of the original region. In this local bioequivalence study, the generic copy of the original region serves as the reference formulation. On the other hand, the generic copy of the original region is the test formulation in the bioequivalence study conducted in the original region. As a result, average bioequivalence of the generic copy manufactured by the local sponsor in the new region to the original reference formulation in the original region can be evaluated through the generic copy of the original region. Therefore, the local bioequivalence study in the new region is referred to as the bridging bioequivalence study (BBES). The generic copy made by the local sponsor in the new region is designated as the test formulation, and the generic copy of the original region is referred to as the bridging reference formulation. We also call the bioequivalence study conducted in the original region for comparing the bridging reference formulation with the original reference formulations as the original bioequivalence study (OBES). However, to avoid bias, it is very crucial that both bioequivalence studies have the same inclusion/exclusion criteria, the same design, the same sampling time points, the same amount of blood drawn at each time point, and most important of all, the same analytical procedures for the determination of the plasma concentrations of active ingredients.

For the assessment of biosimilarity in foreign countries, it is suggested that the concept of bridging bioequivalence studies be considered.

17.3.7 Assessing Biosimilarity Using Biomarker

For some drug products, the FDA indicates that in vitro dissolution testing may serve as a surrogate for an in vivo bioequivalence testing by comparing the dissolution profiles between drug products. Two drug products are considered, in some cases, to have a similar drug absorption profile if their dissolution profiles are similar. These drug products include (1) pre-1962 classified "AA" drug products, (2) lower-strength products, (3) scale-up and post-approval change, and (4) products demonstrating in vitro and in vivo correlation (Chow and Shao, 2002). Along this line, Chow et al. (2004) proposed assessing bioequivalence using genomic data. In other words, under the assumption that two drug products will have a similar drug absorption profile if their genomic profiles are similar provided that there is a well-established relationship between the PK parameters and the genomic data. This concept is useful in establishing bioequivalence especially between a new (or modified) formulation and a reference formulation of an innovative drug product going off patent protection if it is accepted by the regulatory agencies.

Let x be a genomic prediction of a PK response under consideration. Typically, x is a function of genomic data such as genetic markers, DNA sequence, mRNA transcription profiling, linkage and physical maps, gene location, and quantitative trait loci (QTL) mapping. Chow et al. (2004) attempted to use the genomic prediction x as a surrogate for the PK response in assessing bioequivalence. More specifically, if we can claim bioequivalence between two drug products using x in place of the PK response but the same statistical test designed for PK data, can we claim bioequivalence between the two drug products without a bioavailability/bioequivalence study? The answer is affirmative if x is a perfect prediction of the PK response. In practice, however, genomic prediction is usually not perfect, because of the existence of variability, model misspecification, and/or missing important genomic variables. The idea of Chow et al. (2004) is to evaluate the impact of the differences between the distribution of the genomic prediction and PK response on the assessment of bioequivalence. For ABE, a tolerance limit for this difference is derived so that if the difference is within the tolerance limits, then ABE can be assessed by using the genomic prediction. For PBE and IBE, Chow et al. (2004) considered a sensitivity analysis of prediction bias and variation difference within some predetermined limits.

Similarly, under certain assumptions, we may use biomarker data to assess biosimilarity.

17.3.8 Stepwise Approach and Totality-of-the-Evidence

The concept of the stepwise approach is easy to comprehend. However, the term "stepwise approach" can be easily mistaken for "stepwise regression" in statistics. Thus, it is suggested that the term "stepwise approach" be changed to "step-by-step approach" in order to clarify the confusion.

One of the major concerns of the step-by-step approach proposed for the demonstration of evidence of biosimilarity is the control of the overall type I error rate for achieving the needed totality-of-the-evidence. In practice, the evidence obtained at different steps could carry different weights of clinical importance, which may or may not achieve statistical significance. In addition, the order of the step-by-step testing procedures may have an impact on the final test results. Also, the possible multiplicity of the variables could affect the type I error rate; this calls for clarification. At each step of the approach, the "residual uncertainty" is to be evaluated, which is still needed to demonstrate biosimilarity satisfactorily. At the end of the series of steps, the draft guidance presents clinical studies and thereby appears to leave the impression that the clinical program and its data are needed only if there is still "residual uncertainty" after evaluating the preceding steps (including structural analysis, functional assays, and studies in animals). On the other hand, the BPCI Act requires, not in a sequential manner, "a clinical study or studies (including the assessment of immunogenicity and PK/PD) that are sufficient to demonstrate safety, purity and potency." It would be important to clarify the differing interpretations.

The concept of totality-of-the-evidence is, in effect, global biosimilarity across different domains. FDA seems to suggest that similarity should be demonstrated across different domains. The degree of biosimilarity in different domains, however, may have different degrees of impact on the clinical outcomes (i.e., safety and effectiveness). Therefore, it is suggested that different criteria for biosimilarity in different domains should be considered. Thus, the criteria and degrees of biosimilarity in different domains will have an impact on the totality-of-the-evidence for global similarity. Chow et al. (2011) proposed a totality biosimilarity index based on reproducibility probability, which may be helpful in achieving the totality-of-the-evidence for the assessment of biosimilarity. However, several questions regarding the selection of biosimilarity criteria at different functional areas or domains and the assignment of different weights at different domain remain unsolved.

17.3.9 Contamination in a Manufacturing Process

In practice, virus contamination of the cell culture during the manufacturing process is possible. Virus contamination could raise potential safety concern. It usually begins with the advent of recombinant continuous cell lines, which replicate indefinitely and can be cultured in large bioreactors. Continuous cell lines are derived from tumors. Some continuous cell lines produce large quantities of endogenous retrovirus-like particles. Continuous cell lines support the replication and amplification of some viruses that can potentially contaminate cell culture processes. A typical example of virus contamination in the manufacturing process is the recent incidence of Genzyme Corp., which is briefly described in the following.

As reported by the Boston Globe, June 17, 2009, Genzyme, the state's largest biotechnology company, has halted production of two drugs

(Cerezyme and Fabrazyme) for rare genetic disorders after a virus was discovered in the production equipment at its Allston plant. Cerezyme is used to treat Gaucher disease, an enzyme deficiency in which fatty substances accumulate in the spleen, liver, lungs, bone marrow, and—sometimes—the brain. It can cause bruising, enlarged organs, and lung and kidney ailments. Fabrazyme treats Fabry disease, in which a missing or faulty enzyme prevents the body from breaking down oils, waxes, and fatty acids that build up in the eyes and kidneys, as well as the nervous and cardiovascular systems.

The drugs are used by 8000 people worldwide and cost about $200,000 per patient annually. The diseases treated by these enzyme replacement drugs are rare. About 5500 people worldwide, for example, depend on Cerezyme, the best-selling Genzyme drug, while about 2500 use Fabrazyme. Fabrazyme treats Fabry disease, which prevents the body from breaking down oils and fats that build up in the eyes and kidneys. As a result of the plant's shutdown, Cerezyme patients could go without one or two treatments, while those taking Fabrazyme may need to skip up to four doses. Patients usually receive the drugs intravenously every two weeks. The missed doses will not cause significant health problems because most patients' bodies have been cleansed of the fatty substances, and it takes more than a few skipped treatments for them to return.

Since an FDA inspection of the Allston plant found "significant deviations from current good manufacturing practice in the manufacture of licensed therapeutic drug products, bulk drug substances, and drug components," Genzyme has spent a lot of effort scrambling to regain its footing after detecting a virus at its Allston plant. Federal regulators warned doctors to look for foreign particles in five Genzyme drugs used to treat rare genetic disorders, including two—Cerezyme and Fabrazyme—that have been rationed because of the viral contamination detected in the Allston Landing plant last summer. The five drugs represent roughly half of Genzyme's $4.6 billion in annual sales. In addition, Genzyme receives an FDA consent decree including an up-front disgorgement fee of $175 million.

As the result of Genzyme's disaster, WHO cell substrate guidance document is being revised. More biotechnology companies are implementing viral process barriers (see Figure 17.2) and recognize that emergency preparedness is important. In addition, new innovative virus detection and identification technologies are being developed and implemented. Biotechnology companies seem to be more open about their virus contamination experience than in the past. However, sharing the database of contamination experience still maintains corporate confidentiality.

17.3.10 Meta-Analysis for Biosimilarity Review

As indicated in Chapter 1, no generic copies of the brand-name drug can be made unless the FDA determines that they work as well as the brand-name drug

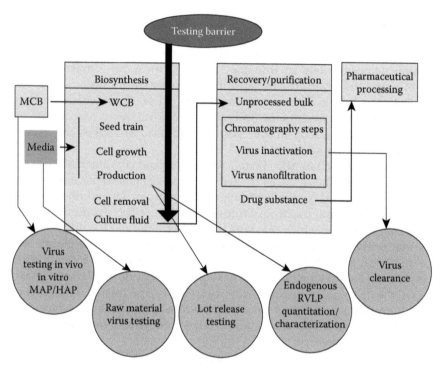

FIGURE 17.2
Virus process barrier. (Reproduced from a presentation slide of M. E. Wiebe, Quantum Consulting, Redwood City, CA.)

based on bioequivalence testing. When a generic drug is claimed bioequivalent to the brand-name drug, it is assumed that they will reach the equivalent therapeutic effect, or that they are therapeutically equivalent. This statement is true only under the *Fundamental Bioequivalence Assumption*. A patient may be switched, in many cases, from the brand-name drug to its generic copy, provided that the generic copy has been shown to be bioequivalent to the brand-name drug. An interesting question for physicians and patients is whether the brand-name drug and its generic copies can be used interchangeably, especially when different generic copies of the same innovator drug product are available and competition among generic copies is fierce. The same question arises, but in different context, and in view of the statements of the BPCI Act, about the interchangeability of biosimilars and brand-name biologics.

As more generic drugs become available, the quality, safety, and efficacy of generic drugs have become a public concern because it is very likely that a patient may switch from one generic drug to another. This situation is particularly true in developing countries where only cheaper generic copies are available. There is a tremendous debate on the quality, safety, and efficacy of generic drugs because they are not identical in terms of inactive ingredients that are binded and bulked, coated and colored, and may vary from one version to another. The current FDA guidance and many regulatory agencies around the world require only that evidence of equivalence in average bioavailabilities between the brand-name drug and its generic copies be provided. Bioequivalence between generic copies of the brand-name drug is not required. Therefore, whether the brand-name drug and its generic copies can be used interchangeably has become a safety concern. To address this issue, Chow and Liu (1997) proposed the performance of a meta-analysis based on average bioequivalence for bioequivalence review. The idea of a meta-analysis is to provide an overview of bioequivalence among generic drugs based on data from independent bioequivalence trials (or submissions). The purpose is not only to assess bioequivalence among generic drugs of the same brand-name drug but also to provide a tool to monitor the performance of the approved generic copies of the same brand-name drug. In Chow and Liu's approach, a rather restricted, yet strong, assumption of inter-subject and intra-subject variances is made, which limits its practical use. To overcome this problem, Chow and Shao (1999) proposed an alternative method for meta-analysis that relaxes the assumption. The proposed alternative meta-analysis increases statistical power when the inter-subject variability is not too large.

Note that the concept of meta-analysis for bioequivalence review for small-molecule drug products can be applied to drug interchangeability of biosimilar products since the concepts of switching and alternating for interchangeability involve the reference product (R) and a number of biosimilar products (i.e., a number of Ts which have been demonstrated to be highly similar to the reference product). Meta-analysis based on data from approved biosimilar products provides the opportunity for the regulatory agency to monitor whether there is a potential risk of switching and/or alternating between the approved biosimilar products and the reference product.

17.3.11 Profile Analysis

The bootstrap procedure described in Section 4.2.3 has received much attention and criticisms since it was introduced by the FDA. Major criticisms are described later.

First, the statistical properties of this procedure are unknown. It includes two aspects. One is that the statistical model, which should be used to describe the profile data, is not clearly defined in the FDA draft guidances. In addition, even under an appropriate statistical model, the statistical properties of the bootstrap procedure are still unknown. More specifically, it is not clear whether the bootstrap sample mean is a consistent estimator for $E(rd)$. As a result, the 95% percentile of the bootstrap samples may not be an appropriate 95% upper bound for $E(rd)$. These questions are not addressed in the FDA draft guidances.

Second, no criteria are given regarding the passage or failure of the bioequivalence/biosimilarity study. This is the issue that confuses most researchers/scientists in practice. After the conduct of a valid trial and an appropriate statistical analysis following the FDA draft guidance, the sponsor still cannot tell if its product has passed or failed the bioequivalence/biosimilarity test. This is a direct consequence of our first point (i.e., the statistical properties of the recommended bootstrap procedure are unknown).

Third, the simulation study using different random number generation schemes may produce contradictory results. It is possible for a good product to fail the bioequivalence/biosimilarity test simply because of *bad luck*. It is also possible for a bad product to pass the bioequivalence/biosimilarity test with an "appropriate" choice of random number generation scheme. As a result, researchers/scientists tend to rely more on the descriptive statistics of the two products in order to assess their bioequivalence/biosimilarity instead of the bootstrap procedure. The proposed bootstrap procedure recommended by the FDA is not as reliable as it should be.

As a result, further research of profile analysis becomes a problem of interest in practice. More specifically, the questions of interest include (1) What statistical model should be used to describe the profile data? (2) Is $E(rd)$ defined by the FDA a good parameter for characterizing the bioequivalence between test and reference products? (Can we define the test-to-reference distance and reference-to-reference variability differently?) and (3) What bioequivalence/biosimilarity limits should we use to evaluate the in vitro bioequivalence between two products based on appropriate model, parameter, and bioequivalence criterion?

17.4 Concluding Remarks

For the assessment of bioequivalence of small-molecule drug products, we claim that a test drug product is bioequivalent to a reference (innovative) drug product if the 90% confidence interval for the ratio of means (in%) of a primary PK parameter is completely within the bioequivalence limits of (80%, 125%). This one size-fits-all criterion focuses only on average bioavailability and ignores the heterogeneity of variability. Thus, it is not scientifically/statistically justifiable for the assessment of biosimilarity. In practice, it is then suggested that appropriate criteria, which can take the heterogeneity of variability into consideration be developed since biosimilars are known to be variable and sensitive to small variations in environmental conditions.

At the FDA public hearing, commonly asked questions were: "How similar is considered similar?" and "How the degree of similarity should be measured and translated to clinical outcomes (e.g., safety and efficacy)?" These questions are closely related to drug interchangeability of biosimilars or follow-on biologics which had been shown to be biosimilar to the innovative product. For the assessment of bioequivalence for chemical drug products, a crossover design is often considered, except for drug products with relatively long half-lives. Since most biosimilar products have relatively long half-lives, it is suggested that a parallel-group design should be considered. However, a parallel-group design does not provide independent estimates of variance components such as the inter- and intra-subject variabilities and the variability due to subject-by-product interaction. Thus, it is a major challenge for assessing biosimilars under a parallel-group design. Although EMA of the EU has published several product-specific guidances based on the concept papers, it has been criticized that there are no objective *standards* for the assessment of biosimilars because it depends upon the nature of the products. Product-specific standards seem to suggest that a *flexible* biosimilarity criterion should be considered and the flexible criterion should be adjusted for variability and/or the therapeutic index of the innovative (or reference) product. As described earlier, there are many uncertainties for the assessment of biosimilarity and interchangeability of biosimilars. As a result, it is a major challenge to both clinical scientists and biostatisticians to develop valid and robust clinical/statistical methodologies for the assessment of biosimilarity and interchangeability under the uncertainties. In addition, how to address the issues of quality and comparability in the manufacturing process is another challenge to both the pharmaceutical scientists and the biostatisticians. The proposed general approach using the biosimilarity index (derived based on the concept of reproducibility probability) may be useful. However, further research on the statistical properties of the proposed biosimilarity index is required.

Although FDA has circulated three draft guidances to assist the sponsors for demonstrating biosimilarity of biosimilar products, many scientific factors and statistical issues remain unanswered. In addition, many other issues such as manufacturing and marketing need to be addressed (Simoens et al. 2011).

References

Aitchison, J. and Dunsmore, I.R. (1975). *Statistical Prediction Analysis*. Cambridge University Press, New York.

Anderson, S. and Hauck, W.W. (1990). Consideration of individual bioequivalence. *J. Pharmacokinet. Biopharm.*, 18, 259–273.

Arnold, B. and Groeneveld, R. (1979). Bound on expectations of linear systematic statistics based on dependent samples. *Ann. Statist.*, 7, 220–223.

Berger, R.L. (1982). Multiparametric hypothesis testing and acceptance sampling. *Technometrics*, 24, 295–300.

Boddy, A.W., Snikeris, F.C., Kringle, R.O., Wei, G.C.G., Opperman, J.A., and Midha, K.K. (1995). An approach for widening the bioequivalence limits in the case of highly variable drugs. *Pharm. Res.*, 12, 1865–1868.

Box, G.E.P. and Tiao, G.C. (1973). *Bayesian Inference in Statistical Analysis*. Addison-Wesley, Reading, MA.

Brown, M.B. and Forsythe, A.B. (1974). Robust tests for the equality of variances. *J. Am. Statist. Assoc.*, 69, 364–367.

Carrasco, J.L. and Jover, L. (2003). Assessing individual bioequivalence using structural equation model. *Stat. Med*, 22, 901–912.

Carstenson, J.T., Franchini, M., and Ertel, K. (1992). Statistical approaches to stability protocol design. *J. Pharm. Sci.*, 81, 303–308.

Casella, G. and Berger, R. (2002). *Statistical Inference*, 2nd edn. Duxbury, Pacific Grove, CA.

CBER/FDA. (1993). Points to consider in the characterization of cell lines to produce biologicals. Center for Biologic Evaluation and Research, Food and Drug Administration, Rockville, MD.

CBER/FDA. (1999). *Summary of CBER Considerations on Selected Aspects of Active Controlled Trial Design and Analysis for the Evaluation of Thrombolytics in Acute MI*, Center for Biological Evaluation and Research, Food and Drug Administration, Rockville, MD.

CD. (2003). Commission Directive 2003/63/EC of 25 June 2003 amending Directive 2001/83/EC of the European Parliament and of the Council on the Community code relating to medicinal products for human use. *Off. J. Eur. Union* L 159/46.

Chen, B.L. (2009). CMC issues and regulatory requirements for biosimilars. *Trends Bio/Pharm. Ind.*, 5, 19–26.

Chen, C. (1996). FDA's views on bracketing and matrixing. *EFPIA Symposium: Advanced Topics in Pharmaceutical Stability Testing—Building in the ICH Guideline*, Brussels, Belgium, October 1996.

Chen, K.W., Chow, S.C., and Li, G. (1997). A note on sample size determination for bioequivalence studies with higher-order crossover designs. *J. Pharm. Biopharm.*, 25, 753–765.

Chen, K.W., Li, G., Sun, Y., and Chow, S.C. (1996). A confidence region approach for assessing equivalence in variability of bioavailability. *Biom. J.*, 4, 475–487.

Chen, M.L. (1995). Individual bioequivalence. Invited Presentation at *International Workshop: Statistical and Regulatory Issues on the Assessment of Bioequivalence*, Dusseldorf, Germany, October 19–20, 1995.

Chen, M.L. (1997). Individual bioequivalence—A regulatory update. *J. Biopharm. Stat.*, 7, 5–11.

Chen, M.L., Shah, V., Patnaik, R., Adams, W., Hussain, A., Conner, D., Mehta, M., Malinowski, H., Lazor, J., Huang, S.M., Hare, D., Lesko, L., Sporn, D., and Williams, R. (2001). Bioavailability and bioequivalence: A FDA regulatory overview. *Pharm. Res.*, 18, 1645–1650.

Chinchilli, V.M. and Esinhart, J.D. (1996). Design and analysis of intra-subject variability in cross-over experiments. *Stat. Med.*, 15, 1619–1634.

Chirino, A.J. and Mire-Sluis, A. (2004). Characterizing biological products and assessing comparability following manufacturing changes. *Nat. Biotechnol.*, 22, 1383–1391.

Chiu, S.T., Chen, C., Chow, S.C., and Chi, E. (2013). Assessing biosimilarity using the method of generalized Pivotal quantities. Generics Biosimilars Initiatives to appear.

Chow, S.C. (1988). A new procedure for the estimation of variance components. *Stat. Prob. Lett.*, 6, 349–355.

Chow, S.C. (1992). Statistical design and analysis of stability studies. *Proceedings of the 48th Annual Conference on Applied Statistics*, Atlantic City, NJ, 1992.

Chow, S.C. (1999). Individual bioequivalence-A review of the FDA draft guidance. *Drug Inf. J.*, 33, 435–444.

Chow, S.C. (2007). *Statistical Design and Analysis of Stability Studies*, Chapman and Hall/CRC Press/Taylor & Francis Group, New York.

Chow, S.C. (2010). On Scientific factors of biosimilarity and interchangeability. Presented at *FDA Public Hearing on Approval Pathway for Biosimilar and Interchangeable Biological Products*. Silver Spring, MD, November 2–3, 2010.

Chow, S.C. (2011). Quantitative evaluation of bioequivalence/biosimilarity. *J. Bioequiv. Bioavailab.*, Suppl. 1-002, 1–8, http://dx.doi.org/10.4172/jbbs1-002.

Chow, S.C. (2013). Assessing biosimilarity and drug interchangeability of biosimilar products. *Stat. Med.*, 32, 361–363.

Chow, S.C., Endrenyi, L., and Lachenbruch, P.A. (2013a). Comments on FDA draft guidances on biosimilar products. *Stat. Med.*, 32, 364–369.

Chow, S.C., Endrenyi, L., Lachenbruch, P.A., Yang, L.Y., and Chi, E. (2011). Scientific factors for assessing biosimilarity and drug interchangeability of follow-on biologics. *Biosimilars*, 1, 13–26.

Chow, S.C., Hsieh, T.C., Chi, E., and Yang, J. (2010a). A comparison of moment-based and probability-based criteria for assessment of follow-on biologics. *J. Biopharm. Stat.*, 20, 31–45.

Chow, S.C., Lu, Q., Tse, S.K., and Chi, E. (2010b). Statistical methods for assessment of biosimilarity using biomarker data. *J. Biopharm. Stat.*, 20, 90–105.

Chow, S.C., Shao, J., and Ho, H.C. (2000). Statistical analysis for placebo-challenging design in clinical trials, *Stat. Med.*, 19, 1029–1037.

Chow, S.C., Shao, J., and Li, L. (2004). Assessing bioequivalence using genomic data. *J. Biopharm. Stat.*, 14, 869–880.

Chow, S.C., Shao, J., and Wang, H. (2002). Individual bioequivalence testing under 2×3 crossover designs. *Stat. Med.*, 21, 629–648.

Chow, S.C., Shao, J., and Wang, H. (2008). *Sample Size Calculation in Clinical Research*, 2nd edn., Chapman & Hall/CRC Press/Taylor & Francis Group, New York.

Chow, S.C., Wang, J., Endrenyi, L., and Lachenbruch, P.A. (2013b). Scientific considerations for assessing biosimilar products. *Stat. Med.*, 32, 370–381.

Chow, S.C., Yang, L.Y., Starr, A, and Chiu, S.T. (2013c). Statistical methods for assessing interchangeability of biosimilars. *Stat. Med.*, 32, 442–448.

Chow, S.C. and Chang, M. (2011). *Adaptive Design Methods in Clinical Trials*, 2nd edn., Chapman and Hall/CRC Press/Taylor & Francis Group, New York.

Chow, S.C. and Chiu, S.T. (2013). Sample size and data monitoring for clinical trials with extremely low incidence rate. *Therapeutic Innovation of Regulatory Science*, In press.

Chow, S.C. and Ki, F. (1997). Statistical comparison between dissolution profiles of drug products. *J. Biopharm. Stat.*, 7, 241–258.

Chow, S.C. and Liu, J.P. (1995). *Statistical Design and Analysis in Pharmaceutical Science*. Marcel Dekker, Inc., New York.

Chow, S.C. and Liu, J.P. (1997). Meta-analysis for bioequivalence review. *J. Biopharm. Stat.*, 7, 97–111.

Chow, S.C. and Liu, J.P. (2008). *Design and Analysis of Bioavailability and Bioequivalence Studies*, 3rd edn. Chapman and Hall/CRC Press/Taylor & Francis Group, New York.

Chow, S.C. and Liu, J.P. (2010). Statistical assessment of biosimilar products. *J. Biopharm. Stat.*, 20, 10–30.

Chow, S.C. and Shao, J. (1991). Estimating drug shelf-life with random batches. *Biometrics*, 47, 1071–1079.

Chow, S.C. and Shao, J. (1997). Statistical methods for two-sequence dual crossover designs with incomplete data. *Stat. Med.*, 16, 1031–1039.

Chow, S.C. and Shao, J. (1999). Bioequivalence review for drug interchangeability. *J. Biopharm. Stat.*, 9, 485–497.

Chow, S.C. and Shao, J. (2002a). *Statistics in Drug Research*. Marcel Dekker, Inc., New York.

Chow, S.C. and Shao, J. (2002b). A note on statistical methods for assessing therapeutic equivalence. *Controll. Clin. Trials*, 23, 515–520.

Chow, S.C. and Shao, J. (2006). On non-inferiority margin and statistical test in active control trials. *Stat. Med.*, 25, 1101–1113.

Chow, S.C. and Tse, S.K. (1990). A related problem in bioavailability/bioequivalence studies—Estimation of intrasubject variability with a common CV. *Biomet. J.*, 32, 597–607.

Chow, S.C. and Tse, S.K. (1991). On the estimation of total variability in assay validation. *Stat. Med.*, 10, 1543–1553.

Church, J.D. and Harris, B. (1970). The estimation of reliability from stress–strength relationships. *Technometrics*, 12, 49–54.

Conover, W.J. (1973). Rank tests for one sample, two samples, and k samples without the assumption of a continuous distribution function. *Ann. Stat.*, 1, 1105–1125.

Conover, W.J. (1999). *Practical Nonparametric Statistics*, 3rd edn., Wiley, New York.

Cornell, R.G. (1990). The evaluation of bioequivalence using nonparametric procedures. *Commun. Stat.: Theory Methods*, 19, 4153–4169.

CPMP. (1997). Reduced stability testing plan—Bracketing and matrixing. CPMP/QWP/157/96. London, U.K.

CPMP. (2001). Guideline on comparability of medicinal products containing biotechnology-derived proteins as active substance: Non-clinical and clinical issues. EMEA/CPMP/3097/02/Final8. London, U.K.

Crommelin, D., Bermejo, T., Bissig, M., Damianns, J., Kramer, I., Rambourg, P., Scroccaro, G., Strukelj, B., Tredree, R., and Ronco, C. (2005). Biosimilars, generic versions of the first generation of therapeutic proteins: Do they exist? *Contrib. Nephrol.*, 149, 287–294.

David, H. (1981). *Order Statistics*. Wiley, New York.

David, H. and Nagaraja, H. (2003). *Order Statistics*. John Wiley & Sons, New York.

Davis, G.C., Beals, J.M., Johnson, C., Mayer, M.H., Meiklejohn, B.I., Mitlak, B.H., Roth, J.L., Towns, J.K., and Veenhuizen, M. (2009). Recommendations regarding technical standards for follow-on biologics: Comparability, similarity, interchangeability. *Curr. Med. Res. Opin.*, 25, 1655–1661.

Davit, B.M., Conner, D.P., Fabian-Fritsch, B. et al. (2008). Highly variable drugs: Observations from bioequivalence data submitted to the FDA for new generic drug applications. *AAPS J*, 10, 148–156.

De Weck, A.L. (1974). Low molecular weight antigens. In: *The Antigens*, Vol. 2, Sela, M., Ed. Academic Press, New York, pp. 141–248.

DeWoody, K. and Raghavarao, D. (1997). Some optimal matrix designs in stability studies. *J. Biopharm. Stat.*, 7, 205–213.

Dragalin, V., Fedorov, V., Patterson, S. et al. (2003). Kullback-Leibler divergence for evaluating bioequivalence. *Stat. Med.*, 22, 913–930.

Edwards, W., Lindman, H., and Savage, L.J. (1963). Bayesian statistical inference for psychological research. *Psycol. Rev.*, 70, 193.

EMA. (2001). Note for guidance on the investigation of bioavailability and bioequivalence. The European Medicines Agency Evaluation of Medicines for Human Use. EMEA/EWP/QWP/1401/98, London, U.K.

EMA. (2003a). Note for guidance on comparability of medicinal products containing biotechnology-derived proteins as drug substance—Non clinical and clinical issues. The European Medicines Agency Evaluation of Medicines for Human Use. EMEA/CHMP/3097/02, London, U.K.

EMA. (2003b). Rev. 1 guideline on comparability of medicinal products containing biotechnology-derived proteins as drug substance—Quality issues. The European Medicines Agency Evaluation of Medicines for Human Use. EMEA/CHMP/BWP/3207/00/Rev 1, London, U.K.

EMA. (2006a). Guideline on similar biological medicinal products. The European Medicines Agency Evaluation of Medicines for Human Use. EMEA/CHMP/437/04, London, U.K.

EMA. (2006b). Draft guideline on similar biological medicinal products containing biotechnology-derived proteins as drug substance: Quality issues. The European Medicines Agency Evaluation of Medicines for Human Use. EMEA/CHMP/49348/05, London, U.K.

EMA. (2006c). Draft annex guideline on similar biological medicinal products containing biotechnology-derived proteins as drug substance—Non clinical and clinical issues—Guidance on biosimilar medicinal products containing recombinant erythropoietins. The European Medicines Agency Evaluation of Medicines for Human Use. EMEA/CHMP/94526/05, London, U.K.

EMA. (2006d). Draft annex guideline on similar biological medicinal products containing biotechnology-derived proteins as drug substance—Non clinical and clinical issues—Guidance on biosimilar medicinal products containing recombinant granulocyte-colony stimulating factor. The European Medicines Agency Evaluation of Medicines for Human Use. EMEA/CHMP/31329/05, London, U.K.

EMA. (2006e). Draft annex guideline on similar biological medicinal products containing biotechnology-derived proteins as drug substance—Non-clinical and clinical issues—Guidance on biosimilar medicinal products containing somatropin. The European Medicines Agency Evaluation of Medicines for Human Use. EMEA/CHMP/94528/05, London, U.K.

EMA. (2006f). Draft annex guideline on similar biological medicinal products containing biotechnology-derived proteins as drug substance—Non clinical and clinical issues—Guidance on biosimilar medicinal products containing recombinant human insulin. The European Medicines Agency Evaluation of Medicines for Human Use. EMEA/CHMP/32775/05, London, U.K.

EMA. (2006g). Guideline on the clinical investigating of the pharmacokinetics of therapeutic proteins. The European Medicines Agency Evaluation of Medicines for Human Use. EMEA/CHMP/89249/04, London, U.K.

EMA. (2006h). Guideline on similar biological medicinal products containing biotechnology-derived proteins as active substance: Non-clinical and clinical issues. EMEA/CHMP/BMWP/42832, London, U.K.

EMA. (2007). Guideline on immunogenicity assessment of biotechnology-derived therapeutic proteins. The European Medicines Agency Evaluation of Medicines for Human Use. EMEA/CHMP/MWP/14327/2006, London, U.K.

EMA. (2009a). Guideline on non-clinical and clinical development of similar biological medicinal products containing low-molecular-weight-heparins. EMEA/CHMP/BMWP/118264/2007. London, U.K., 19 March.

EMA. (2009b). Non-clinical and clinical development of similar medicinal products containing recombinant interferon alfa. EMEA/CHMP/BMWP/102046/06, London, U.K.

EMA. (2010a). Draft guideline on similar biological medicinal products containing monoclonal antibodies. EMA/CHMP/BMWP/403543/2010, London, U.K.

EMA. (2010b). Concept paper on similar biological medicinal products containing recombinant follicle stimulation hormone. EMA/CHMP/BMWP/94899/2010, London, U.K.

EMA. (2010c). Guideline on the investigation of bioequivalence. CPMP/EWP/QWP/1401/98 Rev. 1/Corr, London, U.K.

EMA. (2011a). Concept paper on the revision of the guideline on similar biological medicinal product. EMA/CHMP/BMWP/572643, London, U.K.

EMA. (2011b). Concept paper on the revision of the guideline on similar biological medicinal products contain biotechnology-derived proteins as active substance: Quality issues. EMEA/CHMP/BWP/617111, London, U.K.

EMA. (2011c). Concept paper on the revision of the guideline on similar biological medicinal products containing biotechnology-derived proteins as active substance: Non-clinical and clinical issues. EMEA/CHMP/BMWP/572828, London, U.K.

EMA. (2011d). Guideline on similar biological medicinal products containing interferon beta. EMA/CHMP/BMWP/652000/2010, London, U.K.

Endrenyi, L., Chang, C., Chow, S.C., and Tothfalusi, L. (2013). On the interchangeability of biologic drug products. *Stat. Med.*, 32, 434–441.

Endrenyi, L., Fritsch, S., and Wei, Y. (1991). C_{max}/AUC is a clearer measure than C_{max} for absorption rates in investigations of bioequivalence. *Int. J. Clin. Pharm. Ther. Toxicol.*, 29, 394–399.

Endrenyi, L. and Tothfalusi, L. (2009). Regulatory and study conditions for the determination of bioequivalence of highly variable drugs. *J. Pharm. Pharm. Sci.*, 12, 138–149.

Enis, P. and Geisser, S. (1971). Estimation of the probability that Y < X. *J. Am. Stat. Assoc.,* 66, 162–168.

Fairweather, W.R., Lin, T.D., and Kelly, R. (1994). Regulatory and design aspects of complex stability studies. *Proceedings of the Biostatistics Subsection/Clinical Data Management Group of Pharmaceutical Research and Manufacturers of America,* Washington, DC, October 1994.

Fairweather, W.R., Lin, T.D., and Kelly, R. (1995). Regulatory, design, and analysis aspects of complex stability studies. *J. Pharm. Sci.,* 84, 1322–1326.

FDA. (1987). *Guideline for Submitting Documentation for the Stability of Human Drugs and Biologics.* Center for Drugs and Biologics, Office of Drug Research and Review, Food and Drug Administration, Rockville, MD.

FDA. (1988). *Guideline for the Format and Content of the Clinical and Statistical Sections of New Drug Application.* U.S. Food and Drug Administration, Rockville, MD.

FDA. (1992). *Guidance on Statistical Procedures for Bioequivalence Using a Standard Two-treatment Crossover Design.* Division of Bioequivalence, Office of Generic Drugs, Center for Drug Evaluation and Research, U.S. Food and Drug Administration, Rockville, MD.

FDA. (1996). FDA guidance concerning demonstration of comparability of human biological products, including therapeutic biotechnology-derived products, the U.S. Food and Drug Administration, Rockville, MD.

FDA. (1997). Guidance for industry: Dissolution testing of immediate release solid oral dosage forms. The U.S. Food and Drug Administration, Rockville, MD.

FDA. (1998). Data sets of bioequivalence for individual and population bioequivalence. www.fda.gov/cder/bioeuivdata/index.htm.

FDA. (1999). *Guidance for Industry on Nasal Spray and Inhalation Solution, Suspension and Spray Drug Products.* Center for Drug Evaluation and Research, U.S. Food and Drug Administration, Rockville, MD.

FDA. (2001). Guidance on statistical approaches to establishing bioequivalence. Center for Drug Evaluation and Research, the U.S. Food and Drug Administration, Rockville, MD.

FDA. (2002). Guidance for industry—Immunotoxicology evaluation of investigational new drugs. Center for Drug Evaluation and Research, the U.S. Food and Drug Administration, Rockville, MD.

FDA. (2003). Guidance on bioavailability and bioequivalence studies for orally administrated drug products—General considerations. Center for Drug Evaluation and Research, the U.S. Food and Drug Administration, Rockville, MD.

FDA. (2004). *Guidance for Industry—Botanical Drug Products.* The United States Food and Drug Administration, Rockville, MD.

FDA. (2005). Q5E comparability of biotechnological/biological products subject to changes in their manufacturing process. The U.S. Food and Drug Administration, Rockville, MD.

FDA. (2010). Guidance for industry—Non-inferiority clinical trials. Center for Drug Evaluation and Research, Center for Biologics Evaluation and Research, the U.S. Food and Drug Administration, Siler Spring, MD.

FDA. (2012a). Scientific considerations in demonstrating biosimilarity to a reference product. The U.S. Food and Drug Administration, Silver Spring, MD.

FDA. (2012b). Quality considerations in demonstrating biosimilarity to a reference protein product. The U.S. Food and Drug Administration, Silver Spring, MD.

FDA. (2012c). Biosimilars: Questions and answers regarding implementation of the Biologics Price Competition and Innovation Act of 2009. The U.S. Food and Drug Administration, Silver Spring, MD.

Fieller, E. (1954). Some problems in interval estimation. *J. R. Stat. Soc., Series B*, 16, 175–185.

Finney, D.J. (1979). *Statistical Method in Biological Assay*, 3rd edn. Oxford University Press, New York.

Fleming, T.R. (2000). Design and interpretation of equivalence trials. *Am. Heart J.*, 139, S172–S176.

Fox, A. (2010). Biosimilar medicines—New challenges for new class of medicine. *J. Biopharm. Stat.*, 20, 1–9.

GaBI Online. (2012a). Generics and biosimilars initiative. Generics grab 80% share of US market and fill 78% of prescriptions [www.gabionline.net]. Mol, Belgium: Pro Pharma Communications International. www.gabionline.net/Reports/Generics-grab-80-share-of-US-marketand-fill-78-of-prescriptions. Accessed on March 23, 2012.

GaBI Online. (2012b). Generics and Biosimilars Initiative. Biosimilars approved in Europe [www.gabionline.net]. Mol, Belgium: Pro Pharma Communications International. www.gabionline.net/Biosimilars/General/Biosimilars-approved-in-Europe. Accessed on March 23, 2012.

Goodman, S.N. (1992). A common on replication, p-values and evidence. *Stat. Med.*, 11, 875–879.

Gould, A.L. (1995). Group sequential extensions of Standard bioequivalence testing procedure. *J. Pharmacokinet. Biopharm.*, 23, 57–85.

GPhA. (2004). Biopharmaceuticals (follow-on protein products): Scientific considerations for an abbreviated approval pathway. Generic Pharmaceutical Association, December 8, 2004. Docket No. 2004N-0355 Scientific Considerations Related to Developing Follow-on Protein Products, U.S. Food and Drug Administration, Rockville, MD.

Graybill, F. and Wang, C.M. (1980). Confidence intervals on nonnegative linear combinations of variances. *J. Am. Stat. Assoc.*, 75, 869–873.

Gumbel, E.J. (1954). The maxima of the mean largest value and of the range. *Ann. Math. Statist.*, 25, 76–84.

Haidar, S.H., Davit, B.M., Chen, M.L. et al. (2008). Bioequivalence approaches for highly variable drugs and drug products. *Pharm. Res.*, 25, 237–241.

Haidar, S.H., Makhlouf, F., Schuirmann, D.J., Hyslop, T., Davit, B., Conner, D., and Yu, L.X. (2008). Evaluation of a scaling approach for the bioequivalence of highly variable drugs. *AAPS J.*, 10, 450–454.

Hartley, H.O. and David, H.A. (1954). Universal bounds for mean range and extreme observation. *Ann. Math. Statist.*, 25, 85–99.

Hauschke, D., Steinijans, V.W., Diletti, E., and Burke, W. (1992). Sample size determination for bioequivalence assessment using a multiplicative model. *J. Pharmacokinet. Biopharm.*, 20, 557–581.

Hauschke, D., Steinijians, V.W., and Diletti, E. (1990). A distribution-free procedure for the statistical analyses of bioequivalence studies. *Int. J. Clin. Pharmacol. Ther. Toxicol.*, 28, 72–78.

Health Canada. (1992). Guidance for industry: Conduct and analysis of bioavailability and bioequivalence studies—Part A: Oral dosage formulation used for systemic effects. Ottawa, Ontario, Canada.

Health Canada. (2006). *Guidance for Industry, Bioequivalence Requirements: Critical Dose Drugs.* Health Canada, Ottawa, Ontario, Canada.

Health Canada. (2010). Guidance for sponsors: Information and submission requirements for subsequent entry biologics (SEBs). Ottawa, Ontario, Canada.

Health Canada. (2012). Guidance document: Comparative bioavailability standards: Formulations used for systemic effects. Ottawa, Ontario, Canada.

Helboe, P. (1992). New designs for stability testing programs: Matrix or factorial designs. Authorities' viewpoint on the predictive value of such studies. *Drug Inform. J.*, 26, 629–634.

Howe, W.G. (1974). Approximate confidence limits on the mean of $X + Y$ where X and Y are two tabled independent random variables. *J. Am. Stat. Assoc.*, 69, 789–794.

Hsieh, T.C., Chow, S.C., Liu, J.P., Hsiao, C.F., and Chi, E. (2010). Statistical test for evaluation of biosimilarity of follow-on biologics. *J. Biopharm. Stat.*, 20, 20, 75–89.

Hsieh, T.C., Chow, S.C., Yang, L.Y., and Chi, E. (2013). The evaluation of biosimilarity index based on reproducibility probability for assessing follow-on biologics. *Stat. Med.*, 32, 406–414.

Hung, H.M.J., Wang, S.J., Tsong, Y., Lawrence, J., and O'Neil, R.T. (2003). Some fundamental issues with non-inferiority testing in active controlled trials. *Stat. Med.*, 22, 213–225.

Hyslop, T., Hsuan, F., and Holder, K.J. (2000). A small-sample confidence interval approach to assess individual bioequivalence. *Stat. Med.*, 19, 2885–2897.

ICH. (1993). Stability testing of new drug substances and products. *Tripartite International Conference on Harmonization Guideline*, Q1A, Geneva, Switzerland.

ICH. (1996). Q5C guideline on quality of biotechnological products: Stability testing of biotechnological/biological products. Center for Drug Evaluation and Research, Center for Biologics Evaluation and Research, the U.S. Food and Drug Administration, Rockville, MD.

ICH. (1997). Guidance for industry—S6 preclinical safety evaluation of biotechnology-derived pharmaceuticals. Center for Drug Evaluation and Research, Center for Biologics Evaluation and Research, the U.S. Food and Drug Administration, Rockville, MD.

ICH. (1998). E5 guideline on ethnic factors in acceptability of foreign data. *The U.S. Federal Register*, 83, 31790–31796.

ICH. (1999). Q6B guideline on test procedures and acceptance criteria for biotechnological/biological products. Center for Drug Evaluation and Research, Center for Biologics Evaluation and Research, the U.S. Food and Drug Administration, Rockville, MD.

ICH. (2000). Guideline E-10. International Conference on Harmonization Guideline: Guidance on choice of control group and related design and conduct issues in clinical trials. Food and Drug Administration, DHHS, Rockville, MD.

ICH. (2003). Guidance for industry. Q1A(R2) stability testing of new drug substances and products. Center for Drug Evaluation and Research, Center for Biologics Evaluation and Research, the U.S. Food and Drug Administration, Rockville, MD, November 2003.

ICH. (2003). Guidance for industry. Q1D bracketing and matrixing designs for stability testing of new drug substances and products. Center for Drug Evaluation and Research, Center for Biologics Evaluation and Research, the U.S. Food and Drug Administration, Rockville, MD, November 2003.

ICH. (2004). Guidance for industry. Q1E evaluation of stability data. Center for Drug Evaluation and Research, Center for Biologics Evaluation and Research, the U.S. Food and Drug Administration, Rockville, MD, June 2004.

ICH. (2005). Q5E guideline on comparability of biotechnological/biological products subject to changes in their manufacturing process. Center for Drug Evaluation and Research, Center for Biologics Evaluation and Research, the U.S. Food and Drug Administration, Rockville, MD.

Ju, H.L. and Chow, S.C. (1995). On stability designs in drug shelf-life estimation. *J. Biopharm. Stat.*, 5, 210–214.

Kang, S.H. and Chow, S.C. (2013). Statistical assessment of biosimilarity based on relative distance between follow-on biologics. *Stat. Med.*, 32, 382–392.

Karalis, V., Symillides, M., and Macheras, P. (2004). Novel scaled average bioequivalence limits based on GMR and variability considerations. *Pharm. Res.*, 21, 1933–1942.

Karalis, V., Symillides, M., and Macheras, P. (2004). Novel scaled average bioequivalence limits based on GMR and variability considerations. *Pharm. Res.*, 21, 1933–1942.

Kendrick, B.S., Chrimes, G., Cockrill, S.L., Gabrielson, J.P., Arthur, K.K. et al. (2009). Comparability of biotechnological/biological products subject to changes in their manufacturing. *BioPharm Int.*, 22, 32–44.

KFDA. (2011). Korean guidelines on the evaluation of similar biotherapeutic products (SBPs). Korean Food and Drug Administration, South Korea.

Kimber, I., Kerkvliet, N.I., Taylor, S.L., Astwood, J.D., Sarlo, K., and Dearman, R.J. (1999). Toxicology of protein allergenicity: Prediction and characterization. *Toxicol. Sci.*, 48, 157–162.

Korn, E.L., Albert, P.S., and McShane, L.M. (2005). Assessing surrogated as trial endpoints using mixed models, *Stat. Med.*, 24, 163–182.

Kozlowski, S. (2007). FDA policy on follow on biologics. *Proceedings of the Biosimilars 2007*, George Washington University, Washington, DC.

Kuhlmann, M. and Covic, A. (2006). The protein science of biosimilars. *Nephrol. Dial. Transplant.*, 21, Suppl 5: v4–v8.

Lanthier, M., Behrman, R., and Nardinelli, C. (2008). Economic issues with follow-on protein products. *Nat. Rev. Drug Discov.*, 7, 733–737.

Laster, L.L. and Johnson, M.F. (2003). Non-inferiority trials: the 'at least as good as' criterion. *Stat. Med.*, 22, 187–200.

Lee, M.S., Chen, M.C., Liao, Y.C., and Hsiung, A.G. (2007). Identifying potential immunodominant positions and predicting antigenic variants of influenza A/H3N2 viruses. *Vaccine*, 25, 8133–8139.

Lee, M.S. and Chen, M.C. (2004). Predicting antigenic variants of influenza A/H3N2 viruses. *Emerg. Infect. Dis.*, 10, 1385–1390.

Lee, Y., Shao, J., and Chow, S.C. (2004). Modified large-sample confidence intervals for linear combinations of variance components: Extension, theory, and application. *J. Am. Stat. Assoc.*, 99, 467–478.

Lee, Y., Shao, J., Chow, S.C., and Wang, H. (2002). Test for inter-subject and total variabilities under crossover designs. *J. Biopharm. Stat.*, 12, 503–534.

Leeson, L.J. (1995). In vitro/in vivo correlation. *Drug Inform. J.*, 29, 903–915.

Lei, L. and Olson, K. (2010). Evaluating statistical methods to establish clinical similarity of two biologics. *J. Biopharm. Stat.*, 20, 62–74.

Levene, H. (1960). Robust tests for the equality of variances. In: *Contributions to Probability and Statistics*. Olkin, I., Ed. Stanford University Press, Palo Alto, CA, pp. 278–292.

Levy, N.W. (1986). Bioequivalence of Solid oral dosage forms. A presentation to the *U.S. Food and Drug Administration Heaving on Bioequivalence of Solid Oral Dosage Forms*, September 29–October 1, Pharmaceutical Manufacturer Association, Section II, pp. 9–11.

Li, Y., Liu, Q., Wood, P., and Johri, A. (2013). Statistical considerations in biosimilar clinical efficacy trials with asymmetrical margins. *Stat. Med.*, 32, 393–405.

Liang, B.A. (2007). Regulating follow-on biologics. *Harvard J. Legis.*, 44, 363–373.

Liao, J.J.Z. and Darken, P.F. (2013). Comparability of critical quality attributes for establishing biosimilarity. *Stat. Med.*, 32, 462–469.

Liao, J.J.Z and Heyse, J.F. (2011). Biosimilarity for follow-on biologics. *Stat. Biopharm. Res.*, 3, 445–455.

Liao, Y.C., Lee, M.S., Ko, C.Y., and Hsiung, C.A. (2008). Bioinformatics models for predicting variants of influenza A/H3N2 viruses. *Bioinformatics*, 24, 505–512.

Lin, D. (1997). Stability studies at the FDA. PERI Course: Non-Clinical Statistics for Drug Discovery and Development, Arlington, VI, March 1997.

Lin, J.R., Chow, S.C., Chang, C.H., Lin, Y.C., and Liu, J.P. (2013). Application of the parallel line assay to assessment of biosimilar products based on binary endpoints. *Stat. Med.*, 32, 449–461.

Lin, T.D. (1994). Applicability of matrix and bracket approach to stability study design. *Proceedings of the Biopharmaceutical Section of the American Statistical Association*, Alexandria, VA, pp. 142–147.

Lindley, D.V. (1965). *Introduction to Probability and Statistics for a Bayesian Viewpoint, Part II Inference*. Cambridge University Press, Cambridge, U.K.

Liu, J.P. (1998). Statistical evaluation of individual bioequivalence. *Commun. Stat.: Theory Methods*, 27, 1433–1451.

Liu, J.P., Lin, J.R., and Chow, S.C. (2009). Inference on treatment effects for targeted clinical trials under enrichment design. *Pharm. Stat.*, published on line. DOI: 10.1002/pst.364.

Liu, J.P. and Chow, S.C. (1992). On assessment of bioequivalence in variability of bioavailability. *Comm. Stat. Theory Methods*, 21, 2591–2608.

Liu, J.P. and Chow, S.C. (2008). Statistical issues on the diagnostic multivariate index assay and targeted clinical trials, *J. Biopharm. Stat.*, 18, 167–182.

Liu, J.P. and Lin, J.R. (2008). Statistical methods for targeted clinical trials under enrichment design. *J. Formosan Med. Assoc.*, 107, S34–S41.

Liu, J.P. and Weng, C.S. (1992). Estimation of direct formulation effect under lognormal distribution in bioavailability/bioequivalence studies. *Stat. Med.*, 11, 881–896.

Liu, J.P. and Weng, C.S. (1994). Estimation of log-transformation in assessing bioequivalence. *Comm. Stat. Theory Methods*, 23, 421–434.

Liu, J.P. and Weng, C.S. (1995). Bias of two one-sided tests procedures in assessment of bioequivalence. *Stat. Med.*, 14, 853–861.

Liu, J.P., Ma, M.C., and Chow, S.C. (1997). Statistical evaluation of similarity factor f_2 as a criterion for assessment of similarity between dissolution profiles. *Drug Inf. J.*, 31, 1255–1271.

Los, M., Roodhart, J.M., and Voest, E.E. (2007). Target practice: Lessons from phase III trials with bevacizumab and vatalanib in the treatment of advanced colorectal cancer. *Oncologist*, 12, 443–450.

Lu, Q., Chow, S.C., and Tse, S.K. (2007). Statistical quality control process for traditional Chinese medicine with multiple correlative components. *J. Biopharm. Stat.*, 17, 791–808.

Lu, Q., Tse, S.K., Chow, S.C., and Yang, J. (2009). On assessing bioequivalence using genomic data with model misspecification. *J. Biopharm. Stat.*, 19, 571–579.

Ma, M.C., Lin, R.P., and Liu, J.P. (1999). Statistical evaluation of dissolution similarity. *Stat. Sin.*, 9, 1011–1027.

Mann, H.B. and Whitney, D.R. (1947). On a test of whether one or two random variables is stochastically larger than the other. *Ann. Math. Stat.*, 18, 50–60.

Markovic, I. (2007). Chemistry, manufacturing and control issues in production of therapeutic biologic protein products. Presented at *NCI Biological Resources Branch Workshop "Working with FDA: Biological Products and Clinical Development"*. National Cancer Institute, Bethesda, MD.

Markovic, I. (2009). Chemistry, manufacturing and control issues in production of therapeutic biologic protein products. *Proceedings of the Working with FDA: Biological Products and Clinical Development*, Rockville, MD.

McCamish, M. and Woollett, G. (2011). Worldwide experience with biosimilar development. *mAbs*, 3, 209–217.

MHLW. (2009). Guidelines for the quality, safety and efficacy assurance of follow-on biologics (Yakushoku shinsahatu 0304007). Japan.

Moore, J.W. and Flanner, H.H. (1996). Mathematical comparison of curves with an emphasis on dissolution profiles. *Pharm. Technol.*, 20, 64–74.

Morgan, W.A. (1939). A test for the significance of the difference between the two variances in a sample from a normal bivariate population. *Biometrika*, 31, 13–19.

Murphy, J.R. (1996). Uniform matrix stability study designs. *J. Biopharm. Stat.*, 6, 477–494.

Nordbrock, E. (1989). Statistical study design. *Proceedings of the National Stability Discussion Group*; October 1989, Washington, DC.

Nordbrock, E. (1991). Statistical comparison of NDA stability study designs. *Proceedings of the Midwest Biopharmaceutical Statistics Workshop*, Chelsea, MI, May 1991.

Nordbrock, E. (1992). Statistical comparison of stability study designs. *J. Biopharm. Stat.*. 2, 91–113.

Nordbrock, E. (1994a). Computing power details. PERI: Training Course in Non-Clinical Statistics, Dallas, TX, February 1994.

Nordbrock, E. (1994b). Design and analysis of stability studies. *Proceedings of the Biopharmaceutical Section of the American Statistical Association*, Alexandria, VA, pp. 291–294.

Nordbrock, E. (1994c). Statistically designed stability studies, an industry perspective. *Proceedings of the Biostatistics Subsection/Clinical Data Management Group of Pharmaceutical Research and Manufacturers of America*, Washington, DC, October 1994.

Nordbrock, E. (2003). Stability matrix designs. In *Encyclopedia of Biopharmaceutical Statistics*, 2nd Edn., Ed. Chow, S.C., Marcel Dekker, Inc., New York, pp. 934–939.

Nordbrock, E. (2009). Use of statistics to establish a stability trend: Matrixing. In: *Pharmaceutical Testing to Support Global Markets*. Kim Kuynh-Ba Ed. Springer, New York, 2009.

Nordbrock, E. and Valvani, S. (1995). PhRMA Stability Working Group. In: *Guideline for Matrix Designs of Drug Product Stability Protocols*, January 1995.

Owen, D.B. (1965). A special case of a noncentral t distribution. *Biometrika*, 52, 437–446.

Papadatos, N. (1995). Maximum variance of order statistics. *Ann. Inst. Stat. Math*, 47, 185–193.

Patel, H.I. (1994). Dose-response in pharmacokinetics. *Comm. Stat. Theory Methods*, 23, 451–465.

Phillips, K.F. (1990). Power of the two one-sided tests procedure in bioequivalence. *J. Pharm. Biopharm.*, 18, 137–144.

Phillips, K.F. (2003). A new test of non-inferiority for anti-infective trials. *Stat. Med.*, 22, 201–212.

PIC/S. (2009). *Guide to Good Manufacturing Practice for Switzerland Annexes.* Pharmaceutical Inspection Convention Pharmaceutical Inspection Co-operation Scheme, Geneva, Switzerland.

Pitman, E.J.G. (1939). A note on normal correlation. *Biometrika*, 31, 9–12.

Pocock, S.J. (1983). *Clinical Trials—A Practical Approach.* John Wiley & Sons, New York.

Pong, A. and Raghavarao, D. (2000). Comparison of bracketing and matrixing designs for a two-year stability study, *J. Biopharm. Stat.*, 10, 217–228.

Quan, H. and Shih, W.J. (1996). Assessing reproducibility by the within-subject coefficient of variation with random effects models. *Biometrics*, 52, 1195–1203.

Raines, L.J. (2002). Bad medicine: Why the generic drug regulatory paradigm is inapplicable to biotechnology products. *Biolaw. Bus.*, 5, 6–13.

Rodda, B.E. and Davis, R.L. (1980). Determining the probability of an important difference in bioavailability. *Clin. Pharmacol. Ther.*, 28, 247–252.

Roger, S.D. (2006). Biosimilars: How similar or dissimilar are they? *Nephrology*, 11, 341–346.

Roger, S.D. and Mikhail, A. (2007). Biosimilars: Opportunity or cause for concern? *J. Pharm. Sci.*, 10, 405–410.

Sargent, D.F., Wieand, S., Haller, D.G. et al. (2005). Disease-free survival versus overall survival as a primary end point for adjuvant colon cancer studies. *J. Clin. Oncol.*, 23, 8864–8670.

Schall, R. and Luus, H.G. (1993). On population and individual bioequivalence. *Stat. Med.*, 12, 1109–1124.

Schellekens, H. (2003). Relationship between biopharmaceutical immunogenicity of epoetin alfa and pure red cell aplasia. *Curr. Med. Res. Opin.*, 19, 433–434.

Schellekens, H. (2004). How similar do 'biosimilar' need to be? *Nat. Biotechnol.*, 22, 1357–1359.

Schellekens, H. (2005). Follow-on biologics: Challenges of the "next generation." *Nephrol. Dial. Transplant.*, 20(Suppl 4), 31–36.

Schuirmann, D.J. (1981). On hypothesis testing to determine if the mean of a normal distribution is continued in a known interval. *Biometrics*, 37, 617.

Schuirmann, D.J. (1987). A comparison of the two one-sided tests procedure and the power approach for assessing the equivalence of average bioavailability. *J. Pharmacokinet. Biopharm.*, 15, 657–680.

Serfling, R.J. (1980). *Approximation Theorems of Mathematical Statistics*, John Wiley, New York.

Shah, V.P., Tsong, Y., Sathe, P., and Liu, J.P. (1998). In Vitro dissolution profile comparison—Statistics and analysis of the similarity factor f_2. *Pharm. Res.*, 15, 889–896.

Shah, V.P., Yacobi, A., Barr, W.H. et al. (1996). Evaluation of orally administered highly variable drugs and drug formulations. *Pharm. Res.*, 13, 1590–1594.

Shao, J. and Chen, L. (1997). Prediction bounds for random shelf-lives. *Stat. Med.*, 16, 1167–1173.

Shao, J. and Chow, S.C. (1994). Statistical inference in stability analysis. *Biometrics*, 50, 753–763.

Shao, J. and Chow, S.C. (2002). Reproducibility probability in clinical trials. *Stat. Med.*, 21, 17727–1742.

Simoens, S., Verbeken, G., and Huys, I. (2011). Market access of biosimilars: Not only a cost issue. *Oncologie*, 13(5), 218–221.

Suh, S.K. and Park, Y. (2011). Regulatory guideline for biosimilar products in Korea. *Biologicals*, 39, 336–338.

SUPAC-IR. (1995). *The United States Food and Drug Administration Guideline Immediate Release Solid Oral Dosage Forms: Scale-Up and Postapproval Changes: Chemistry, Manufacturing, and Controls, In Vitro Dissolution Testing, and In Vivo Bioequivalence Documentation.* Rockville, MD.

Ting, N., Burdick, R.K., Graybill, F.A., Jeyaratnam, S., and Lu, T.-F.C. (1990). Confidence intervals on linear combinations of variance components that are unrestricted in sign. *J. Stat. Comput. Simul.*, 35, 135–143.

Torti, F. (2008). FDA response to house subcommittee on health. Letter to the House on biosimilar issues. FDA, Rockville, MD, September 2008.

Tothfalusi, L., Endrenyi, L., and Arieta, A.G. (2009). Evaluation of bioequivalence for highly variable drugs with scaled average bioequivalence. *Clin. Pharmacokinet.*, 48, 725–743.

Tothfalusi, L., Endrenyi, L., Midha, K.K., Rawson, M.J., and Hubbard, J.W. (2001). Evaluation of the bioequivalence of highly variable drugs and drug products. *Pharm. Res.*, 18, 728–733.

Tothfalusi, L., Speidl, S., and Endrenyi, L. (2008). Exposure-response analysis reveals that clinically important toxicity difference can exist between bioequivalent carbamazepine tablets. *Br. J. Clin. Pharmacol.*, 65, 110–122.

Tothfalusi, L. and Endrenyi, L. (2003). Limits for the scaled average bioequivalence of highly variable drugs and drug products. *Pharm. Res.*, 20, 382–389.

Tse, S.K., Chang, J.Y., Su, W.L., Chow, S.C., Hsiung, C., and Lu, Q. (2006). Statistical quality control process for traditional Chinese medicine. *J. Biopharm. Stat.*, 16, 861–874.

Tsong, Y., Chen, W.J., and Chen, C.W. (2008). ANCOVA approach for shelf life analysis of stability study of multiple factor designs. *J. Biopharm. Stat.*, 13, 375–393.

Tsong, Y., Higgins, K., Wang, S.J., and Hung, H.M.J. (1999). An overview of equivalence testing—CDER reviewers' perspective. *Proceedings of the Biopharmaceutical Section of American Statistical Association*, Alexandria, VA, pp. 214–219.

Tsou, H.H., Chien, T.Y., Liu, J.P., and Hsiao, C.F. (2011). A consistency approach to evaluation of bridging studies and multiregional trials. *Stat. Med.*, 30, 2171–2186.

USP/NF XXI. (2000). *United States Pharmacopeia 24 and National Formulary 19.* United States Pharmacopeial Convention, Inc., Rockville, MD.

Wang, J. and Chow, S.C. (2012). On regulatory approval pathway of biosimilar products. *Pharmaceuticals*, 5, 353–368.

Wang, Y.M. and Chow, A.T. (2010). Development of biosimilars—Pharmacokinetic and pharmacodynamic considerations. *J. Biopharm. Stat.*, 20, 46–61.

Webber, K.O. (2007). Biosimilars: Are we there yet? *Proceedings of the Biosimilars 2007*, George Washington University, Washington, DC.

WHO. (1992). World Health Organization technical report series, No. 822. Geneva, Switzerland.

WHO. (2005). World Health Organization draft revision on multisource (generic) pharmaceutical products: Guidelines on registration requirements to establish interchangeability. Geneva, Switzerland.

WHO. (2009). Guidelines on evaluation of similar biotherapeutic products (SBPs). Geneva, Switzerland.

WHO. (2010). Guideline for the production and control of specified starting materials. Geneva, Switzerland.

Wilcoxon, F. (1945). Individual comparisons by ranking methods. *Biometrics*, 1, 80–83.

Wolff, R. (2011). CMC requirements for biological products. *Proceedings of the Workshop Sponsored by Korean Food and Drug Administration*, Seoul, South Korea, June 1, 2011.

Woodcock, J. (2007). The FDA's assessment of follow-on protein products: A historical perspective. *Nat. Rev. Drug Discov.*, 6, 437–442.

Woodcock, J., Griffin, J., Behrman, R. et al. (2007). The FDA's assessment of follow-on protein products: A historical perspective. *Nat. Rev. Drug Discov.*, 6, 437–442.

Yang, J., Zhang, N., Chow, S.C., and Chi, E. (2013). An extended F-test for heterogeneity of variability in follow-on biological products. *Stat. Med.*, 32, 415–423.

Zhang, N., Yang, J., Chow, S.C., Endrenyi, L., and Chi, E. (2013). Impact of variability on the choice of biosimilarity limits in assessing follow-on biologics. *Stat. Med.*, 32, 424–433.

Index

Milton Keynes UK
Ingram Content Group UK Ltd.
UKHW021842071024
449327UK00021B/1531

9 780367 379728